THE ultimate diabetes
diabetes
MEAL PLANNER

A Complete System for
Eating Healthy with Diabetes

Jaynie F. Higgins, A.C., C.P.T.,
and David Groetzinger

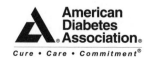

American
Diabetes
Association®

Cure • Care • Commitment®

Director, Book Publishing, Robert Anthony; *Managing Editor, Book Publishing,* Abe Ogden; *Editor,* Greg Guthrie; *Production Manager,* Melissa Sprott; *Composition,* Circle Graphics, Inc.; *Cover Design,* Jody Billert; *Printer,* R.R. Donnelley.

Nutritional Consulting: Clara Schneider, MS, RD, RN, LD, CDE

Printed in the United States of America
3 5 7 9 10 8 6 4 2

The suggestions and information contained in this publication are generally consistent with the *Clinical Practice Recommendations* and other policies of the American Diabetes Association, but they do not represent the policy or position of the Association or any of its boards or committees. Reasonable steps have been taken to ensure the accuracy of the information presented. However, the American Diabetes Association cannot ensure the safety or efficacy of any product or service described in this publication. Individuals are advised to consult a physician or other appropriate health care professional before undertaking any diet or exercise program or taking any medication referred to in this publication. Professionals must use and apply their own professional judgment, experience, and training and should not rely solely on the information contained in this publication before prescribing any diet, exercise, or medication. The American Diabetes Association—its officers, directors, employees, volunteers, and members—assumes no responsibility or liability for personal or other injury, loss, or damage that may result from the suggestions or information in this publication.

♾ The paper in this publication meets the requirements of the ANSI Standard Z39.48-1992 (permanence of paper).

ADA titles may be purchased for business or promotional use or for special sales. To purchase more than 50 copies of this book at a discount, or for custom editions of this book with your logo, contact the American Diabetes Association at the address below, at booksales@diabetes.org, or by calling 703-299-2046.

American Diabetes Association
1701 North Beauregard Street
Alexandria, Virginia 22311

Library of Congress Cataloging-in-Publication Data
Higgins, Jaynie.
  The ultimate diabetes meal planner / Jaynie Higgins with David Groetzinger.
    p. cm.
  Includes index.
  ISBN 978-1-58040-299-6 (alk. paper)
  1. Diabetes—Diet therapy—Recipes. I. Groetzinger, David. II. Title.

RC662.H54 2008
641.5′6314—dc22
                    2008033680

Contents

Acknowledgments

Thanks are due to my friends and my clients. I couldn't have completed this book without the support of my folks, Victor and Joan Hanington; my two girls, Geneva-Beth and Haleigh; and my husband, Hal Higgins, Jr., who persevered with me for more than eight years. I must also thank God, who gave me the gifts and talents to help others through the example I set in my life with diabetes.

Thanks also go to my dear friend, David Groetzinger. Without him, the *Ultimate Diabetes Meal Planner* would never have become a reality.

Lastly, special thanks go to the staff of the American Diabetes Association for their collaboration and support in publishing this book.

—*Jaynie Higgins*
www.Jaynie.me

Thanks go to Jaynie Higgins, who has been a tireless and supportive partner in bringing this book to publication. It's been a long, excellent adventure.

I must also acknowledge Greg Guthrie, our editor at the American Diabetes Association, whose professionalism and expertise led us from a wonderful idea to a tremendous book.

I owe a deep and loving thanks to my wife. Without her vigorous and endless encouragement, I would have never stopped procrastinating and eventually finished this project. It only took 10 years, Vix!

—*David Groetzinger*
www.ResidentialCareSolutions.weebly.com

Preface

Although diabetes can be treated, it still has no cure. Turning this obstacle into opportunity goes beyond having a vision. It is more like having a mission. Your quality of life does not have to suffer because of diabetes, disability, or age. Proper nutrition and exercise can help you manage diabetes and bringing wellness into your life. Through proper fitness and diet, I have been able to not only improve my life with diabetes, but I've also been able to pass on the secrets of my success to other people with diabetes.

I never imagined that I'd be where I am today. At first, my chosen career was in gerontology, and I was the owner of a licensed assisted-living facility. But life took me in a different direction when my evening job as a certified fitness instructor turned into a full-time career.

I got involved in teaching fitness and weight training when my daily exercise routine became stale and burdensome. Because I have type 1 diabetes, exercise is something that I have to accomplish to stay healthy. One night, after crying through my entire five-mile run, I decided that variety and change needed to become a priority. I designed my own free-weight program, and after a few months of strength training (and running two to three times a week), people started asking me how I did it. I began training people in my home, but my client list quickly grew so large that I found myself scouting for a larger location for my gym.

In order to keep fit, I was also eating healthfully. Soon, people were asking me about my nutrition, too. Before I knew it, I was spending endless hours writing meal plans to help others transform their lives. Seeing the fruits of their success reminded me of something that I learned at my assisted-living facility—the menu is always number one! It's always easier to follow a healthy meal plan if the menus include variety and taste. The fruits of those years of labor are now here in your hands, the *Ultimate Diabetes Meal Planner*.

Diabetes ABCs (and Ds)

The content of this manual is based on what worked for me in getting my diabetes under control, but I also think it's important to keep in mind the Diabetes ABCs.

A **is for A1C.** This test measures your average blood glucose levels over the previous three months. You should have an A1C test regularly.

B **is for Blood Pressure.** Diabetes and high blood pressure (hypertension) often go hand in hand. High blood pressure can lead to kidney damage, heart attacks, and stroke.

C **is for Cholesterol.** There are two kinds of cholesterol you'll want to watch: LDL (or bad) cholesterol and HDL (or good) cholesterol. LDL cholesterol can build up and clog your blood vessels, leading to heart attacks and stroke. HDL cholesterol can remove other cholesterol from your blood vessels.

It is important to keep these care goals in mind and to speak with your health care providers about where to set your goals. However, my own experiences taught me that many diabetes self-care problems revolved around the plate. By eating healthfully and exercising regularly, I began bringing health into my life. You can, too! It was my goal of following a nutritious diet and getting regular exercise that changed my diabetes story into a life-abetes success journey.

That's why I like to add another letter to these ABCs: *D* **for Diet.** The *Ultimate Diabetes Meal Planner* should give you most of the information and guidance you need to bring healthful meals into the lives of you and your loved ones.

Even better, if you've picked up this book, you're already on your way there. Remember these ABCs, and know that by following the D for Diet, you can begin to make all of those other building blocks of strong diabetes self-care fall into place. It'll take work and a lot of time, but you have a long life in front of you to enjoy.

Living life-abetes,
Jaynie Higgins, A.C./C.P.T.

Introduction

Being diagnosed with diabetes does not mean your life is over or even that your entire life will be radically different. The diagnosis is a wake-up call that from now on you may need to make some lifestyle changes, such as eating healthy foods and being physically active. You may need to watch what you eat, how much you eat, and when you eat. And really, all of us need to do that.

This book has been designed to make eating much simpler for people with diabetes. The menus are designed so that everyone in your family eats the same meal. Each meal has different calorie levels, but the menus are the same, so the only difference for people at the table is how much food they're getting, depending on their daily calorie allowance.

There are thousands and thousands of food choices and an equal number of diet books promising quick fixes and making questionable claims about the miraculous power of following their diets…this book isn't one of them. This book is all about helping you make the right choices in the foods that you eat and is based solely on the established principles of healthy nutrition.

Despite all the books on diets, we remain a society that is undernourished and overweight. Obviously, the quick fixes and unrealistic promises are not working, so let's get back to the tried-and-true basics. This book is not about trying to follow a "diet" of only grapefruit or cabbage or some other food or food group while excluding all of the other food groups. It is unrealistic to think people could follow such a diet for a lifetime and still enjoy themselves. We need all the varieties of the food groups to live well, and we should enjoy eating.

One of the main themes of this book is that "live foods" (grains, fruits, and vegetables) are very good for you. All of the scientific research shows us that plant-based foods and whole grains should be the foundation of a healthy diet. The great thing is that all three of these are low in calories and dense in nutrients. They pack a wallop nutritionally without adding a lot of calories or fat.

There are two ways in which you can approach using the *Ultimate Diabetes Meal Planner*. After following the menu plans, you can simply start over again or you can strike out on your own because you may feel more comfortable making your own healthy food choices. You will likely begin to recognize what a healthy serving size is and how it fits into a sensible meal plan. And, if you feel that you need more work, you can easily go back and reference the meal plans in this book.

HOW TO USE THIS BOOK

The *Ultimate Diabetes Meal Planner* has been designed to take the heavy lifting of meal planning out of your hands and to give you some help in bringing a healthy meal plan to your lifestyle. For that purpose, there are 16 weeks of meal plans.

Step 1: Meet with Your Health Care Team

Before you begin anything that will affect your diabetes self-care routine, you should meet with your health care providers and tell them that you are planning on using the meal plans contained in this book. Ask them how many calories you should be eating daily and whether this is a good approach for you to take. Your health care team should include a registered dietitian (or RD); if not, now is the time to ask your primary care physician or diabetes educator for a referral to a dietitian with experience in diabetes. An RD is an expert in nutrition who can help you create a healthy and safe meal plan.

Find out if it will be safe for you to begin following the healthy meal plans included in this book and if there are any specific foods or activities that you should avoid. For example, some people with diabetes will have to eat more snacks than others and people with high blood pressure may need to reduce their sodium intake. If these apply to you, you can still use the meal plans contained in the *Ultimate Diabetes Meal Planner*, but you'll need to use a little more care in choosing your recipes. Some people can't drink milk or eat dairy products; if this applies to you, you may have to use soy products or something else. For those with special dietary needs, the expertise of an RD will be very helpful.

Step 2: Choose a Calorie Level

During the meeting with your health care team, you should ask how many calories you should be eating per day. The meal plans in the *Ultimate Diabetes Meal Planner* fall into four daily calorie levels: 1,500, 1,800, 2,000, and 2,200 calories per day. Find out which of these levels will work best for your health needs.

The meal plans in this book have been developed with a keen eye toward carbohydrate intake and also use the exchange list/food choices system, so if your dietitian or educator suggests that you use these methods of meal planning, you can still use the *Ultimate Diabetes Meal Planner*. You'll find complete nutrition and exchange list information for each individual serving of a recipe on that recipe's page. In some cases, you may have to adjust the daily meal plans; however, in most cases, you'll find that the plans in this book will meet the needs of most people with diabetes.

> ### "But…I'm cooking for a family of four!"
>
> Not a problem. If you are cooking for two or more, you can still use the meal plans in this book! Most of the recipes in this book yield four servings. You'll simply change how much of a certain dish each person gets. In many cases, the only difference will be the portion sizes of the side dishes.

Planning Snacks

You will notice that each daily meal plan comes with a number of snacks, labeled A and B. For most people, the A snack will be eaten during the middle of the day and the B snack will be eaten before bedtime. You'll also see that the 1,500-calorie plan doesn't include snacks, whereas the 2,200-calorie plan consists of the biggest snacks. It is important that you discuss with your health care team how many snacks you should be having every day and when you should be eating these snacks, especially if you're taking medications to treat your diabetes. To keep things simple, the snacks are listed together in the *Ultimate Diabetes Meal Planner*, so you can find them easily.

Step 3: Become Familiar with the *Ultimate Diabetes Meal Planner*

Now that you've chosen your calorie level, you're ready to get started using the *Ultimate Diabetes Meal Planner*. You'll notice that this book is divided into four seasons: winter, spring, summer, and fall. Don't worry about starting your healthy meal plan in January; start with the season that you're currently in. It's never too early or too late to get your eating on a healthier track.

Further, each season is divided into four weeks of meal plans. You've probably already recognized that a season contains more than four weeks. What you will need to do is repeat each week a few times each month. You probably won't become bored with the same dishes over and over because there are four weeks separating each meal, but if you do, try swapping out days from other weeks. For example, if you don't want the Whole-Grain Waffle for breakfast on the first Sunday of Week 1 of the Winter Cycle, use the Whole-Grain Muffin from Tuesday of that week or the Whole-Wheat Pancakes from Sunday of Week 2 of the Winter Cycle. The thing to remember is that you'll need to use the entire day's meal plan to keep your nutritional levels carefully balanced. As you become more accustomed to using this book, substitutions and improvisations will become natural and easy.

If you don't want to follow a Winter Cycle meal plan and prefer a Spring Cycle meal plan instead, go ahead and do it. Just remember to stick with the whole day's meals and you will be fine.

Also note how this book is organized. Each section begins with a week of meal plans, which includes pages of daily meal plans broken down into calorie levels, followed by a shopping list, and then the recipes in the order that they are used. After you have finished with that week's meal plans, the next week's meal plan is presented, along with its daily meal plans, the shopping list, and the recipes. This structure repeats itself throughout the book, so you won't have to flip through the whole book when you're preparing meals. It's that easy!

How do I make individual recipe substitutions?

Maybe you have a food allergy or condition that prevents you from having a specific food, such as milk, fish, nuts, or wheat gluten. Maybe you're really tired of having waffles for breakfast. Or maybe you really can't handle eating anything with mayonnaise in it. If any of this applies to you, there is a tool out there that can help you make healthy substitutions: the food choice/exchange lists found in *Choose Your Foods: Exchange Lists for Diabetes* (APPENDIX 1).

The food choice/exchange list system is an easy way of making healthy, nutritionally sound meal substitutions. Put simply, this system categorizes a single serving of a food item based on its nutritional content. Foods in the same exchange list have about the same amount of calories, carbohydrates, and other nutrients. So, if you want to change a recipe or a food item in your daily meal plan, determine the exchange list that the food is in and swap it out with another food from the same list. Foods with the same exchanges will generally affect your blood glucose levels in the same manner.

However, not every recipe or meal has the same exchange value. If this is the case, you can adjust your exchanges through the day's meals to fit in the recipe you want. The table on page xiii provides the number of exchanges in every meal of this book. If your recipe uses more exchanges than the previous one, all you need to do is "borrow" an exchange from somewhere else in that day's meal plan and use it for the recipe you want to prepare. What you cannot do is "borrow" exchanges from one day and add them to another.

You can find the choice/exchange value for each recipe in this book with its nutrition data. Also, every cookbook published by the American Diabetes Association provides the choice/exchange value for its recipes. So, if you don't want to substitute a recipe from the *Ultimate Diabetes Meal Planner*, you can use any of the recipes from other American Diabetes Association cookbooks.

To take full advantage of the choice/exchange system, you may want to pick up a nutrition guide that provides exchanges for common foods, such as *The Diabetes Carb & Fat Gram Guide* by Lea Ann Holzmeister (available at http://store.diabetes.org; order #4708-03), so that you can make substitutions with all of the items in your daily meal plan. As always, it won't hurt to discuss exchange lists with your dietitian or diabetes educator, too. He or she will be able to give you valuable guidance in bringing balanced meal plans into your lifestyle.

Step 4: Go Grocery Shopping

Now that you know what you'll be cooking throughout the week, you'll need to pick up the ingredients for your meals. For each week, you'll find a shopping list containing the names of each ingredient you'll need to have on hand to prepare all of those meals.

These shopping lists don't contain the precise amounts of each ingredient—everyone's needs will be different—but they do give you a pretty complete list of items to make sure that you have everything on hand for the week's meals. When it comes time to go shopping, take out the upcoming week's shopping list, look closely at the meal plans and recipes, and write down how much of each item you'll need in the space provided. *It is important to note that snacks are not included in the shopping lists, because snacks will vary greatly for every person.* Also, the shopping lists were built on the items in the 2,000-calorie plans, so not every item from the list may apply to

---

Example Substitution Using the Food Choice/Exchange System

Don is on the 1,800-calorie meal plan, and he's on Tuesday of Winter Week 1. Don is allergic to peanuts, so he can't eat **Spicy Whole-Grain Rice with Peanuts** for lunch. Rather than just replace the peanuts with a different type of nut that he can eat, Don decides to prepare something else. He will have to use the exchange list to do this. Looking at the recipe for Spicy Whole-Grain Rice with Peanuts, he sees that it has the following exchanges: 2 Starch and 2 Fat. So he looks around the recipes for something that will use these exchanges. He decides that the **Parmesan Potatoes** look good. This recipe has 2 Starch and 1 1/2 Fat exchanges. That leaves him with 1/2 Fat exchange left over for the day.

Looking at the rest of the meal plan, Don sees that he's assigned 10 peanuts for his A Snack. He refers to APPENDIX 1—*Choose Your Foods: Exchange Lists for Diabetes*—and sees that 10 peanuts are equal to 1 Fat exchange. He can't eat that, either. However, Don loves black olives, and he sees that 8 large black olives are equal to 1 Fat exchange, too. He also knows that he's going to have an additional 1/2 Fat exchange left over from his lunch. So, for his A Snack, he has 12 large black olives (8 olives [1 Fat] + 4 olives [1/2 Fat] = 12) instead of the peanuts. Don's daily meal plan is still balanced, and he gets to eat the foods he wants.

DAILY MEAL PLANS Choice/Exchange Values

Meal	1,500 calories	1,800 calories	2,000 calories	2,200 calories
Breakfast	2 Carbohydrate/Starch 1 Fruit 1 Fat-Free Milk 1 Lean Meat 2 Fat	2 Carbohydrate/Starch 1 Fruit 1 Fat-Free Milk 1 Lean Meat 2 Fat	2 Carbohydrate/Starch 1 Fruit 1 Fat-Free Milk 1 Lean Meat 2 Fat	2 Carbohydrate/Starch 1 Fruit 1 Fat-Free Milk 2 Lean Meat 2 Fat
Lunch	3 Carbohydrate/Starch 1 Fruit 1 Vegetable 2 Lean Meat 1 Fat	3 Carbohydrate/Starch 1 Fruit 1 Vegetable 2 Lean Meat 2 Fat	3 Carbohydrate/Starch 2 Fruit 2 Vegetable 2 Lean Meat 2 Fat	3 Carbohydrate/Starch 2 Fruit 2 Vegetable 2 Lean Meat 2 Fat
Snack A		1 Fat 1 Fruit	1 Vegetable 1 Fat 1 Fruit	1 Vegetable 1 Fat 1 Fruit
Snack B		1 Fat-Free Milk	1 Carbohydrate/Starch 1 Fat 1 Fat-Free Milk	1 Carbohydrate/Starch 1 Fat 1 Fat-Free Milk
Dinner	2 Carbohydrate/Starch 1 Fruit 1 Fat-Free Milk 2 Vegetable 2 Lean Meat 2 Fat	2 Carbohydrate/Starch 1 Fruit 1 Fat-Free Milk 2 Vegetable 3 Lean Meat 2 Fat	2 Carbohydrate/Starch 1 Fruit 1 Fat-Free Milk 2 Vegetable 3 Lean Meat 2 Fat	3 Carbohydrate/Starch 1 Fruit 1 Fat-Free Milk 2 Vegetable 3 Lean Meat 2 Fat

you if you're on the 1,500- or 1,800-calorie plans; the same applies to you if you're on the 2,200-calorie plan, because these plans sometimes have a few extra items over the course of the week.

It is best to purchase most of your food on a weekly basis; doing this will ensure that very little of your food will spoil and save you money. When you first begin using the *Ultimate Diabetes Meal Planner*, you may have to pick up several staple items, such as spices, nonstick cooking spray, and sauces. You won't have to buy these every week. After a while, you will have a fully stocked, healthy pantry!

Reading Food Labels

An excellent tool for keeping your shopping smart and healthy is printed on just about everything you will buy at the grocery store—the Nutrition Facts label. With this little label, you can find out just about anything you need to know about a food before you put it in your shopping cart. Here's a short breakdown of what you should be looking at.

- *Serving Size.* This is the first thing you should look at when picking up a food product. Does the serving size seem realistic? The nutrition information on the food label corresponds directly to the size of the serving. For example, a jar of pasta sauce may say that it has 6 servings in it and each serving is 1/2 cup. What happens if you have 1 cup of pasta sauce? Well, instead of getting 12 grams of total carbohydrate for that serving (as it says on the label), you'll be getting 24 grams, because you're having two

How do I shop smart?

First off, don't shop when you're hungry. When you are hungry, you're more liable to make impulse purchases because something looks good at the moment. Save yourself some extra calories and some money, and avoid the grocery store when you haven't eaten.

Another great shopping rule is to approach a grocery store by circling the outside walls first and then moving to the interior aisles. Foods that perish require refrigeration, and those foods tend to be along the walls of a grocery store because that's where they plug in the refrigerators. Also, foods that perish have fewer additives and preservatives, which means that they are healthier and pack fewer hidden calories. So, when you hit the store, start at the edges.

When you've finished picking up your perishable goods, head toward the aisles. Remember to stick with your shopping list and avoid last-minute purchases. With the meal plans in the *Ultimate Diabetes Meal Planner*, you won't eat or need those foods anyway, so save the money you might spend on those items for a healthier gift to yourself—like a trip to the spa or a visit to a museum. Try to buy the best-quality ingredients you can find (remember that a high price does not always mean high quality), so you can get the best taste out of your dishes.

servings of the sauce. That's a big difference!

- *Servings.* This is another handy tool that gives you tons of information about whether a food will fit into your meal plan. This item tells you how many servings are in the package. Every other bit of data in the food label is based on *one serving*. If a small bag of potato chips says it has 2 1/2 servings and you eat the entire package, then you're taking in *two and a half times* the amount of calories, fat, and carbohydrate listed in the food label. If you look at that bag of chips and can see yourself eating the whole thing in one sitting, it may be best to avoid temptation and not purchase it.
- *Calories.* Keep an eye on the number of calories in the foods you buy. The meal plans in this book are based on calorie levels throughout the day, so you'll want to purchase foods that will fit into your daily calorie limit. It's also important to note how many of the food's calories come from fat, which is listed right below the entry for

calories. If most of the calories come from fat, then it's probably not a good choice for a healthy diet. If you're trying to lose weight, paying attention to the number of calories in a food is essential.

- *Total Fat.* This entry shows you how much total fat is contained in the food you're thinking about buying. There are several types of fat that can be found in food, including monounsaturated, polyunsaturated, saturated, and trans fat. In general, try to avoid foods that contain a lot of saturated and trans fat in each serving. None of the recipes in the *Ultimate Diabetes Meal Planner* contain more than 3 grams of saturated fat and most contain almost no trans fat. Fat packs more calories per gram than any other nutrient, so if you're aiming to lose weight, it is especially important to lower the amount of fat in your daily meals.
- *Total Carbohydrate.* Because you have diabetes, it is very important to take a look at how much carbohydrate is included

in every food you buy, especially if you're counting your carbohydrates. You should pay more attention to this than to the amount of sugar in a food, because total carbohydrate is what ultimately affects your blood glucose levels the most. Also make it a point to check out how much dietary fiber is included in each food. Dietary fiber is an essential part of a healthy diet, and Americans don't get nearly enough of it. You don't need a lot of it (about 25–30 grams a day), so make this a daily goal.

- **Ingredient list.** Ingredients are listed in descending order by weight, so the first ingredient comprises the majority of any food item. Check out the ingredient list for things you're trying to avoid, such as coconut or palm oil, which is high in saturated fat. Also try to avoid hydrogenated oils that are high in trans fats. The ingredient list is also a good place to look for heart-healthy ingredients, such as whole-wheat flour and oats.

Each recipe in the *Ultimate Diabetes Meal Planner* has its own Nutrition Facts label printed on the same page. Just like when you're buying foods at the grocery store, you'll need to look at these details when preparing your meals. Keep an eye out for the number of servings that each recipe yields, so you know how much of the dish you should be eating. And just like with a packaged food item, the nutritional information for each recipe applies to *one serving only.*

Nutrition Facts

Serving Size 1 cup (53g/1.9 oz)
Servings Per Container About 8

Amount Per Serving

Calories 190	Calories from Fat 25

	% Daily Value**
Total Fat 3g*	**5%**
Saturated Fat 0g	**0%**
Trans Fat 0g	
Cholesterol 0mg	**0%**
Sodium 95mg	**4%**
Potassium 300mg	**9%**
Total Carbohydrate 36g	**12%**
Dietary Fiber 8g	**32%**
Soluble Fiber 3g	
Sugars 13g	
Protein 9g	**14%**

Vitamin A 0%	•	Vitamin C 0%
Calcium 4%	•	Iron 10%
Phosphorus 10%	•	Magnesium 10%
Copper 8%		

*Amount in Cereal. One half cup of fat free milk contributes an additional 40 calories, 65mg sodium, 6g total carbohydrates (6g sugars), and 4g protein.
**Percent Daily Values are based on a 2,000 calorie diet. Your Daily Values may be higher or lower depending on your calorie needs.

		Calories:	2,000	2,500
Total Fat	Less than		65g	80g
Sat Fat	Less than		20g	25g
Cholesterol	Less than		300mg	300mg
Sodium	Less than		2,400mg	2,400mg
Potassium			3,500mg	3,500mg
Total Carbohydrate			300g	375g
Dietary Fiber			25g	30g

Calories per gram:
Fat 9 • Carbohydrate 4 • Protein 4

Also, there are a lot of similar products out there with differing nutritional contents. We don't want you to go out and feel that you can buy only one kind of sugar-free jam, because that makes grocery shopping difficult and it's unnecessary. Diabetes is difficult enough to manage without having to worry about which store carries that one specific brand of canola oil mayonnaise called for in the recipe. So please be aware that the nutritional information for each recipe is a very close approximation to what you'll be getting from your cooking, but it may not be exactly the same.

Step 5: Start Cooking

Now it's time to get started with cooking. If you've become a take-out meal addict, then now is the time to reconnect with cooking at home. In our busy workaday world, it's nice to take a breather at the end of the day and spend some quality time with yourself preparing meals. Sharing meals with family and friends can be a great way to bring everyone closer and take pause at the end of a long day. Give it a chance—you may find that you like it quite a bit. If you've been cooking at home and loving it, then you may have to make a few changes to your current cooking habits.

The recipes in the *Ultimate Diabetes Meal Planner* use the healthiest cooking methods and ingredients available and still offer great taste. With these recipes—and definitely on the first time through—try to avoid substitutions or adding ingredients because you feel that it needs more flavor. An extra dash of oil or another pat of butter dramatically increases the amount of fat and calories in each dish you prepare. Give the recipes a chance to stand on their own, especially if you're using fresh, high-quality ingredients. You may find that you've been relying on salt and butter in the past when you didn't really need it.

Step 6: Repeat Cycles as Desired

It's generally best if you follow the weekly cycles as they are written during your first time through the book. Following a healthy meal plan takes practice and experience, so let the *Ultimate Diabetes Meal Planner* gradually teach you how to do this. As you become more comfortable with meal planning and making healthy food choices, you'll be able to create your own meal plans and adjust your own favorite recipes. In the meantime, let this book do all of the hard work for you.

If you do come across recipes that don't quite suit your fancy, swap out that day with another one in the book. Be sure to use the entire day's meal plan, so you can keep your diet balanced and your nutrient intake consistent. In some cases, an entire week's worth of meals may not appeal to you. If that's the case, then swap out the entire week with a different one. If you feel like eating a summer meal and it's only spring, go ahead and do it! Following a healthy meal plan should be fun and flexible, so don't feel like there are rules carved in stone with this book.

Remember, your goal in using this book is to bring a healthy, diabetes-friendly meal plan into your life. Don't get discouraged or frustrated. It is a tool to help you, so make changes as you see fit to make it work for you.

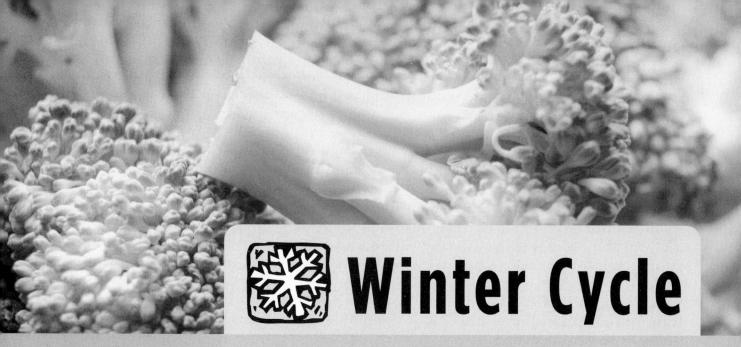

Winter Cycle

WEEK 1

FEATURED RECIPES

Whole-Wheat Pancakes or Waffles

Sweet and Sour Green Beans

Pineapple Pudding Parfait

Friendship Stew

Splendid Blueberry Crisp

Spicy Whole-Grain Rice with Peanuts

Broccoli Floret Salad

Creole Fish Fillets

Red Beans and Brown Rice

Sugar-Free Raspberry Bars

Whole-Grain Muffins

Pizza Muffins

Sizzlin' Fruit Salad

Apricot-Glazed Chicken

Chicken Salad Roll-Up

Lentil Stroganoff

Zucchini Carrot Muffins

Chicken Cucumber Salad

Cajun Pork Chops

Potatoes Au Gratin

Banana Bran Muffin

No Egg, Egg Salad Sandwich

Seasoned Chilled Vegetables

Savory Sirloin

Lemon Parsley Carrots

Granola, Oats, Blackberry, and Raspberry Bake

French Toast

Fried Bananas

Barbecued Pork Sandwich

Oven-Roasted Tomatoes

Skewered Chicken and Shrimp

Cold Pasta Salad

Carrots in Sherry Wine

1500 calorie MEAL PLAN WINTER WEEK 1

	Sunday	Monday	Tuesday	Wednesday	Thursday	Friday	Saturday
Breakfast	Whole-Wheat Pancakes or Waffles (2) 1/4 cup sugar-free syrup 1 small orange 1 cup nonfat milk 1 oz lean turkey ham 5 peanuts 2 tsp margarine	1/2 whole-wheat bagel 1/2 large grapefruit 1 cup nonfat milk 1/4 cup egg substitute 2 tsp light jam	Whole-Grain Muffins (2) 1 cup nonfat milk 4 tsp tahini (sesame paste)	3/4 cup bran cereal 1 slice multigrain toast 1 kiwi fruit 1/2 cup nonfat milk 1/4 cup low-fat cottage cheese 2 tsp margarine 2 tsp light jam	Zucchini Carrot Muffins 3/4 cup strawberries 1 cup nonfat milk 1/2 tsp margarine	Banana Bran Muffin 1/2 cup Kashi cereal 1 cup nonfat milk 3 mixed nuts	French Toast Fried Bananas 4 oz nonfat milk
Lunch	Sweet and Sour Green Beans Pineapple Pudding Parfait 1/2 cup mashed potatoes 1 slice whole-wheat low-calorie bread 2 oz roasted chicken, skin removed 2 tsp margarine	Spicy Whole-Grain Rice with Peanuts Broccoli Floret Salad 2 small plums 2 oz cheese (3 grams of fat or less per slice)	Pizza Muffins Sizzlin' Fruit Salad	Chicken Salad Roll-Up 10 baked tortilla chips 1/2 cup corn kernels 1 small apple 1 cup green pepper slices 4 black olives	Chicken Cucumber Salad 2/3 cup baked beans 1 small roll 1/2 large pear 1 tsp margarine	No Egg, Egg Salad Sandwich Seasoned Chilled Vegetables 15 fat-free potato chips 1/2 cup fruit cocktail in sugar-free syrup 1 oz reduced-fat cheese	Barbecued Pork Sandwich Oven-Roasted Tomatoes 1/2 ear corn on the cob 1/2 cup unsweetened plums 1/2 tsp margarine
Snack A							
Snack B							
Dinner	Friendship Stew Splendid Blueberry Crisp 1/2 slice whole-wheat low-calorie bread 1/8 cup fat-free salad dressing 1 cup nonfat milk 2 cups salad made from nonstarchy vegetables 2 oz baked haddock seasoned with paprika	Creole Fish Fillets Red Beans and Brown Rice Sugar-free Raspberry Bars 6 walnut halves	Apricot-Glazed Chicken Scalloped Jack Potatoes 1 slice whole-wheat bread 1 cup nonfat milk 1 cup nonstarchy stir-fry vegetables 1 1/2 tsp canola oil (for stir-fry)	Lentil Stroganoff 1 cup grilled or sautéed nonstarchy vegetables 2 tsp canola oil (to cook vegetables) 1 oz reduced-fat cheese	Cajun Pork Chops Potatoes Au Gratin 1 slice rye bread 3/4 cup blueberries 1 cup nonfat milk 1/2 cup Harvard beets 1/2 cup cooked spinach 2 tsp margarine	Savory Sirloin Lemon Parsley Carrots Granola Oats Blackberry Raspberry Bake 3-inch cube low-fat corn bread 1 cup nonfat milk 1 cup salad made from dark greens 1 1/2 Tbsp reduced-fat salad dressing	Skewered Chicken and Shrimp Cold Pasta Salad Carrots in Sherry Wine 6 mixed nuts

*Indicates that the recipe has been used previously.

	Sunday	Monday	Tuesday	Wednesday	Thursday	Friday	Saturday
Breakfast	Whole-Wheat Pancakes or Waffles (2) 1/4 cup sugar-free syrup 1 small orange 1 cup nonfat milk 1 oz lean turkey ham 5 peanuts 2 tsp margarine	1/2 whole-wheat bagel 1/2 large grapefruit 1 cup nonfat milk 1/4 cup egg substitute 1/2 Tbsp almond butter 2 tsp light jam	Whole-Grain Muffins (2) 1 cup nonfat milk 1/4 cup egg substitute 4 tsp tahini (sesame paste)	3/4 cup bran cereal 1 slice multigrain toast 1 kiwi fruit 1/2 cup nonfat milk 1/4 cup low-fat cottage cheese 2 tsp margarine 2 tsp light jam	Zucchini Carrot Muffins 3/4 cup strawberries 1 cup nonfat milk 1/2 tsp margarine	Banana Bran Muffin 1/2 cup Kashi cereal 1 cup nonfat milk 1 oz reduced-fat cheese 9 mixed nuts	French Toast Fried Bananas 4 oz nonfat milk
Lunch	Sweet and Sour Green Beans Pineapple Pudding Parfait 1/2 cup mashed potatoes 1 slice whole-wheat low-calorie bread 2 oz roasted chicken, skin removed 1 Tbsp 30–50% vegetable oil margarine	Spicy Whole-Grain Rice with Peanuts Broccoli Floret Salad 2 small plums 2 oz cheese (3 grams of fat or less per slice)	Pizza Muffins Sizzlin' Fruit Salad 16 pistachios	Chicken Salad Roll-Up 10 baked tortilla chips 1/2 cup corn kernels 1 small apple 1 cup green pepper slices 4 black olives 3 macadamia nuts	Chicken Cucumber Salad 2/3 cup baked beans 1 small roll 1/2 large pear 1 tsp margarine 10 dry roasted peanuts	No Egg, Egg Salad Sandwich Seasoned Chilled Vegetables 15 fat-free potato chips 1/2 cup fruit cocktail in sugar-free syrup 1 oz reduced-fat cheese	Barbecued Pork Sandwich Oven-Roasted Tomatoes 1/2 ear corn on the cob 1/2 unsweetened plums 1 1/2 tsp margarine
Snack A	1/2 Tbsp peanut butter 1 small apple	10 dry roasted peanuts 2 Tbsp raisins 1/4 cup low-fat cottage cheese	2 Brazil nuts 3/4 cup blackberries	1 1/2 tsp cashew butter 1/2 large pear	5 hazelnuts 1 cup raspberries	4 pecan halves 2 Tbsp raisins	6 almonds 3/4 cup blueberries
Snack B	6 oz fat-free yogurt (100 calories or less)	1 cup nonfat milk	6 oz fat-free yogurt	1 cup nonfat milk	1 cup fat-free yogurt	1 cup nonfat milk	1 cup fat-free yogurt
Dinner	Friendship Stew Splendid Blueberry Crisp 1/2 slice whole-wheat low-calorie bread 1/8 cup fat-free salad dressing 1 cup nonfat milk 2 cups salad made from nonstarchy vegetables 3 oz baked haddock seasoned with paprika	Creole Fish Fillets Red Beans and Brown Rice Sugar-free Raspberry Bars 6 walnut halves	Apricot-Glazed Chicken Scalloped Jack Potatoes 1 slice whole-wheat bread 1 cup nonfat milk 1 cup nonstarchy stir-fry vegetables 1 1/2 tsp canola oil (for stir-fry)	Lentil Stroganoff 1 cup grilled or sautéed nonstarchy vegetables 2 tsp canola oil (to cook vegetables) 2 oz reduced-fat cheese	Cajun Pork Chops Potatoes Au Gratin 1 slice rye bread 3/4 cup blueberries 1 cup nonfat milk 1/2 cup beets 1/2 cup cooked spinach 2 tsp margarine	Savory Sirloin Lemon Parsley Carrots Granola Oats Blackberry Raspberry Bake 3-inch cube low-fat corn bread 1 cup nonfat milk 1 cup salad made from dark greens 1 1/2 Tbsp reduced-fat salad dressing	Skewered Chicken and Shrimp Cold Pasta Salad Carrots in Sherry Wine 6 mixed nuts

*Indicates that the recipe has been used previously.

2000 calorie MEAL PLAN WINTER WEEK 1

	Sunday	Monday	Tuesday	Wednesday	Thursday	Friday	Saturday
Breakfast	**Whole-Wheat Pancakes or Waffles** (2) 1/4 cup sugar-free syrup 1 small orange 1 cup nonfat milk 1 oz lean turkey ham 5 peanuts 2 tsp margarine	1/2 whole-wheat bagel 1/2 large grapefruit 1 cup nonfat milk 1/4 cup egg substitute 1/2 Tbsp almond butter 2 tsp light jam	**Whole-Grain Muffins** (2) 1 small banana 1 cup nonfat milk 1/4 cup egg substitute, scrambled 4 tsp tahini (sesame paste)	3/4 cup bran cereal 1 slice multigrain toast 1 kiwi fruit 1/2 cup nonfat milk 1/4 cup low-fat cottage cheese 2 tsp margarine 2 tsp light jam	**Zucchini Carrot Muffins** 3/4 cup strawberries 1 cup nonfat milk 1/2 tsp margarine	**Banana Bran Muffin** 1/2 cup Kashi cereal 1 cup nonfat milk 1 oz reduced-fat cheese 9 mixed nuts	**French Toast Fried Bananas** 4 oz nonfat milk
Lunch	**Sweet and Sour Green Beans Pineapple Pudding Parfait** 1/2 cup mashed potatoes 1 slice whole-wheat low-calorie bread 1 1/4 cup strawberries 2 oz roasted chicken, skin removed 1 Tbsp 30–50% vegetable oil margarine	**Spicy Whole-Grain Rice with Peanuts Broccoli Floret Salad** 2 large plums 2 oz cheese (3 grams of fat or less per slice)	**Pizza Muffins Sizzlin' Fruit Salad** 16 pistachios	**Chicken Salad Roll-Up** 10 baked tortilla chips 1/2 cup corn kernels 1 small apple 1 cup green pepper slices 8 small grape tomatoes 4 black olives 3 macadamia nuts	**Chicken Cucumber Salad** 2/3 cup baked beans 1 small roll 1 large pear 1 cup raw cauliflower and broccoli 1 tsp margarine 10 dry roasted peanuts	**No Egg, Egg Salad Sandwich Seasoned Chilled Vegetables** 15 fat-free potato chips 1/2 cup fruit cocktail in sugar-free syrup 1 cup green pepper slices 1 oz reduced-fat cheese	**Barbecued Pork Sandwich Oven-Roasted Tomatoes** 1/2 ear corn on the cob 1 cup unsweetened plums 1 cup vegetable sticks 1 1/2 tsp margarine
Snack A	1 cup raw vegetables 1/2 Tbsp peanut butter 1 small apple	1 cup raw celery sticks 1 1/2 Tbsp reduced-fat cream cheese 2 Tbsp raisins 1/4 cup low-fat cottage cheese	1 cup nonstarchy vegetable sticks 2 Brazil nuts 3/4 cup blackberries	1 cup raw broccoli 1 1/2 tsp cashew butter 1/2 large pear	1 cup raw mixed vegetables 5 hazelnuts 1 cup raspberries	4 pecan halves 2 Tbsp raisins 1 cup raw vegetables	6 almonds 3/4 cup blueberries 1 cup raw carrot sticks
Snack B	8 animal crackers 2 Tbsp reduced-fat salad dressing 6 oz fat-free yogurt (100 calories or less)	3 ginger snaps 6 dry roasted almonds 1 cup nonfat milk	2 (4-inch) rice cakes 1/2 Tbsp peanut butter 6 oz fat-free yogurt	3 cups popcorn 1 tsp margarine 1 cup nonfat milk	1/2 English muffin 1 tsp margarine 1 cup fat-free yogurt	1/2 English muffin 1 tsp margarine 1 cup nonfat milk	1 cup fat-free yogurt 3 macadamia nuts 3/4 cup shredded wheat
Dinner	**Friendship Stew Splendid Blueberry Crisp** 1/2 slice whole-wheat low-calorie bread 1/8 cup fat-free salad dressing 1 cup nonfat milk 2 cups salad made from nonstarchy vegetables 3 oz baked haddock seasoned with paprika	**Creole Fish Fillets Red Beans and Brown Rice Sugar-free Raspberry Bars** 6 walnut halves	**Apricot-Glazed Chicken Scalloped Jack Potatoes** 1 slice whole-wheat bread 1 cup nonfat milk 1 cup nonstarchy stir-fry vegetables 1 1/2 tsp canola oil (for stir-fry)	**Lentil Stroganoff** 1 cup grilled or sautéed nonstarchy vegetables 2 tsp canola oil (to cook vegetables) 2 oz reduced-fat cheese	**Cajun Pork Chops Potatoes Au Gratin** 1 slice rye bread 3/4 cup blueberries 1 cup nonfat milk 1/2 cup beets 1/2 cup cooked spinach 2 tsp margarine	**Savory Sirloin Lemon Parsley Carrots Granola Oats Blackberry Raspberry Bake** 3-inch cube low-fat corn bread 1 cup nonfat milk 1 cup salad made from dark greens 1 1/2 Tbsp reduced-fat salad dressing	**Skewered Chicken and Shrimp Cold Pasta Salad Carrots in Sherry Wine** 6 mixed nuts

*Indicates that the recipe has been used previously.

	Sunday	Monday	Tuesday	Wednesday	Thursday	Friday	Saturday
Breakfast	**Whole-Wheat Pancakes or Waffles** (2) 1/4 cup sugar-free syrup 1 small orange 1 cup nonfat milk 2 oz lean turkey ham 5 peanuts 2 tsp margarine	1/2 whole-wheat bagel 1/2 large grapefruit 1 cup nonfat milk 1/2 cup egg substitute 1 Tbsp almond butter 2 tsp light jam	**Whole-Grain Muffins** (2) 1 small banana 1 cup nonfat milk 1/2 cup egg substitute, scrambled 4 tsp tahini (sesame paste)	3/4 cup bran cereal 1 slice multigrain toast 1 kiwi fruit 1 cup nonfat milk 1/2 cup low-fat cottage cheese 2 tsp margarine 2 tsp light jam	**Zucchini Carrot Muffins** 3/4 cup strawberries 1 cup nonfat milk 1 oz lean sausage 1/2 tsp margarine	**Banana Bran Muffin** 1/2 cup Kashi cereal 1 cup nonfat milk 2 oz reduced-fat cheese 9 mixed nuts	**French Toast Fried Bananas** 4 oz nonfat milk 1 oz lean sausage
Lunch	**Sweet and Sour Green Beans Pineapple Pudding Parfait** 1/2 cup mashed potatoes 1 slice whole-wheat low-calorie bread 1 1/4 cup strawberries 2 oz roasted chicken, skin removed 1 Tbsp 30–50% vegetable oil margarine	**Spicy Whole-Grain Rice with Peanuts Broccoli Floret Salad** 2 large plums 2 oz cheese (3 grams of fat or less per slice)	**Pizza Muffins Sizzlin' Fruit Salad** 16 pistachios	**Chicken Salad Roll-Up** 10 baked tortilla chips 1/2 cup corn kernels 1 large apple 1 cup green pepper slices 8 small grape tomatoes 4 black olives 3 macadamia nuts	**Chicken Cucumber Salad** 2/3 cup baked beans 1 small roll 1 large pear 1 cup raw cauliflower and broccoli 1 tsp margarine 10 dry roasted peanuts	**No Egg, Egg Salad Sandwich Seasoned Chilled Vegetables** 15 fat-free potato chips 1/2 cup fruit cocktail in sugar-free syrup 1 cup green pepper slices 1 oz reduced-fat cheese	**Barbecued Pork Sandwich Oven-Roasted Tomatoes** 1/2 ear corn on the cob 1 cup unsweetened plums 1 cup vegetable sticks 1 1/2 tsp margarine
Snack A	1 cup raw vegetables 1/2 Tbsp peanut butter 1 small apple	1 cup raw celery 1 1/2 Tbsp reduced-fat cream cheese 2 Tbsp raisins 1/4 cup low-fat cottage cheese	2 Brazil nuts 3/4 cup blackberries	1 cup raw broccoli 1 1/2 tsp cashew butter 1/2 large pear	1 cup raw mixed vegetables 5 hazelnuts 1 cup raspberries	4 pecan halves 2 Tbsp raisins 1 cup raw vegetables	6 almonds 3/4 cup blueberries 1 cup raw carrot sticks
Snack B	8 animal crackers 2 Tbsp reduced-fat salad dressing 6 oz fat-free yogurt (100 calories or less)	3 ginger snaps 6 dry roasted almonds 1 cup nonfat milk	6 oz fat-free yogurt	3 cups popcorn 1 tsp margarine 1 cup nonfat milk	1/2 English muffin 1 tsp margarine 1 cup fat-free yogurt	1/2 English muffin 1 tsp margarine 1 cup nonfat milk	1 cup fat-free yogurt 3 macadamia nuts 3/4 cup shredded wheat
Dinner	**Friendship Stew Splendid Blueberry Crisp** 1 1/2 slices whole-wheat low-calorie bread 1/8 cup fat-free salad dressing 1 cup nonfat milk 2 cups salad made from nonstarchy vegetables 3 oz baked haddock seasoned with paprika	**Creole Fish Fillets Red Beans and Brown Rice Sugar-free Raspberry Bars** 1 cup nonfat milk 6 walnut halves	**Apricot-Glazed Chicken Scalloped Jack Potatoes** 1 1/2 slices whole-wheat bread 1 cup nonfat milk 1 cup nonstarchy stir-fry vegetables 1 1/2 tsp canola oil (for stir-fry)	**Lentil Stroganoff** 1 cup fresh cantaloupe cubes 1 cup grilled or sautéed nonstarchy vegetables 2 tsp canola oil (to cook vegetables) 2 oz reduced-fat cheese	**Cajun Pork Chops Potatoes Au Gratin** 2 slices rye bread 3/4 cup blueberries 1 cup nonfat milk 1/2 cup beets 1/2 cup cooked spinach 2 tsp margarine	**Savory Sirloin Lemon Parsley Carrots Granola Oats Blackberry Raspberry Bake** 3-inch cube low-fat corn bread 1 cup nonfat milk 1 cup salad made from dark greens 1 1/2 Tbsp reduced-fat salad dressing	**Skewered Chicken and Shrimp Cold Pasta Salad Carrots in Sherry Wine** 1 cup nonfat milk 6 mixed nuts

*Indicates that the recipe has been used previously.

VEGETABLES

_____ beets
_____ bell peppers, green
_____ bell peppers, red
_____ broccoli
_____ carrots or baby carrots
_____ cauliflower
_____ celery
_____ corn kernels
_____ corn on the cob
_____ cucumbers
_____ garlic
_____ grape tomatoes
_____ green beans
_____ green onions
_____ mushrooms
_____ onions, yellow or white
_____ potatoes, red or russet
_____ purple onions
_____ red onions
_____ spinach
_____ tomatoes
_____ zucchini

MEATS

_____ chicken breasts, boneless, skinless
_____ cod fish fillets
_____ haddock fillets
_____ pork tenderloin
_____ sausage, lean
_____ shrimp
_____ sirloin pork chops, boneless
_____ turkey ham, lean

FRUITS

_____ apples
_____ bananas
_____ blackberries
_____ blueberries
_____ cantaloupe
_____ cherries
_____ dried apricot halves
_____ grapefruit
_____ kiwi fruit
_____ lemons
_____ oranges
_____ pears
_____ pineapple, crushed/cubed
_____ plums
_____ raisins
_____ raspberries
_____ strawberries

DAIRY

_____ egg substitute
_____ egg whites
_____ nonfat milk
_____ yogurt, plain, fat-free
_____ Smart Balance Light margarine

CHEESE

_____ cheddar, fat-free and reduced-fat, shredded
_____ mozzarella, fat-free and reduced-fat, shredded
_____ cottage cheese, reduced-fat

BREAD, GRAINS, & PASTA

_____ bagels, whole-wheat
_____ bread, rye
_____ bread, whole-wheat, whole-grain
_____ brown rice
_____ corn bread, low-fat
_____ dinner rolls
_____ English muffins, multigrain
_____ hamburger buns, whole-wheat
_____ pasta/noodles, whole-grain

BEANS

_____ baked beans
_____ kidney beans
_____ lentils
_____ Northern mixed dried beans

NUTS

_____ almonds
_____ dates, chopped
_____ macadamia nuts
_____ peanuts, dry roasted
_____ pistachios
_____ walnuts

CONDIMENTS

_____ almond butter
_____ canola mayonnaise
_____ catsup, no-salt
_____ Dijon mustard
_____ Italian salad dressing, reduced-fat or fat-free
_____ jam, light
_____ maple syrup, sugar-free
_____ peanut butter
_____ prepared mustard
_____ raspberry preserves, sugar-free
_____ soy sauce, light
_____ tahini

SPICES & HERBS

_____ allspice
_____ basil
_____ bay leaves
_____ black pepper
_____ cayenne pepper
_____ chili powder
_____ cilantro
_____ cinnamon, ground
_____ cloves
_____ cumin seeds
_____ dill seeds
_____ dill weed
_____ dried rosemary
_____ dried thyme
_____ dry mustard
_____ garlic powder
_____ ginger, ground
_____ gingerroot
_____ nutmeg, ground
_____ paprika
_____ parsley
_____ red pepper flakes
_____ rubbed sage
_____ turmeric

OTHER

_____ animal crackers
_____ black olives
_____ cereal, bran
_____ cereal, Kashi
_____ corn tortillas (6 inches)
_____ diced tomatoes, no-added-salt
_____ fruit cocktail in sugar-free syrup
_____ instant mashed potatoes
_____ old-fashioned (rolled) oats
_____ orange juice
_____ potato chips, fat-free
_____ spaghetti/tomato sauce, no-added-salt
_____ tofu
_____ tomato paste, no-added-salt
_____ tortilla chips, baked
_____ unsweetened applesauce
_____ vanilla pudding, instant, sugar-free
_____ water chestnuts
_____ whipped topping, fat-free

STAPLES

_____ baking powder
_____ baking soda
_____ canola oil
_____ cornstarch
_____ honey
_____ lemon juice
_____ lime juice
_____ nonstick cooking spray
_____ sherry, dry cooking
_____ Smart Balance Omega oil
_____ sodium-free chicken bullion
_____ Splenda
_____ Splenda Brown Sugar Blend
_____ vanilla extract
_____ vinegar, apple cider
_____ vinegar, rice wine
_____ vinegar, white
_____ wheat germ
_____ whole-wheat flour
_____ Worcestershire sauce

Whole-Wheat Pancakes or Waffles

Serves 4   Serving size: 2 pancakes or waffles

1/2   **cup** rolled oats

1/2   **cup** whole-wheat flour, sifted

2   **tsp** baking powder

2   **Tbsp** Splenda

1/2   **cup** egg substitute, beaten well

3/4   **cup** nonfat milk

2   **Tbsp** Smart Balance Omega oil

Nonstick cooking spray

Stir together dry ingredients. Combine egg substitute, milk, and oil; stir into flour mixture. Cook on a griddle lightly coated with nonstick spray until golden brown, then turn. Can also be made in a waffle iron.

Exchanges/Choices

1 1/2 Starch
1 1/2 Fat

Basic Nutritional Values

Calories	185
Calories from Fat	70
Total Fat	8.0 g
Saturated Fat	0.7 g
Trans Fat	0.0 g
Cholesterol	0 mg
Sodium	265 mg
Total Carbohydrate	22 g
Dietary Fiber	3 g
Sugars	3 g
Protein	8 g

Sweet and Sour Green Beans

Serves 4   Serving size: 1/4 recipe

16   **oz** fresh green beans, cut into 1 1/2-inch pieces, or 16 oz frozen cut green beans

3   **Tbsp** white vinegar

2   **Tbsp** Splenda

3   **Tbsp** Splenda Brown Sugar Blend, packed

3   **Tbsp** no-salt catsup

2   **Tbsp** Smart Balance Omega oil

1   **tsp** Worcestershire sauce

1/4   **tsp** dry mustard

5   **oz** water chestnuts sliced, drained

1/3   red onion, small, thinly sliced

1. Boil or steam the green beans for 5–15 minutes until done as desired. Drain and chill.

2. In a medium bowl, whisk together the vinegar, Splenda, catsup, oil, Worcestershire sauce, and dry mustard until blended. Add the green beans, water chestnuts, and onion, stirring until coated. Serve hot. Dish can stand at room temperature for up to 2 hours, but requires occasional stirring.

Exchanges/Choices

1 Carbohydrate
2 Vegetable
1 Fat

Basic Nutritional Values

Calories	170
Calories from Fat	65
Total Fat	7.0 g
Saturated Fat	0.6 g
Trans Fat	0 g
Cholesterol	0 mg
Sodium	30 mg
Total Carbohydrate	26 g
Dietary Fiber	4 g
Sugars	16 g
Protein	2 g

Pineapple Pudding Parfait

Serves 4   Serving size: 1/4 recipe

4 oz fat-free whipped topping

1 oz pkg sugar-free instant vanilla pudding

1 (8-oz) can no-sugar-added crushed pineapple

Thaw the whipped topping and mix with dry pudding mix. Add crushed pineapple with juice and refrigerate. Serve in large parfait glasses. If desired, add maraschino cherries to decorate. Peach slices can be used instead of pineapple.

Exchanges/Choices

1 1/2 Carbohydrate

Basic Nutritional Values

Calories 100
 Calories from Fat 0
Total Fat . . . . 0.0 g
 Saturated Fat . . . . 0.0 g
 Trans Fat . . . . 0.0 g
Cholesterol . . . . 0 mg
Sodium . . . . 315 mg
Total Carbohydrate . . . 22 g
 Dietary Fiber . . . . 0 g
 Sugars . . . . 10 g
Protein . . . . 0 g

Friendship Stew

Serves 10   Serving size: 1 cup

1/2 cup Northern mixed dried beans

1 large onion, chopped fine

3 celery stalks, chopped fine

1 large clove garlic, pressed

3 medium fresh tomatoes, diced

2 Tbsp sodium-free chicken bullion

2 quarts boiling water

Black pepper, to taste

Pinch dill weed

Soak the beans overnight in 1 quart of water. Drain and add to a large crock pot. Add all other ingredients and simmer on low for 3–4 hours.

Exchanges/Choices

1/2 Starch
1 Vegetable

Basic Nutritional Values

Calories 55
 Calories from Fat 0
Total Fat . . . . 0.0 g
 Saturated Fat . . . . 0.1 g
 Trans Fat . . . . 0.0 g
Cholesterol . . . . 0 mg
Sodium . . . . 25 mg
Total Carbohydrate . . . 11 g
 Dietary Fiber . . . . 3 g
 Sugars . . . . 4 g
Protein . . . . 3 g

Splendid Blueberry Crisp

Serves 9   Serving size: 1/9 recipe

Nonstick cooking spray

4 Tbsp Splenda

1 1/2 Tbsp whole-wheat flour

1 1/2 tsp ground cinnamon

1 tsp pure vanilla extract

6 cups fresh or frozen (partially thawed) blueberries

1 cup old-fashioned oats, uncooked

1/3 cup coarsely chopped almonds

1/3 cup chopped walnuts

4 Tbsp melted Smart Balance Light margarine

1. Lightly coat an 8-inch baking dish with nonstick cooking spray.

2. Combine 2 Tbsp Splenda, flour, 1 tsp cinnamon, and vanilla. Mix well. Fold in blueberries until fruit is evenly coated. Spoon into baking dish.

3. Combine all remaining ingredients; mix well. Sprinkle evenly over fruit. Preheat oven to 350°F. Bake for 35–40 minutes or until topping is golden and filling is bubbly. Serve warm.

Exchanges/Choices

1 1/2 Carbohydrate
1 1/2 Fat

Basic Nutritional Values

Calories 170
  Calories from Fat 70
Total Fat . . . . 8.0 g
  Saturated Fat . . . . 1.2 g
  Trans Fat . . . . 0.0 g
Cholesterol . . . . 0 mg
Sodium . . . . 40 mg
Total Carbohydrate . . . 23 g
  Dietary Fiber . . . . 4 g
  Sugars . . . . 11 g
Protein . . . . 4 g

Spicy Whole-Grain Rice with Peanuts

Serves 4   Serving size: 1/4 recipe

2	**Tbsp** Smart Balance Omega oil	1/2	**cup** onion, minced
2	**tsp** cumin seed	1	medium garlic clove, minced
1	**tsp** whole cloves	2/3	**cup** whole-grain rice, uncooked
1	bay leaf	2 1/2	**cups** water
1	**tsp** red pepper flakes	1/4	**cup** dry roasted peanuts

1. In a large heavy saucepan, heat the oil over moderate heat until it is hot. Add cumin seed, cloves, and bay leaf; cook, stirring constantly, for 5–10 seconds or until the cumin seed is a few shades darker and fragrant. Add the red pepper flakes, onion, and garlic; cook, stirring constantly, until the onion has softened. Add the rice and cook, while stirring, for 2 minutes or until it is well coated with the mixture. Add water; bring to a boil. Simmer covered for 35–40 minutes or until the water is absorbed and the rice is fluffy and tender.

2. Put the peanuts in a blender and grind for a few seconds. Fluff the rice with a fork, remove the pan from the heat, and discard the bay leaf. Let the rice stand, covered, for 10 minutes. Stir in the peanuts and serve.

Exchanges/Choices

2 Starch
2 Fat

Basic Nutritional Values

Calories 245
  Calories from Fat 115
Total Fat . . . . 13.0 g
  Saturated Fat . . . . 1.3 g
  Trans Fat . . . . 0.0 g
Cholesterol . . . . 0 mg
Sodium . . . . 80 mg
Total Carbohydrate . . . 29 g
  Dietary Fiber . . . . 3 g
  Sugars . . . . 2 g
Protein . . . . 5 g

Broccoli Floret Salad

Serves 4   Serving size: 1/4 recipe

2	**cups** fresh or frozen broccoli florets, cut small		Black pepper, to taste
2	**Tbsp** chopped parsley	1	small purple onion, diced
1	**Tbsp** fresh basil	2/3	**cup** light Italian salad dressing
1	medium red pepper, thinly sliced		

Combine all ingredients (except dressing) in a large bowl. Add dressing. Stir well and chill for 2 hours before serving.

Exchanges/Choices

1/2 Carbohydrate
1 Vegetable
1/2 Fat

Basic Nutritional Values

Calories 80
  Calories from Fat 25
Total Fat . . . . 3.0 g
  Saturated Fat . . . . 0.3 g
  Trans Fat . . . . 0.0 g
Cholesterol . . . . 0 mg
Sodium . . . . 480 mg
Total Carbohydrate . . . 12 g
  Dietary Fiber . . . . 2 g
  Sugars . . . . 9 g
Protein . . . . 2 g

Creole Fish Fillets

Serves 4   Serving size: 1/4 recipe

1 (16-oz) can no-added-salt diced tomatoes

1/2 **cup** celery, diced

1/2 **cup** onion, diced

1/4 **cup** green pepper, diced

1 clove garlic, minced

1 bay leaf

1 **tsp** thyme

1/2 **tsp** red pepper flakes

Black pepper, to taste

1 **lb** fresh cod fish fillets

1. Preheat oven to 400°F. Combine all ingredients, except the fish, in a saucepan. Bring to a boil. Cover and reduce heat; simmer for about 20 minutes, stirring occasionally. Remove pan from heat and discard the bay leaf.

2. Meanwhile, place fish in a baking dish. Bake uncovered for about 15 minutes, until fish flakes easily when tested with a fork. Pour sauce over fish and serve.

Exchanges/Choices

2 Vegetable
2 Lean Meat

Basic Nutritional Values

Calories	130
Calories from Fat	10
Total Fat	1.0 g
Saturated Fat	0.2 g
Trans Fat	0.0 g
Cholesterol	50 mg
Sodium	125 mg
Total Carbohydrate	9 g
Dietary Fiber	3 g
Sugars	5 g
Protein	21 g

Red Beans and Brown Rice

Serves 4   Serving size: 1/4 recipe

1 **Tbsp** sodium-free chicken bouillon

1 **cup** water

1 **cup** whole-grain brown rice

1/4 **cup** no-added-salt tomato paste

1/4 **tsp** chili powder

1 **Tbsp** light soy sauce

1/2 **cup** onion, chopped

1 **cup** kidney beans, drained

1. In a medium pot over medium heat, combine bouillon and water. Add rice and cover.

2. When the rice has finished cooking, stir in the tomato paste, chili powder, soy sauce, and onions. Add kidney beans; continue to cook over low heat until all is thoroughly cooked.

Exchanges/Choices

3 Starch
1 Vegetable

Basic Nutritional Values

Calories	260
Calories from Fat	20
Total Fat	2.0 g
Saturated Fat	0.3 g
Trans Fat	0.0 g
Cholesterol	0 mg
Sodium	225 mg
Total Carbohydrate	53 g
Dietary Fiber	6 g
Sugars	4 g
Protein	9 g

Sugar-Free Raspberry Bars

Serves 16   Serving size: 1 bar

1 **cup** Splenda

1 **cup** whole-wheat flour

1/2 **cup** Smart Balance margarine, melted

Nonstick cooking spray

1 **(20-oz)** jar sugar-free raspberry preserves

1. Combine the Splenda, flour, and melted margarine in a bowl.

2. Lightly spray a 9-inch baking dish with nonstick cooking spray. Spread half of the crumb mixture in the bottom of the dish. Layer the preserves on top of the crumb mixture. Sprinkle remaining crumb mixture over the preserves. Bake at 375°F for about 25 minutes. Cut into 16 individual bars.

Exchanges/Choices

1 Carbohydrate
1/2 Fat

Basic Nutritional Values

Calories 90
  Calories from Fat 40
Total Fat . . . . .4.5 g
  Saturated Fat . . . . .1.3 g
  Trans Fat . . . . .0.0 g
Cholesterol . . . . .0 mg
Sodium . . . . .45 mg
Total Carbohydrate . . .17 g
  Dietary Fiber . . . . .1 g
  Sugars . . . . .7 g
Protein . . . . .1 g

TUESDAY

Whole-Grain Muffins
Serves 8   Serving size: 1 muffin

Nonstick cooking spray

3/4 **cup** whole-wheat flour

2 **tsp** baking powder

1 1/2 **Tbsp** Splenda

2/3 **cup** rolled oats cereal

1 **cup** nonfat milk

1/4 **cup** egg substitute

1/4 **cup** unsweetened applesauce

Exchanges/Choices
1 Carbohydrate

Basic Nutritional Values
Calories 85
  Calories from Fat 5
Total Fat . . . . 0.5 g
  Saturated Fat . . . . 0.1 g
  Trans Fat . . . . 0.0 g
Cholesterol . . . . 0 mg
Sodium . . . . 120 mg
Total Carbohydrate . . . 16 g
  Dietary Fiber . . . . 2 g
  Sugars . . . . 3 g
Protein . . . . 5 g

1. Lightly spray muffin pan cups with nonstick cooking spray; set aside.

2. Stir together the flour, baking powder, and Splenda; set aside.

3. Combine rolled oats and milk in a large mixing bowl; let stand until oats are softened, about 1–2 minutes. Add egg substitute and applesauce; beat well. Add whole-wheat flour mixture; gently stir to combine. Divide batter evenly among prepared muffin cups. Bake at 400°F for 25 minutes or until lightly browned.

Pizza Muffins
Serves 4   Serving size: 1 muffin

4 light multigrain English muffins

1 **cup** no-salt-added spaghetti sauce

4 **oz** fat-free shredded mozzarella cheese

4 **oz** reduced-fat shredded mozzarella cheese

1/4 **cup** sliced fresh mushrooms

1 small onion, sliced into thin rings

4 green bell pepper rings

Exchanges/Choices
2 Starch
2 Vegetable
2 Lean Meat

Basic Nutritional Values
Calories 305
  Calories from Fat 65
Total Fat . . . . 7.0 g
  Saturated Fat . . . . 2.4 g
  Trans Fat . . . . 0.0 g
Cholesterol . . . . 15 mg
Sodium . . . . 660 mg
Total Carbohydrate . . . 42 g
  Dietary Fiber . . . . 12 g
  Sugars . . . . 8 g
Protein . . . . 25 g

1. Preheat the oven to 400°F.

2. Split the English muffins in half and put on a baking sheet, cut sides up. Spread spaghetti sauce over muffins. Top with 1 ounce of each of the cheeses. Top with mushrooms, onion rings, and pepper rings. Place pizzas in oven and bake for about 5 minutes or until cheese melts.

This recipe is high in sodium.

Sizzlin' Fruit Salad

Serves 4   Serving size: 1/4 recipe

1/2 **cup** sliced pears (can use fresh, frozen, or canned light, drained)

1/2 **cup** fresh cherries (or canned light, drained)

1/2 **cup** fresh cubed pineapple (or canned light, drained)

2 medium oranges, peeled and cut into cubes

1 **cup** water

1/2 **cup** Splenda

2 **Tbsp** Smart Balance margarine

1 **Tbsp** cornstarch

1 **Tbsp** lemon juice

1/4 **cup** dry cooking sherry

1/2 **cup** raisins

Exchanges/Choices

3 Fruit
1 Fat

Basic Nutritional Values

Calories	205
Calories from Fat	45
Total Fat	5.0 g
Saturated Fat	1.3 g
Trans Fat	0.0 g
Cholesterol	0 mg
Sodium	55 mg
Total Carbohydrate	42 g
Dietary Fiber	4 g
Sugars	34 g
Protein	2 g

1. Combine pears, cherries, and pineapple in an ovenproof glass bowl.

2. Combine orange cubes and water in a saucepan. Heat to boiling and simmer 5–10 minutes or until oranges are tender. Strain; add to pears, cherries, and pineapple. Sprinkle the Splenda on top.

3. Melt the margarine and combine with cornstarch in a saucepan. Add lemon juice, sherry, and raisins; cook, stirring consistently, until thickened. Pour over fruit and bake at 350°F for 30–45 minutes. Cool slightly before serving.

Apricot-Glazed Chicken

Serves 4   Serving size: 1/4 recipe

2 **Tbsp** lemon juice

1 clove garlic, minced

1/4 **tsp** pepper

1 **lb** boneless, skinless chicken breast halves

3/4 **cup** orange juice

12 dried apricot halves

1 **Tbsp** vinegar

1 **tsp** Splenda

1 **tsp** prepared mustard

1/4 **tsp** ground ginger

1. Preheat oven to 400°F.

2. Combine lemon juice, garlic, and pepper. Brush chicken with the mixture. Arrange chicken on a rack in a baking dish. Cover and bake for 45 minutes.

3. Combine the orange juice and apricots in a small saucepan. Simmer uncovered for 10 minutes or until apricots are tender. Stir in the vinegar, Splenda, mustard, and ginger. Simmer 2 minutes longer. Remove from heat and pour into blender jar. Puree apricots for about 15 seconds.

4. Spread half of the glaze on one side of the chicken; bake 3 minutes longer. Turn chicken and spread with remaining glaze. Bake for 3 minutes more or until chicken is tender.

Exchanges/Choices

1 Fruit
3 Lean Meat

Basic Nutritional Values

Calories 180
  Calories from Fat 25
Total Fat . . . . .3.0 g
  Saturated Fat . . . . .0.8 g
  Trans Fat . . . . .0.0 g
Cholesterol . . . . .65 mg
Sodium . . . . .75 mg
Total Carbohydrate . . .13 g
  Dietary Fiber . . . . .1 g
  Sugars . . . . .11 g
Protein . . . . .25 g

Chicken Salad Roll-Up

Serves 4   Serving size: 1 roll-up

- **8 oz** boneless, skinless chicken breast (trimmed of all visible fat)
- **1 Tbsp** lemon juice
- **1/2 cup** celery, diced
- **1/2 cup** onion, diced
- **1/2 cup** crushed pineapple (fresh or canned light, drained)
- Black pepper, to taste
- **1/4 cup** canola mayonnaise
- **1/2 cup** plain fat-free yogurt
- **4 (6-inch)** corn tortillas

Exchanges/Choices

1 Starch
2 Lean Meat
1/2 Fat

Basic Nutritional Values

Calories 205
  Calories from Fat 65
Total Fat . . . . 7.0 g
  Saturated Fat . . . . 0.5 g
  Trans Fat . . . . 0.0 g
Cholesterol . . . . 35 mg
Sodium . . . . 155 mg
Total Carbohydrate . . . 20 g
  Dietary Fiber . . . . 2 g
  Sugars . . . . 7 g
Protein . . . . 15 g

Place chicken breasts in boiling water and thoroughly cook. When done, put chicken in the refrigerator to cool while preparing the other ingredients. Combine all other ingredients in a large bowl; mix well. When the chicken has cooled, cut the breasts into small chunks. Add to the other ingredients; mix well. Refrigerate mixture for 2 hours before serving. Spoon equal amounts of the chicken salad in each tortilla and roll up. Pin closed with a toothpick.

Lentil Stroganoff

Serves 4   Serving size: 1/4 recipe

1 **cup** dry lentils	1/2 **cup** red or green pepper, cut into strips
4 1/2 **cups** water	
8 **oz** whole-wheat noodles, cooked	1/2 medium onion, chopped
	2 **Tbsp** whole-wheat flour
1 **tsp** Smart Balance Omega oil	2 **tsp** dry mustard
	1/4 **tsp** black pepper
1/2 **cup** fresh mushrooms, sliced	8 **oz** plain fat-free yogurt

Exchanges/Choices

4 1/2 Starch
1 Lean Meat

Basic Nutritional Values

Calories 405	
Calories from Fat 30	
Total Fat . . . . 3.5 g	
Saturated Fat . . . . 0.6 g	
Trans Fat . . . . 0.0 g	
Cholesterol . . . . 5 mg	
Sodium . . . . 50 mg	
Total Carbohydrate . . . 78 g	
Dietary Fiber . . . . 18 g	
Sugars . . . . 9 g	
Protein . . . . 23 g	

1. Combine the lentils and water in a large saucepan. Bring to a boil; cover, simmer until water is reduced and lentils are tender, about 30 minutes. Drain, set aside, and keep warm.

2. Cook the pasta according to the package instructions.

3. Heat the oil in a large frying pan. Add mushrooms, peppers, and onion. Cook until vegetables are just tender. Mix in the flour, mustard, and pepper; stirring constantly, cook over medium heat until mixture is smooth and thickened. Add lentils; mix well. Heat to desired serving temperature. Just before serving, stir in yogurt. Serve over noodles.

Zucchini Carrot Muffins

Serves 8   Serving size: 1 muffin

3/4	**cup** rolled oats		2	**tsp** ground nutmeg
2 1/2	**cups** whole-wheat flour		3	**Tbsp** Smart Balance Omega oil
2/3	**cup** nonfat milk		3	egg whites, beaten
1/2	**cup** wheat germ, toasted		1	**cup** carrots, finely shredded
3	**tsp** baking powder		1/2	**cup** zucchini, stemmed and grated
3/4	**cup** Splenda			
1	**Tbsp** ground cinnamon			

Preheat oven to 350°F. Combine all ingredients and mix well; pour into muffin liners in muffin pans. Bake for about 1 hour. Let cool for about 30 minutes before removing.

Exchanges/Choices

2 1/2 Carbohydrate
1 1/2 Fat

Basic Nutritional Values

Calories	260
Calories from Fat	65
Total Fat	7.0 g
Saturated Fat	0.9 g
Trans Fat	0.0 g
Cholesterol	0 mg
Sodium	180 mg
Total Carbohydrate	42 g
Dietary Fiber	7 g
Sugars	5 g
Protein	11 g

Chicken Cucumber Salad

Serves 4   Serving size: 1/4 recipe

1	**lb** boneless, skinless chicken breasts (trimmed of all visible fat)		2	medium cucumbers
			1	**Tbsp** apple cider vinegar
1	medium red pepper		1/4	**tsp** pepper
			4	**oz** plain fat-free yogurt

Place chicken breasts in boiling water and cook thoroughly. When done, transfer chicken to the refrigerator to cool while preparing the other ingredients. Chop red pepper, and peel and cube cucumbers; mix together in a medium bowl. Sprinkle with vinegar and pepper. Let sit about 5 minutes. When the chicken has cooled, cut the breasts into small chunks. Stir chicken and yogurt into pepper and cucumber mixture; toss gently. Cover and refrigerate until completely chilled.

Exchanges/Choices

1 Vegetable
3 Lean Meat

Basic Nutritional Values

Calories	165
Calories from Fat	25
Total Fat	3.0 g
Saturated Fat	0.9 g
Trans Fat	0.0 g
Cholesterol	70 mg
Sodium	80 mg
Total Carbohydrate	7 g
Dietary Fiber	1 g
Sugars	5 g
Protein	26 g

Cajun Pork Chops

Serves 4   Serving size: 1/4 recipe

1 **Tbsp** paprika	1/2 **tsp** garlic powder
1 **tsp** rubbed sage	3/4 **lb** boneless sirloin pork chops (trimmed of all visible fat)
1/2 **tsp** cayenne pepper	
1/2 **tsp** black pepper	2 **tsp** Smart Balance margarine

Combine paprika, sage, cayenne pepper, black pepper, and garlic powder; coat chops with seasoning mixture on both sides. Heat margarine over high heat, just until it starts to brown. Put chops in pan, reduce heat to medium. Fry on both sides until golden brown, about 3–4 minutes each side. Serve hot.

Exchanges/Choices

2 Lean Meat

Basic Nutritional Values

Calories 100
  Calories from Fat 35
Total Fat. . . . . 4.0 g
  Saturated Fat . . . . 0.8 g
  Trans Fat. . . . . 0.0 g
Cholesterol . . . . 40 mg
Sodium. . . . . 225 mg
Total Carbohydrate . . . 2 g
  Dietary Fiber. . . . . 1 g
  Sugars . . . . 1 g
Protein . . . . 15 g

Potatoes Au Gratin

Serves 4   Serving size: 1/4 recipe

Nonstick cooking spray	3/16 **tsp** pepper
2 **cups** red or russet potatoes, peeled and cubed	2 **oz** fat-free shredded cheddar cheese
1/2 **cup** nonfat milk	1 1/2 **oz** reduced-fat shredded cheddar cheese
1/2 **Tbsp** whole-wheat flour	

1. Preheat oven to 375°F. Lightly spray a 9-inch baking dish with nonstick cooking spray.

2. In a mixing bowl, add potato cubes, cover with cold water, and set aside.

3. In a saucepan, whisk together the milk, flour, and pepper until well blended. Stirring constantly over medium-high heat, bring to a full boil. Reduce heat to low and stir in the cheeses; simmer until cheese is melted.

4. Drain potatoes and place in baking dish. Pour cheese mixture on top of potatoes. Bake for 1 hour or until potatoes are tender.

Exchanges/Choices

1 Starch
1 Lean Meat

Basic Nutritional Values

Calories 135
  Calories from Fat 20
Total Fat. . . . . 2.5 g
  Saturated Fat . . . . 1.4 g
  Trans Fat. . . . . 0.0 g
Cholesterol . . . . 10 mg
Sodium. . . . . 245 mg
Total Carbohydrate . . . 19 g
  Dietary Fiber. . . . . 2 g
  Sugars . . . . 3 g
Protein . . . . 10 g

Banana Bran Muffin

Serves 8   Serving size: 1 muffin

2/3 **cup** bran cereal	3/16 **tsp** ground nutmeg
2/3 **cup** plain fat-free yogurt	2 **cups** bananas, mashed
5/8 **cup** whole-wheat flour	1/4 **cup** unsweetened applesauce
5 **Tbsp** Splenda	1/2 **cup** egg substitute, beaten
1 **tsp** ground cinnamon	
1/2 **tsp** baking soda	

1. Preheat oven to 375°F. Place paper liners in muffin pan cups.

2. In a medium bowl, mix cereal and yogurt. Let stand for 5 minutes or until cereal is softened and breaks up.

3. Meanwhile, in a small bowl, combine the flour, Splenda, cinnamon, baking soda, and nutmeg; set aside.

4. Stir banana, applesauce, and egg substitute into cereal mixture. Stir in flour mixture until moistened. Fill muffin cups to about 2/3 full. Bake for 20–25 minutes or until muffins are lightly browned on top. Remove from pan and let cool on a wire rack before serving.

Exchanges/Choices

1 Starch
1 Fruit

Basic Nutritional Values

Calories 120
 Calories from Fat 5
Total Fat. . . . . .0.5 g
 Saturated Fat . . . . .0.2 g
 Trans Fat. . . . . .0.0 g
Cholesterol. . . . . .0 mg
Sodium. . . . . .135 mg
Total Carbohydrate . . .27 g
 Dietary Fiber. . . . . .5 g
 Sugars . . . . .11 g
Protein . . . . .5 g

No Egg, Egg Salad Sandwich

Serves 4   Serving size: 1 sandwich

12 **oz** tofu	1 celery stalk, minced
1/4 **cup** canola mayonnaise	3 green onions, with tops, minced
2 **tsp** Dijon mustard	3 **Tbsp** fresh chopped parsley
1/2 **tsp** garlic powder	8 slices whole-grain bread
1/4 **tsp** turmeric	
1 green pepper, seeded and minced	

Press tofu to remove liquid; drain and discard liquid. Mash tofu with a fork; then add the rest of the ingredients (except bread). Mix thoroughly. Spread on slices of bread to make sandwiches.

Exchanges/Choices

2 Starch
1 Lean Meat
1 Fat

Basic Nutritional Values

Calories 260
 Calories from Fat 90
Total Fat. . . . . .10.0 g
 Saturated Fat . . . . .1.2 g
 Trans Fat. . . . . .0.0 g
Cholesterol. . . . . .0 mg
Sodium. . . . . .440 mg
Total Carbohydrate . . .29 g
 Dietary Fiber. . . . . .6 g
 Sugars . . . . .6 g
Protein . . . . .15 g

Seasoned Chilled Vegetables

Serves 4   Serving size: 1/4 recipe

- 1/2 **cup** carrots, thinly sliced
- 1/2 **cup** cauliflower florets
- 1/2 **cup** zucchini, quartered and thickly sliced
- 1 **Tbsp** sodium-free chicken bouillon
- 1/2 **cup** water
- 1/4 **cup** sliced celery
- 1/4 **cup** white vinegar
- 2 **Tbsp** red onions, coarsely chopped
- 2 **Tbsp** Smart Balance Omega oil
- 1 **tsp** Splenda
- 1 **tsp** prepared mustard
- 1/2 **tsp** dill seeds
- 1/2 **tsp** dried rosemary, crushed
- 1/2 **tsp** dried thyme, crushed
- 1/2 **tsp** black pepper

Exchanges/Choices

1 Vegetable
1 1/2 Fat

Basic Nutritional Values

Calories 85
 Calories from Fat 65
Total Fat . . . . 7.0 g
 Saturated Fat . . . . 0.5 g
 Trans Fat . . . . 0.0 g
Cholesterol . . . . 0 mg
Sodium . . . . 40 mg
Total Carbohydrate . . . 6 g
 Dietary Fiber . . . . 1 g
 Sugars . . . . 3 g
Protein . . . . 1 g

Place all ingredients in a 3-quart saucepan. Bring to a boil; reduce heat to low, cover, and simmer for 10 minutes or until vegetables are crisp-tender. Pour into a bowl and chill for 2 hours or until cold. Serve.

Savory Sirloin

Serves 4   Serving size: 1/4 recipe

1 clove garlic, minced

1/4 tsp rosemary, crushed

1/4 tsp thyme leaves

1 lb boneless lean sirloin steak (trimmed of any visible fat)

1 tsp Smart Balance Light margarine

1 Tbsp plain fat-free yogurt

1 Tbsp prepared mustard

1 Tbsp Worcestershire sauce

1 Tbsp parsley, chopped

Exchanges/Choices

3 Lean Meat

Basic Nutritional Values

Calories 145
  Calories from Fat 45
Total Fat . . . . 5.0 g
  Saturated Fat . . . . 1.8 g
  Trans Fat . . . . 0.1 g
Cholesterol . . . . 45 mg
Sodium . . . . 150 mg
Total Carbohydrate . . . 2 g
  Dietary Fiber . . . . 0 g
  Sugars . . . . 1 g
Protein . . . . 23 g

1. Combine garlic, rosemary, and thyme; sprinkle over meat.

2. Melt margarine in a nonstick frying pan. Add meat and cook over medium heat, 6 minutes on each side or to desired doneness. Place meat on a serving patter to keep warm.

3. Combine yogurt, mustard, and Worcestershire sauce in small microwave-safe bowl. Cover and microwave on high power for 1 minute. Sprinkle mixture over warm meat. Garnish with parsley. To serve, slice meat diagonally into thin slices.

Lemon Parsley Carrots

Serves 4   Serving size: 1/4 recipe

2 cups carrots, sliced 1/4-inch thick

2 Tbsp water

2 Tbsp Smart Balance margarine

1 Tbsp Splenda

1 Tbsp fresh parsley, chopped

1/2 tsp lemon peels, grated

1 Tbsp lemon juice

Exchanges/Choices

1 Vegetable
1 Fat

Basic Nutritional Values

Calories 70
  Calories from Fat 40
Total Fat . . . . 4.5 g
  Saturated Fat . . . . 1.3 g
  Trans Fat . . . . 0.0 g
Cholesterol . . . . 0 mg
Sodium . . . . 90 mg
Total Carbohydrate . . . 7 g
  Dietary Fiber . . . . 2 g
  Sugars . . . . 3 g
Protein . . . . 1 g

Place carrots and water in a 2-quart covered glass casserole. Microwave, covered, at 100% power (700 watts) for 8–9 minutes until crisp-tender, stirring once after 5 minutes. Drain. Stir in margarine, Splenda, parsley, lemon peels, and lemon juice. Microwave again, covered, at 100% power for 1–2 minutes, until heated through.

Granola, Oats, Blackberry, and Raspberry Bake

Serves 8   Serving size: 1/8 recipe

Blackberry Raspberry Filling

2	**Tbsp**	Splenda
1 1/2	**Tbsp**	whole-wheat flour
1	**tsp**	ground cinnamon
1	**tsp**	pure vanilla extract
3	**cups**	fresh or frozen (partially thawed) blackberries
3	**cups**	fresh or frozen (partially thawed) raspberries
		Nonstick cooking spray

Oats Topping

1	**cup**	old-fashioned oats, uncooked
1/2	**cup**	chopped dates
		Dash allspice
		Dash nutmeg
		Dash cinnamon
2	**Tbsp**	Splenda
4	**Tbsp**	Smart Balance Light margarine

Exchanges/Choices

1/2 Starch
1 Fruit
1/2 Fat

Basic Nutritional Values

Calories 150	
Calories from Fat 35	
Total Fat . . . . 4.0 g	
Saturated Fat . . . . 0.9 g	
Trans Fat . . . . 0.0 g	
Cholesterol . . . . 0 mg	
Sodium . . . . 45 mg	
Total Carbohydrate . . . 28 g	
Dietary Fiber . . . . 8 g	
Sugars . . . . 13 g	
Protein . . . . 3 g	

1. To prepare the filling, mix Splenda, flour, cinnamon, and vanilla. Fold in berries until fruit is evenly coated. Spray an 8-inch glass baking dish with nonstick cooking spray; spoon filling into baking dish.

2. Combine topping ingredients, mixing well. Sprinkle evenly over fruit filling. Preheat oven to 350°F. Bake for 35–40 minutes or until topping is golden and filling is bubbly. Serve warm.

French Toast

Serves 4   Serving size: 2 slices

- 1 **Tbsp** Splenda
- 1/2 **tsp** pure vanilla extract
- 2 **cups** nonfat milk
- 1 **cup** egg substitute
- 8 slices whole-grain bread
- 2 **Tbsp** Smart Balance Light Spread

Beat Splenda, vanilla, milk, and egg substitute with a beater until well blended and smooth. Soak bread in batter. Heat margarine in skillet and carefully transfer bread to the skillet. Cook bread over medium heat until browned and then flip to cook the other side.

Exchanges/Choices

1 1/2 Starch
1/2 Fat-Free Milk
1 Lean Meat
1/2 Fat

Basic Nutritional Values

Calories 240
  Calories from Fat 40
Total Fat . . . . 4.5 g
  Saturated Fat . . . . 1.2 g
  Trans Fat . . . . 0.0 g
Cholesterol . . . . 0 mg
Sodium . . . . 485 mg
Total Carbohydrate . . . 31 g
  Dietary Fiber . . . . 4 g
  Sugars . . . . 10 g
Protein . . . . 18 g

Fried Bananas

Serves 4   Serving size: 1 banana

- 4 small bananas (or plantains)
- 1/4 **cup** nonfat milk
- 1/4 **cup** egg substitute
- 1 **Tbsp** Splenda
- 1/4 **cup** whole-wheat flour
- 1/4 **cup** Smart Balance Omega oil (for frying)

Peel the bananas and cut diagonally into half-inch-thick slices. Mix milk, egg substitute, Splenda, and flour until smooth. Heat oil in large skillet over medium heat. Dip each banana slice into batter and then drop into oil. Fry until browned, about 2 minutes on each side. Drain on paper towels. Serve warm or at room temperature.

Exchanges/Choices

1/2 Starch
1 1/2 Fruit
1 1/2 Fat

Basic Nutritional Values

Calories 190
  Calories from Fat 65
Total Fat . . . . 7.0 g
  Saturated Fat . . . . 0.6 g
  Trans Fat . . . . 0.0 g
Cholesterol . . . . 0 mg
Sodium . . . . 40 mg
Total Carbohydrate . . . 30 g
  Dietary Fiber . . . . 4 g
  Sugars . . . . 14 g
Protein . . . . 4 g

Barbecued Pork Sandwich

Serves 4   Serving size: 1 sandwich

- 3/4 **lb** pork tenderloin, trimmed of all visible fat
- 1 **tsp** Smart Balance Omega oil
- 1/2 **cup** no-salt-added tomato sauce
- 1 1/2 **Tbsp** Splenda
- 2 **Tbsp** water
- 2 **Tbsp** apple cider vinegar
- 2 **Tbsp** Worcestershire sauce
- 1/4 **tsp** dry mustard
- 4 whole-wheat hamburger buns

Cut pork into thin slices and flatten, using a meat mallet or rolling pin. Heat oil in a large nonstick skillet over medium-high heat. Add pork; cook 3 minutes on each side until browned. Drain and coarsely chop. Wipe drippings from pan; add all other ingredients. Bring to a boil; add pork. Cover, reduce heat, and simmer 20 minutes, stirring often. Spoon 3/4 of the pork mixture onto each bun.

Exchanges/Choices

2 Starch
2 Lean Meat

Basic Nutritional Values

Calories 235
 Calories from Fat 45
Total Fat . . . . 5.0 g
 Saturated Fat . . . . 1.2 g
 Trans Fat . . . . 0.0 g
Cholesterol . . . . 45 mg
Sodium . . . . 345 mg
Total Carbohydrate . . . 26 g
 Dietary Fiber . . . . 4 g
 Sugars . . . . 7 g
Protein . . . . 20 g

Oven-Roasted Tomatoes

Serves 6   Serving size: 1 tomato

- 1 **Tbsp** Smart Balance Omega oil
- 6 medium tomatoes, sliced crosswise 1/2- to 3/4-inch thick
- 2 **Tbsp** Splenda
  Dash pepper

Preheat oven to 300°F. Line a baking sheet with aluminum foil; rub with oil. Arrange tomato slices in a single layer on the baking sheet. Sprinkle with Splenda and pepper. Roast until the tomatoes shrivel, the edges start to turn brown, and most of the liquid around the tomatoes has caramelized, about 1 hour. Roasted tomatoes will keep for 4–5 days in the refrigerator.

Exchanges/Choices

1 Vegetable
1/2 Fat

Basic Nutritional Values

Calories 45
 Calories from Fat 20
Total Fat . . . . 2.5 g
 Saturated Fat . . . . 0.2 g
 Trans Fat . . . . 0.0 g
Cholesterol . . . . 0 mg
Sodium . . . . 5 mg
Total Carbohydrate . . . 5 g
 Dietary Fiber . . . . 1 g
 Sugars . . . . 4 g
Protein . . . . 1 g

Skewered Chicken and Shrimp
Serves 4   Serving size: 1 skewer

6 **Tbsp** lime juice

3 **Tbsp** honey

2 **Tbsp** rice wine vinegar

2 **tsp** chopped cilantro

1/4 **oz** gingerroot

1/4 **tsp** red pepper flakes

1 medium red pepper

1 medium onion

1/2 **lb** boneless, skinless chicken breast (trimmed of all visible fat)

4 medium kiwi fruit

1/2 **lb** shrimp

Exchanges/Choices

1 Fruit
1 Carbohydrate
1 Vegetable
3 Lean Meat

Basic Nutritional Values

Calories	295
Calories from Fat	80
Total Fat	9.0 g
Saturated Fat	1.0 g
Trans Fat	0.0 g
Cholesterol	100 mg
Sodium	115 mg
Total Carbohydrate	34 g
Dietary Fiber	4 g
Sugars	25 g
Protein	21 g

1. Combine lime juice, honey, vinegar, cilantro, gingerroot, and pepper flakes to make a marinade.

2. Cut chicken into 1-inch slices. Core and quarter pepper. Cut each quarter into four pieces. Peel and quarter onion. Cut each quarter into four pieces. Toss chicken, pepper, and onion with the lime-ginger marinade. Marinate 2 hours in refrigerator.

3. When ready to cook, peel kiwi fruit and cut into quarters. Peel and devein shrimp. Toss kiwis and shrimp with marinade until coated. Divide ingredients among four skewers. Grill or boil, 3–4 minutes per side, turning skewers once, until chicken and shrimp are cooked through.

Cold Pasta Salad

Serves 4   Serving size: 1/4 recipe

4 **oz** whole-wheat pasta,
elbows or shells

1/2 **cup** diced tomatoes

1/2 **cup** diced cucumber

1/2 **cup** shredded carrot

1/4 **cup** canola mayonnaise

1/2 **cup** plain fat-free yogurt

Cook pasta according to package instructions. Drain and rinse with cold water. Toss all other ingredients together in a bowl with pasta. Refrigerate 3 hours and serve.

Exchanges/Choices

2 Starch
1/2 Fat

Basic Nutritional Values

Calories	170
Calories from Fat	45
Total Fat	5.0 g
Saturated Fat	0.1 g
Trans Fat	0.0 g
Cholesterol	0 mg
Sodium	125 mg
Total Carbohydrate	26 g
Dietary Fiber	3 g
Sugars	5 g
Protein	6 g

Carrots in Sherry Wine

Serves 4   Serving size: 1/4 recipe

2 **cups** baby carrots

2 **Tbsp** Smart Balance
Light margarine

1/2 **cup** dry cooking sherry

Combine all ingredients and cook carrots over medium heat until tender.

Exchanges/Choices

2 Vegetable
1/2 Fat

Basic Nutritional Values

Calories	70
Calories from Fat	20
Total Fat	2.5 g
Saturated Fat	0.8 g
Trans Fat	0.0 g
Cholesterol	0 mg
Sodium	85 mg
Total Carbohydrate	8 g
Dietary Fiber	2 g
Sugars	4 g
Protein	1 g

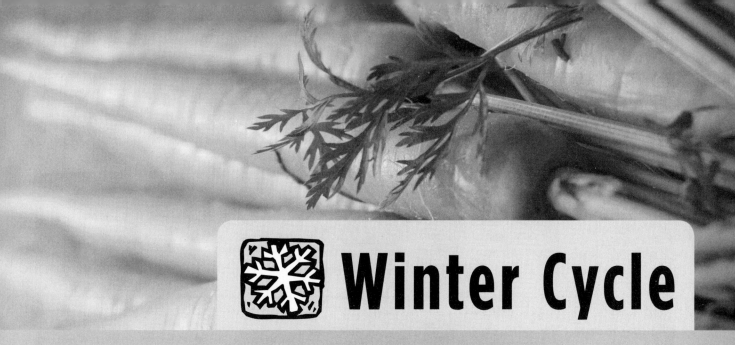

Winter Cycle

WEEK 2

FEATURED RECIPES

Whole-Wheat Pancakes or Waffles*

Pork Chops in Wine Sauce

Lemon-Apple Carrots

Grilled Haddock In Foil

Parmesan Potatoes

Cherry Crisp Dessert

Chicken Gazpacho Salad

Ground Beef Stroganoff

Strawberry Whip Parfaits

Whole-Wheat Cornmeal Muffin

Chilled Cauliflower Salad

Stir-Fry Chicken and Vegetables

Open-Faced Chicken and Almond Sandwich

Sweet and Sour Pork

Pumpkin Spice Muffins

German Potato Salad

Turkey Divan

Broccoli Slaw

Oatmeal and Apple Muffins

Beef and Black Bean Chili

Peas and Cheese Salad

Scalloped Potatoes

Sautéed Zucchini and Red Peppers

Chocolate Zucchini Cake

Sloppy Joes

Cinnamon Apple Yogurt

Veal Parmesan Hoagie

Southwest Tomato Salad

Baked Apples

*Indicates that the recipe has been used previously.

1500 calorie MEAL PLAN WINTER WEEK 2

	Sunday	Monday	Tuesday	Wednesday	Thursday	Friday	Saturday
Breakfast	**Whole-Wheat Pancakes or Waffles*** 1/4 cup sugar-free maple syrup 1 small orange 1 cup nonfat milk 1 1/2 tsp margarine	1 cup Kashi cereal 1 small banana 1 cup nonfat milk 1 Tbsp peanut butter (for the banana)	**Whole-Wheat Corn-meal Muffin** 1/4 cup low-fat granola 1 kiwi fruit 1 cup yogurt 1 tsp margarine	1/2 cup cooked bulgur 1 slice toasted oatmeal bread 1 3/4 cup blueberries 1 cup nonfat milk 1 oz reduced-fat cheese 2 tsp margarine	**Pumpkin Spice Muffins** 1/2 cup shredded wheat 1/2 cup strawberries 1 cup nonfat milk 1 Tbsp peanut butter	**Oatmeal and Apple Muffins** 1 cup nonfat milk 12 cashews	1/2 cup shredded wheat 1 whole-grain waffle 2 Tbsp sugar-free maple syrup 3/4 cup pineapple 1 cup nonfat milk 2 tsp margarine
Lunch	**Pork Chops in Wine Sauce** **Lemon-Apple Carrots** 1/2 cup stuffing 1 dinner roll 1/4 cup cranberry sauce 1 tsp margarine	**Chicken Gazpacho Salad** 3/4 oz baked tortilla chips 4 animal crackers 1 small apple 10 peanuts	**Chilled Cauliflower Salad** (1/2 serving) 2 slices whole-wheat bread 3 cups popcorn 1 small banana 2 oz broiled chicken breast 1/2 tsp margarine	**Open-Faced Chicken and Almond Sandwich** 1 cup mixed peas and corn 1/2 cup fruit cocktail or fruit cup 1/2 cup cooked spinach	**German Potato Salad** 6 saltine crackers 3/4 cup pineapple 1/2 cup broccoli 2 oz lean ham 1 tsp canola mayonnaise	**Beef and Black Bean Chili** (1/2 serving) **Peas and Cheese Salad** 9 round crackers 1 cup cantaloupe 1/2 cup green pepper slices	**Sloppy Joes** **Cinnamon Apple Yogurt** 1 whole-wheat sandwich bun 1/2 cup fruit cocktail or fruit cup 3 cashews
Snack A							
Snack B							
Dinner	**Grilled Haddock in Foil** **Parmesan Potatoes** **Cherry Crisp Dessert** 3 almonds	**Ground Beef Stroganoff** **Strawberry Whip Parfaits** 1/2 cup steamed sugar snap peas 2 Brazil nuts 1 ginger snap	**Stir-Fry Chicken and Vegetables** 2/3 cup brown rice 1/2 pear 1 cup nonfat milk	**Sweet and Sour Pork** 1/3 cup rice 1 cup nonfat milk 2 cups romaine lettuce salad 1 tsp olive oil and vinegar dressing	**Turkey Divan** **Broccoli Slaw** 1 slice whole-grain bread 1/2 cup peas 1 cup raspberries 1/2 cup nonfat milk 2 tsp margarine	**Scalloped Potatoes** **Sautéed Zucchini and Red Peppers** **Chocolate Zucchini Cake** 1/2 cup unsweetened applesauce 2 oz lean steak 1/2 tsp margarine	**Veal Parmesan Hoagie** **Southwest Tomato Salad** **Baked Apples**

*Indicates that the recipe has been used previously.

	Sunday	Monday	Tuesday	Wednesday	Thursday	Friday	Saturday
Breakfast	Whole-Wheat Pancakes or Waffles* 1/4 cup sugar-free maple syrup 1 small orange 1 cup nonfat milk 1 oz Canadian bacon 1 1/2 tsp margarine	1 cup Kashi cereal 1 small banana 1 cup nonfat milk 1 Tbsp peanut butter (for the banana)	Whole-Wheat Cornmeal Muffin 1/4 cup low-fat granola 1 kiwi fruit 1 cup yogurt 1 oz turkey ham 1 tsp margarine	1/2 cup cooked bulgur 1 slice toasted oatmeal bread 1 3/4 cup blueberries 1 cup nonfat milk 2 oz reduced-fat cheese 2 tsp margarine	Pumpkin Spice Muffins 1/2 cup shredded wheat 1/2 cup strawberries 1 cup nonfat milk 1/4 cup egg substitute, scrambled 1 Tbsp peanut butter	Oatmeal and Apple Muffins 1 cup nonfat milk 1/4 cup low-fat cottage cheese 12 cashews	1/2 cup shredded wheat 1 whole-grain waffle 2 Tbsp sugar-free maple syrup 3/4 cup pineapple 1 cup nonfat milk 2 tsp margarine
Lunch	Pork Chops in Wine Sauce Lemon-Apple Carrots 1/2 cup stuffing 1 dinner roll 1/4 cup cranberry sauce 2 tsp margarine	Chicken Gazpacho Salad 3/4 oz baked tortilla chips 4 animal crackers 1 small apple 20 peanuts	Chilled Cauliflower Salad (1/2 serving) 2 slices whole-wheat bread 3 cups popcorn 1 small banana 2 oz broiled chicken breast 1 1/2 tsp margarine	Open-Faced Chicken and Almond Sandwich 1 cup mixed peas and corn 1/2 cup fruit cocktail or fruit cup 1/2 cup cooked spinach 4 pecans	German Potato Salad 6 saltine crackers 3/4 cup pineapple 1/2 cup broccoli 2 oz lean ham 2 tsp canola mayonnaise	Beef and Black Bean Chili (1/2 serving) Peas and Cheese Salad 9 round crackers 1 cup cantaloupe 1/2 cup green pepper slices 2 Tbsp avocado	Sloppy Joes Cinnamon Apple Yogurt 1 whole-wheat sandwich bun 1/2 cup fruit cocktail or fruit cup 9 cashews
Snack A	2 Brazil nuts 1 medium peach	5 hazelnuts 1/2 grapefruit	1 1/2 tsp cashew butter 1 small apple	1 Tbsp toasted pumpkin seeds 1 medium peach	1 Tbsp sunflower seeds 1 cup papaya	6 mixed nuts 2 Tbsp raisins	4 walnut halves 2 small plums
Snack B	1 cup nonfat milk	1 cup yogurt	1 cup nonfat milk	1 cup nonfat milk	1 cup nonfat milk	1 cup nonfat milk	1 cup nonfat milk
Dinner	Grilled Haddock in Foil Parmesan Potatoes Cherry Crisp Dessert 3 almonds	Ground Beef Stroganoff Strawberry Whip Parfaits 1/2 cup steamed sugar snap peas 1/2 cup nonfat milk 2 Brazil nuts 1 ginger snap	Stir-Fry Chicken and Vegetables 2/3 cup brown rice 1/2 pear 1 cup nonfat milk	Sweet and Sour Pork 1/3 cup rice 1 cup nonfat milk 2 cups romaine lettuce salad 1 tsp olive oil and vinegar dressing	Turkey Divan Broccoli Slaw 1 slice whole-grain bread 1/2 cup peas 1 cup raspberries 1/2 cup nonfat milk 2 tsp margarine	Scalloped Potatoes Sautéed Zucchini and Red Peppers Chocolate Zucchini Cake 1/2 cup unsweetened applesauce 3 oz lean steak 1/2 tsp margarine	Veal Parmesan Hoagie Southwest Tomato Salad Baked Apples

*Indicates that the recipe has been used previously.

2000 calorie MEAL PLAN WINTER WEEK 2

	Sunday	Monday	Tuesday	Wednesday	Thursday	Friday	Saturday
Breakfast	Whole-Wheat Pancakes or Waffles* 1/4 cup sugar-free maple syrup 1 small orange 1 cup nonfat milk 1 oz Canadian bacon 1 1/2 tsp margarine	1 cup Kashi cereal 1 small banana 1 cup nonfat milk 1 Tbsp peanut butter (for the banana)	Whole-Wheat Cornmeal Muffin 1/4 cup low-fat granola 1 kiwi fruit 1 cup yogurt 1 oz turkey ham 1 tsp margarine	1/2 cup cooked bulgur 1 slice toasted oatmeal bread 1 3/4 cup blueberries 1 cup nonfat milk 2 oz reduced-fat cheese 2 tsp margarine	Pumpkin Spice Muffins 1/2 cup shredded wheat 1/2 cup strawberries 1 cup nonfat milk 1/4 egg substitute, scrambled 1 Tbsp peanut butter	Oatmeal and Apple Muffins 1 cup nonfat milk 1/4 cup low-fat cottage cheese 12 cashews	1/2 cup shredded wheat 1 whole-grain waffle 2 Tbsp sugar-free maple syrup 3/4 cup pineapple 1 cup nonfat milk 2 tsp margarine
Lunch	Pork Chops in Wine Sauce Lemon-Apple Carrots 1/2 cup stuffing 1 dinner roll 1/4 cup cranberry sauce 1/2 cup unsweetened applesauce 2 tsp margarine	Chicken Gazpacho Salad 3/4 oz baked tortilla chips 4 animal crackers 1 large apple 1 cup raw sliced vegetables 20 peanuts	Chilled Cauliflower Salad 2 slices whole-wheat bread 3 cups popcorn 1 large banana 2 oz broiled chicken breast 1 tsp margarine	Open-Faced Chicken and Almond Sandwich 1 cup mixed peas and corn 1 cup fruit cocktail or fruit cup 1 cup cooked spinach 4 pecans	German Potato Salad 6 saltine crackers 1 1/2 cup pineapple 1 cup broccoli 2 oz lean ham 2 tsp canola mayonnaise	Beef and Black Bean Chili (1/2 serving) Peas and Cheese Salad 9 round crackers 2 cups cantaloupe 1/2 cup green pepper slices 2 Tbsp avocado	Sloppy Joes Cinnamon Apple Yogurt 1 whole-wheat sandwich bun 1 cup fruit cocktail or fruit cup 9 cashews
Snack A	1 cup mixed raw vegetables 2 Brazil nuts 1 medium peach	1 cup raw celery sticks and carrots 5 hazelnuts 1/2 grapefruit	1 cup nonstarchy vegetables 1 1/2 tsp cashew butter 1 small apple	1 cup raw carrots 1 Tbsp toasted pumpkin seeds 1 medium peach	1 cup raw zucchini slices 1 Tbsp sunflower seeds 1 cup papaya	1 cup raw celery 6 mixed nuts 2 Tbsp raisins	1 cup coleslaw 1 Tbsp canola mayonnaise (for making coleslaw) 2 small plums
Snack B	5 vanilla wafers 1 cup skim milk	2 sandwich cookies 1 cup yogurt	6 round crackers 4 walnut halves 1 cup nonfat milk	1 oz dried fruit trail mix 1 cup nonfat milk	1 large sugar-free cookie 1 cup nonfat milk	1 waffle 1 tsp margarine 1 cup nonfat milk	3/4 oz whole-wheat crackers 1 1/2 tsp almond butter 1 cup nonfat milk
Dinner	Grilled Haddock in Foil Parmesan Potatoes Cherry Crisp Dessert 3 almonds	Ground Beef Stroganoff Strawberry Whip Parfaits 1/2 cup nonfat milk 1/2 cup steamed sugar snap peas 2 Brazil nuts 1 ginger snap	Stir-Fry Chicken and Vegetables 2/3 cup brown rice 1/2 pear 1 cup nonfat milk	Sweet and Sour Pork 1/3 cup rice 1 cup nonfat milk 2 cups romaine lettuce salad 1 tsp olive oil and vinegar dressing	Turkey Divan Broccoli Slaw 1 slice whole-grain bread 1/2 cup peas 1 cup raspberries 1/2 cup nonfat milk 2 tsp margarine	Scalloped Potatoes Sautéed Zucchini and Red Peppers Chocolate Zucchini Cake 1/2 cup unsweetened applesauce 3 oz lean steak 1/2 tsp margarine	Veal Parmesan Hoagie Southwest Tomato Salad Baked Apples

*Indicates that the recipe has been used previously.

	Sunday	Monday	Tuesday	Wednesday	Thursday	Friday	Saturday
Breakfast	**Whole-Wheat Pancakes or Waffles*** 1/4 cup sugar-free maple syrup 1 small orange 1 cup nonfat milk 2 oz Canadian bacon 1 1/2 tsp margarine	1 cup Kashi cereal 1 small banana 1 cup nonfat milk 1/4 cup egg substitute, scrambled 1 Tbsp peanut butter (for the banana)	**Whole-Wheat Cornmeal Muffin** 1/4 cup low-fat granola 1 kiwi fruit 1 cup yogurt 2 oz turkey ham 1 tsp margarine	1/2 cup cooked bulgur 1 slice toasted oatmeal bread 1 3/4 cup blueberries 1 cup nonfat milk 2 oz reduced-fat cheese 1 oz low-fat turkey sausage 2 tsp margarine	**Pumpkin Spice Muffins** 1/2 cup shredded wheat 1/2 cup strawberries 1 cup nonfat milk 1/2 cup egg substitute, scrambled 1 Tbsp peanut butter	**Oatmeal and Apple Muffins** 1 cup nonfat milk 1/4 cup low-fat cottage cheese 12 cashews	1/2 cup shredded wheat 1 whole-grain waffle 2 Tbsp sugar-free maple syrup 3/4 cup pineapple 1 cup nonfat milk 1 oz lean ham 2 tsp margarine
Lunch	**Pork Chops in Wine Sauce Lemon-Apple Carrots** 1/2 cup stuffing 1 dinner roll 1/4 cup cranberry sauce 1/2 cup unsweetened applesauce 2 tsp margarine	**Chicken Gazpacho Salad** 3/4 oz baked tortilla chips 4 animal crackers 1 large apple 1 cup raw sliced vegetables 20 peanuts	**Chilled Cauliflower Salad** 2 slices whole-wheat bread 3 cups popcorn 1 large banana 2 oz broiled chicken breast 1 tsp margarine	**Open-Faced Chicken and Almond Sandwich** 1 cup mixed peas and corn 1 cup fruit cocktail or fruit cup 1 cup cooked spinach 4 pecans	**German Potato Salad** 6 saltine crackers 1 1/2 cup pineapple 1 cup broccoli 2 oz lean ham 2 tsp canola mayonnaise	**Beef and Black Bean Chili** (1/2 serving) **Peas and Cheese Salad** 9 round crackers 2 cups cantaloupe 1/2 cup green pepper slices 2 Tbsp avocado	**Sloppy Joes Cinnamon Apple Yogurt** 1 whole-wheat sandwich bun 1 cup fruit cocktail or fruit cup 9 cashews
Snack A	1 cup mixed raw vegetables 2 Brazil nuts 1 medium peach	1 cup raw celery sticks and carrots 5 hazelnuts 1/2 grapefruit	1 cup nonstarchy vegetables 1 1/2 tsp cashew butter 1 small apple	1 cup raw carrots 1 Tbsp toasted pumpkin seeds 1 medium peach	1 cup raw zucchini slices 1 Tbsp sunflower seeds 1 cup papaya	1 cup raw celery 6 mixed nuts 2 Tbsp raisins	1 cup coleslaw 1 Tbsp canola mayonnaise (for making coleslaw) 2 small plums
Snack B	5 vanilla wafers 1 cup nonfat milk	2 sandwich cookies 1 cup yogurt	6 round crackers 4 walnut halves 1 cup nonfat milk	1 oz dried fruit trail mix 1 cup nonfat milk	1 large sugar-free cookie 1 cup nonfat milk	1 waffle 1 tsp margarine 1 cup nonfat milk	3/4 oz whole-wheat crackers 1 1/2 tsp almond butter 1 cup nonfat milk
Dinner	**Grilled Haddock in Foil Parmesan Potatoes Cherry Crisp Dessert** 1 cup nonfat milk 3 almonds	**Ground Beef Stroganoff Strawberry Whip Parfaits** 1 cup nonfat milk 1/2 cup steamed sugar snap peas 2 Brazil nuts 1 ginger snap	**Stir-Fry Chicken and Vegetables** 1 cup brown rice 1/2 pear 1 cup nonfat milk	**Sweet and Sour Pork** 2/3 cup rice 1 cup nonfat milk 2 cups romaine lettuce salad 1 tsp olive oil and vinegar dressing	**Turkey Divan Broccoli Slaw** 1 slice whole-grain bread 1 cup peas 1 cup raspberries 1/2 cup nonfat milk 2 tsp margarine	**Scalloped Potatoes Sautéed Zucchini and Red Peppers Chocolate Zucchini Cake** 1 small roll 1/2 cup unsweetened applesauce 3 oz lean steak 1/2 tsp margarine	**Veal Parmesan Hoagie Southwest Tomato Salad Baked Apples** 1/2 cup corn

*Indicates that the recipe has been used previously.

VEGETABLES

____ bean sprouts
____ bell peppers, green
____ bell peppers, red
____ broccoli
____ carrots
____ cauliflower
____ celery
____ corn
____ cucumber
____ garlic
____ green onions
____ jalapeños
____ mushrooms
____ onions, yellow or white
____ peas, frozen
____ potatoes
____ red onion
____ romaine lettuce
____ spinach
____ sugar snap peas
____ tomatoes
____ zucchini

MEATS

____ bacon, Canadian
____ bacon, turkey
____ beef steak, at least 90% lean
____ chicken breasts, boneless, skinless
____ ground beef, 96% lean
____ haddock fillets
____ ham, lean
____ pork chops, boneless sirloin
____ turkey breast (whole, not sliced)
____ turkey ham
____ turkey sausage, lean
____ veal round steak

FRUITS

____ apples
____ apples, tart, for baking
____ avocado
____ bananas
____ blueberries
____ cantaloupe
____ kiwi fruit
____ oranges
____ pears
____ pineapple, chunks
____ raisins
____ raspberries
____ strawberries

DAIRY

____ buttermilk, fat-free
____ egg substitute
____ eggs (for egg whites)
____ half and half, fat-free
____ milk, nonfat
____ Smart Balance Light margarine
____ sour cream, fat-free
____ whipped topping, fat-free
____ yogurt, fat-free, flavored (if desired) and plain

CHEESE

____ cheddar, sharp, fat-free and reduced-fat
____ cottage cheese, low-fat
____ cream cheese, fat-free
____ mozzarella, fat-free, shredded
____ Parmesan, reduced-fat

BREAD, GRAINS, & PASTA

____ bread, oatmeal
____ bread, whole-grain, whole-wheat
____ bulgur
____ dinner rolls, small
____ English muffins, whole-wheat
____ noodles, whole-wheat
____ rice, brown
____ sandwich/hamburger buns, whole-wheat
____ waffles, whole-grain

BEANS

____ black beans, no-added-salt

NUTS

____ almonds
____ Brazil nuts
____ cashews
____ peanuts, dry roasted
____ pecans

CONDIMENTS

_____ canola mayonnaise
_____ catsup, no-salt
_____ Italian salad dressing, light
_____ maple syrup, sugar-free
_____ prepared mustard
_____ soy sauce, light
_____ sweet pickle relish
_____ Worcestershire sauce

SPICES & HERBS

_____ basil
_____ bay leaves
_____ black pepper
_____ chili seasoning mix
_____ cinnamon, ground
_____ garlic powder
_____ nutmeg, ground
_____ paprika
_____ parsley (fresh)
_____ pumpkin pie spice
_____ salt
_____ thyme

OTHER

_____ angel food cake
_____ apple juice concentrate, frozen, unsweetened
_____ applesauce, unsweetened
_____ black olives, pitted
_____ canned pumpkin
_____ cereal, Kashi
_____ cereal, shredded wheat
_____ cherry pie filling, light
_____ cocoa powder
_____ crackers, animal
_____ crackers, round, reduced-fat, butter-flavor
_____ crackers, saltine
_____ cranberry sauce
_____ croutons, seasoned
_____ fruit cocktail, in light syrup, or fruit cups
_____ ginger snaps
_____ granola, low-fat
_____ peanut butter
_____ popcorn (light or no butter if microwave-style)
_____ poppy seeds
_____ preserves, sugar-free (any flavor)
_____ red pasta sauce, light
_____ salsa, chunky, no-added-salt
_____ stuffing mix
_____ tomato sauce, no-added-salt
_____ tortilla chips, baked
_____ vegetable juice
_____ water chestnuts

STAPLES

_____ almond extract
_____ baking powder
_____ baking soda
_____ bouillon, beef, sodium-free
_____ bouillon, chicken, sodium-free
_____ corn syrup
_____ cornstarch
_____ lemon juice
_____ nonstick cooking spray
_____ old-fashioned oats, rolled
_____ sherry, cooking
_____ Smart Balance Omega oil
_____ Splenda
_____ Splenda Brown Sugar Blend
_____ vanilla extract
_____ vinegar, cider
_____ vinegar, white
_____ vinegar, white wine
_____ whole-wheat flour
_____ wine, dry, white
_____ yellow cornmeal

Whole-Wheat Pancakes or Waffles

Serves 4   Serving size: 2 pancakes or waffles

1/2 **cup** rolled oats

1/2 **cup** whole-wheat flour, sifted

2 **tsp** baking powder

2 **Tbsp** Splenda

1/2 **cup** egg substitute, beaten well

3/4 **cup** nonfat milk

2 **Tbsp** Smart Balance Omega oil

Nonstick cooking spray

Stir together dry ingredients. Combine egg substitute, milk, and oil; stir into flour mixture. Cook on a griddle lightly coated with nonstick spray until golden brown, then turn. Can also be made in a waffle iron.

Exchanges/Choices

1 1/2 Starch
1 1/2 Fat

Basic Nutritional Values

Calories 185
  Calories from Fat 70
Total Fat . . . . 8.0 g
  Saturated Fat . . . . 0.7 g
  Trans Fat . . . . 0.0 g
Cholesterol . . . . 0 mg
Sodium . . . . 265 mg
Total Carbohydrate . . . 22 g
  Dietary Fiber . . . . 3 g
  Sugars . . . . 3 g
Protein . . . . 8 g

Pork Chops in Wine Sauce

Serves 4   Serving size: 1/4 recipe

2 **Tbsp** whole-wheat flour

Black pepper, to taste

3/4 **lb** boneless sirloin pork chops (trimmed of visible fat)

1 **tsp** Smart Balance margarine, melted

3/4 **cup** dry white wine

1/2 **cup** mushrooms

1/2 **cup** fat-free half and half

Combine whole-wheat flour and pepper. Lightly dredge pork chops in flour mixture. Heat margarine in a nonstick skillet; add pork and cook about 2 minutes on each side. Add wine; cook over medium heat, about 4–5 minutes. Remove chops and set aside to keep warm. Add mushrooms and half and half to skillet. Cook over low heat, stirring constantly, just until thickened. Return chops to pan, cook to reheat, and serve immediately.

Exchanges/Choices

1/2 Carbohydrate
2 Lean Meat

Basic Nutritional Values

Calories 135
  Calories from Fat 30
Total Fat . . . . 3.5 g
  Saturated Fat . . . . 0.8 g
  Trans Fat . . . . 0.0 g
Cholesterol . . . . 45 mg
Sodium . . . . 250 mg
Total Carbohydrate . . . 6 g
  Dietary Fiber . . . . 1 g
  Sugars . . . . 2 g
Protein . . . . 16 g

Lemon-Apple Carrots

Serves 4   Serving size: 1/4 recipe

1 tsp Smart Balance
Light margarine

4 cups carrots,
coarsely grated

2 Tbsp frozen unsweetened
apple juice concentrate

1 Tbsp lemon juice

1 tsp poppy seeds

In a nonstick skillet, melt the margarine. Add carrots, apple juice, and lemon juice and cook over medium heat for about 3 minutes or until the carrots are tender, stirring constantly. Sprinkle with poppy seeds just before serving.

Exchanges/Choices

1/2 Fruit
2 Vegetable

Basic Nutritional Values

Calories 70
  Calories from Fat 10
Total Fat . . . . 1.0 g
  Saturated Fat . . . . 0.2 g
  Trans Fat . . . . 0.0 g
Cholesterol . . . . 0 mg
Sodium . . . . 85 mg
Total Carbohydrate . . . 15 g
  Dietary Fiber . . . . 3 g
  Sugars . . . . 9 g
Protein . . . . 1 g

Grilled Haddock In Foil

Serves 4   Serving size: 1/4 recipe

1 **lb** haddock filets
Nonstick cooking spray

2 carrots, pared and sliced
(about 1 cup)

1 medium onion, quartered
and thinly sliced

6 **Tbsp** water

1 green bell pepper, sliced

1/4 **cup** no-added-salt
tomato sauce

2 **Tbsp** Smart Balance
Omega oil

2 **tsp** minced parsley

1/4 **cup** cooking sherry

1. Cut fish crosswise into equal pieces with a serrated knife. Place each portion on separate 12-inch squares of heavy-duty foil lightly sprayed with nonstick cooking spray.

2. In a small saucepan, combine carrots, onion, and water. Bring to a boil; reduce heat. Simmer, covered, for 15–20 minutes or until vegetables are tender. Drain. Top each fish portion with carrot-onion mixture and slices of green pepper.

3. In a small bowl, combine the tomato sauce, oil, sherry, and parsley and mix well.

4. Leaving foil partially open, make a deep fold in each square of foil to hold food and sauce securely, then spoon the sauce over fish and vegetables. Place open packets on a grill. Cook for 25 minutes or until fish flakes easily with a fork.

Exchanges/Choices

2 Vegetable
3 Lean Meat
1/2 Fat

Basic Nutritional Values

Calories 210
 Calories from Fat 70
Total Fat . . . . 8.0 g
 Saturated Fat . . . . 0.7 g
 Trans Fat . . . . 0.0 g
Cholesterol . . . . 65 mg
Sodium . . . . 110 mg
Total Carbohydrate . . . 11 g
 Dietary Fiber . . . . 3 g
 Sugars . . . . 6 g
Protein . . . . 22 g

Parmesan Potatoes

Serves 4   Serving size: 1/4 recipe

2 Tbsp Smart Balance Light margarine, melted

12 reduced-fat butter-flavored crackers, crushed

3 Tbsp reduced-fat grated Parmesan cheese

1 tsp garlic powder

1 tsp paprika

1 tsp pepper

2 cups potatoes, unpeeled and thinly sliced

Combine melted margarine, crushed crackers, cheese, garlic powder, paprika, and pepper in a medium bowl; add potato slices, tossing gently to coat. Arrange coated potato slices in a 9-inch microwave-safe pie plate, sprinkle with remaining crumb mixture. Cover with wax paper and microwave on high power for 7–8 minutes or until potatoes are tender, rotating pie plate a half-turn after 2 minutes.

Exchanges/Choices

2 Starch
1/2 Fat

Basic Nutritional Values

Calories 160
  Calories from Fat 45
Total Fat . . . . 5.0 g
  Saturated Fat . . . . 1.3 g
  Trans Fat . . . . 0.0 g
Cholesterol . . . . 5 mg
Sodium . . . . 235 mg
Total Carbohydrate . . . 26 g
  Dietary Fiber . . . . 2 g
  Sugars . . . . 1 g
Protein . . . . 4 g

Cherry Crisp Dessert

Serves 8   Serving size: 1/8 recipe

1 (20-oz) can light cherry pie filling

3/8 tsp almond extract

3 1/2 Tbsp Smart Balance margarine, melted

2 cups rolled oats, dry

1/4 cup Splenda

Place pie filling and almond extract in a baking dish that has sides about 2 inches high. Stir until blended; set aside. Place melted margarine in a small bowl; add oats and Splenda. Stir until well mixed. Spoon mixture evenly over pie filling. Bake at 350°F for about 30 minutes. Serve warm.

Exchanges/Choices

2 Carbohydrate
1 Fat

Basic Nutritional Values

Calories 165
  Calories from Fat 45
Total Fat . . . . 5 g
  Saturated Fat . . . . 1.3 g
  Trans Fat . . . . 0 g
Cholesterol . . . . 0 mg
Sodium . . . . 55 mg
Total Carbohydrate . . . 27 g
  Dietary Fiber . . . . 3 g
  Sugars . . . . 13 g
Protein . . . . 4 g

Chicken Gazpacho Salad

Serves 4   Serving size: 1/4 recipe

1 lb boneless, skinless chicken breast (trimmed of visible fat)

4 oz pasta

3/4 cup chopped cucumber

3/4 cup chopped red or yellow bell pepper

3/4 cup diced tomato

3/4 cup vegetable juice

1/4 cup lemon juice

1 clove garlic, minced

Exchanges/Choices

1 1/2 Starch
1 Vegetable
3 Lean Meat

Basic Nutritional Values

Calories 265
  Calories from Fat 30
Total Fat . . . . 3.5 g
  Saturated Fat . . . . 0.9 g
  Trans Fat . . . . 0.0 g
Cholesterol . . . . 65 mg
Sodium . . . . 200 mg
Total Carbohydrate . . . 29 g
  Dietary Fiber . . . . 3 g
  Sugars . . . . 6 g
Protein . . . . 29 g

Place chicken breasts in boiling water and thoroughly cook; then transfer chicken to the refrigerator to cool while preparing the other ingredients. Cook pasta according to package directions; drain. When the chicken has cooled to the touch, cut it into small cubes. Mix the pasta with the chicken and remaining ingredients. Serve warm or chilled.

Ground Beef Stroganoff

Serves 4   Serving size: 1/4 recipe

4   **oz** whole-wheat noodles
1   **lb** 96% lean ground beef
1   medium onion, chopped
2   **cups** water
1   **Tbsp** sodium-free beef bouillon

1/2   **cup** fat-free sour cream
1   **cup** mushrooms, sliced
1/4   **tsp** pepper
1/2   **cup** plain fat-free yogurt

Cook noodles according to package directions. In a saucepan, cook the ground beef and the onion. Drain fat. Combine water and bouillon to make a broth; add to the saucepan. Add sour cream, mushrooms, and pepper. Heat to boiling and then lower heat. Simmer uncovered, stirring frequently, for 5 minutes. Stir in yogurt, reheat, and serve hot.

Exchanges/Choices

1 1/2 Starch
1 Vegetable
3 Lean Meat

Basic Nutritional Values

Calories	295
Calories from Fat	45
Total Fat	5.0 g
Saturated Fat	2.2 g
Trans Fat	0.3 g
Cholesterol	65 mg
Sodium	135 mg
Total Carbohydrate	30 g
Dietary Fiber	4 g
Sugars	6 g
Protein	32 g

Strawberry Whip Parfaits

Serves 4   Serving size: 1/4 recipe

2   **cups** sliced strawberries
2   **cups** fat-free whipped topping

4   **(1-oz)** slices angel food cake

Place sliced strawberries in an electric blender. Cover and blend until smooth, stopping once to scrape the sides. Fold strawberry puree into whipped topping. Tear angel food cake into pieces and fold into strawberry mixture. Spoon into parfait glasses, cover, and serve chilled.

Exchanges/Choices

2 Carbohydrate

Basic Nutritional Values

Calories	125
Calories from Fat	15
Total Fat	1.5 g
Saturated Fat	0.6 g
Trans Fat	0.0 g
Cholesterol	5 mg
Sodium	160 mg
Total Carbohydrate	27 g
Dietary Fiber	2 g
Sugars	16 g
Protein	3 g

Whole-Wheat Cornmeal Muffin
Serves 8   Serving size: 1 muffin

2/3 **cup** yellow cornmeal
2/3 **cup** whole-wheat flour
1 **Tbsp** Splenda
2 **tsp** baking powder

2/3 **cup** nonfat milk
1/4 **cup** egg substitute
2 **Tbsp** Smart Balance Omega oil

Preheat oven to 400°F. Place paper liners in muffin trays. Thoroughly mix dry ingredients. Combine milk, egg substitute, and oil; add to dry ingredients. Stir until dry ingredients are just moistened. Batter will be lumpy. Fill muffin tins 2/3 full. Bake until slightly browned, about 20 minutes.

Exchanges/Choices
1 Carbohydrate
1 Fat

Basic Nutritional Values
Calories 120
Calories from Fat 35
Total Fat. . . . . 4.0 g
Saturated Fat . . . . 0.3 g
Trans Fat. . . . . 0.0 g
Cholesterol . . . . 0 mg
Sodium. . . . . 115 mg
Total Carbohydrate . . . 18 g
Dietary Fiber . . . . 2 g
Sugars . . . . 1 g
Protein . . . . 4 g

Chilled Cauliflower Salad
Serves 4   Serving size: 1/4 recipe

1 medium cauliflower head, broken into florets
2 medium tomatoes, cut into wedges
2 **Tbsp** Smart Balance Omega oil
3 **Tbsp** white wine vinegar

3 **Tbsp** black pitted olives, sliced
3 **Tbsp** sweet pickle relish
1/2 **tsp** Splenda
1 **tsp** paprika
1/2 **tsp** black pepper
4 lettuce leaves

1. In a covered saucepan, cook cauliflower in small amount of boiling water, 9–10 minutes or until crisp-tender. Drain. In large bowl, combine the cooked cauliflower and tomato wedges.

2. Combine the oil, vinegar, olives, relish, Splenda, paprika, and pepper. Mix well. Pour dressing over cauliflower and tomatoes. Cover and refrigerate 24 hours, stirring occasionally. To serve, lift vegetables from dressing with slotted spoon; place in a lettuce-lined bowl.

Exchanges/Choices
3 Vegetable
1 Fat

Basic Nutritional Values
Calories 125
Calories from Fat 65
Total Fat. . . . . 7.0 g
Saturated Fat . . . . 0.5 g
Trans Fat. . . . . 0.0 g
Cholesterol . . . . 0 mg
Sodium. . . . . 160 mg
Total Carbohydrate . . . 16 g
Dietary Fiber . . . . 5 g
Sugars . . . . 9 g
Protein . . . . 4 g

Stir-Fry Chicken and Vegetables

Serves 4   Serving size: 1/4 recipe

1 **lb** boneless, skinless chicken breasts (trimmed of visible fat)

1 egg white

3 **tsp** cornstarch

6 **oz** bean sprouts, rinsed

1 celery stalk, thinly sliced

1 medium tomato, cut into wedges

2/3 red or green bell pepper, quartered and cut into 1/2-inch pieces

6 **Tbsp** water chestnuts, sliced

4 green onions, sliced into 1/2-inch pieces

3 **Tbsp** Worcestershire sauce

2 **Tbsp** cooking sherry

2 **Tbsp** Smart Balance Omega oil

Fresh ground pepper, to taste

Exchanges/Choices

2 Vegetable
3 Lean Meat
1 1/2 Fat

Basic Nutritional Values

Calories 255
  Calories from Fat 90
Total Fat . . . . 10.0 g
  Saturated Fat . . . . 1.3 g
  Trans Fat . . . . 0.0 g
Cholesterol . . . . 65 mg
Sodium . . . . 240 mg
Total Carbohydrate . . . 13 g
  Dietary Fiber . . . . 3 g
  Sugars . . . . 7 g
Protein . . . . 28 g

1. Slice chicken breasts diagonally into 1/4-inch slices.

2. In a small bowl, combine egg white and 2 tsp cornstarch. Add chicken slices; set aside.

3. Drain bean sprouts; place in a bowl. Add celery, tomato wedges, and bell pepper; combine and set aside.

4. Place water chestnuts and green onions in a small bowl; add Worcestershire sauce, remaining 1 tsp cornstarch, and sherry.

5. Heat 1 Tbsp oil over high heat in a nonstick or heavy skillet. Add chicken and stir-fry until it loses its pink color, stirring constantly. Remove and set aside. Add 1 Tbsp oil to skillet; add bowl with bean sprouts, celery, tomatoes, and bell pepper; stir-fry for 3–4 minutes or until crisp-tender. Add water chestnuts and onions. Stir-fry for 1 minute; add chicken and stir-fry until heated through. Add pepper to taste.

Open-Faced Chicken and Almond Sandwich

Serves 4   Serving size: 1 sandwich

1 **lb** boneless, skinless chicken breasts (trimmed of visible fat)

1/3 **cup** canola mayonnaise

1/4 **cup** toasted slivered almonds

1 celery stalk, thinly sliced

1 green onion (with top), thinly sliced

1 medium tomato, sliced

2 whole-wheat English muffins, split and toasted

Boil chicken in water until thoroughly cooked; then transfer to refrigerator to chill. When chicken has cooled, dice and mix with mayonnaise, almonds, celery, and onion. Arrange tomato slices on muffin halves. Spoon chicken onto tomato and serve.

Exchanges/Choices

1 Starch
4 Lean Meat
1 Fat

Basic Nutritional Values

Calories 310
  Calories from Fat 125
Total Fat . . . . 14.0 g
  Saturated Fat . . . . 1.2 g
  Trans Fat . . . . 0.0 g
Cholesterol . . . . 65 mg
Sodium . . . . 345 mg
Total Carbohydrate . . . 17 g
  Dietary Fiber . . . . 4 g
  Sugars . . . . 5 g
Protein . . . . 29 g

Sweet and Sour Pork

Serves 4   Serving size: 1/4 recipe

2 **Tbsp** Smart Balance Omega oil

3/4 **lb** boneless sirloin pork chops (trimmed of visible fat)

2 **cups** pineapple chunks, drained

1/4 **cup** corn syrup

1/4 **cup** vinegar

3 **Tbsp** no-salt catsup

1 **Tbsp** light soy sauce

1 **tsp** garlic powder

2 **Tbsp** cornstarch

1/4 **cup** water

1/2 **cup** bell pepper, diced

Heat oil in a skillet and brown the pork. Add pineapple, corn syrup, vinegar, catsup, soy sauce, and garlic powder. Bring to a boil; simmer for 10 minutes. Mix cornstarch with water and stir into the mixture. Add the bell peppers. Boil for 5 minutes until thickened. Serve over rice.

Exchanges/Choices

2 Carbohydrate
2 Lean Meat
1 Fat

Basic Nutritional Values

Calories 275
  Calories from Fat 80
Total Fat . . . . 9.0 g
  Saturated Fat . . . . 0.9 g
  Trans Fat . . . . 0.0 g
Cholesterol . . . . 40 mg
Sodium . . . . 375 mg
Total Carbohydrate . . . 35 g
  Dietary Fiber . . . . 2 g
  Sugars . . . . 22 g
Protein . . . . 16 g

Pumpkin Spice Muffins

Serves 8   Serving size: 2 muffins

1 **cup** whole-wheat flour	1 **cup** canned pumpkin
3 **tsp** baking powder	1/2 **cup** nonfat milk
2 **tsp** ground cinnamon	1/4 **cup** unsweetened applesauce
2 **tsp** ground nutmeg	
1/4 **cup** egg substitute	1/4 **cup** raisins or chopped nuts
2 **Tbsp** Splenda	

Preheat oven to 400°F. Line sixteen muffin-pan cups with paper liners or spray with nonstick cooking spray. In a large bowl, stir together the flour, baking powder, cinnamon, and nutmeg. In a medium bowl, beat egg substitute with a whisk. Add Splenda, pumpkin, milk, and applesauce; stir until well blended. Stir in raisins. Stir into flour mixture until just blended. Fill muffin-pan cups 2/3 full. Bake 20–25 minutes until a wooden toothpick inserted in the center comes out clean. Remove muffins from muffin pans. Serve warm or at room temperature.

Exchanges/Choices

1 1/2 Carbohydrate

Basic Nutritional Values

Calories 95
 Calories from Fat 5
Total Fat . . . . 0.5 g
 Saturated Fat . . . . 0.2 g
 Trans Fat . . . . 0.0 g
Cholesterol . . . . 0 mg
Sodium . . . . 160 mg
Total Carbohydrate . . . 20 g
 Dietary Fiber . . . . 3 g
 Sugars . . . . 6 g
Protein . . . . 4 g

German Potato Salad

Serves 4   Serving size: 1/4 recipe

4 **cups** potatoes	1 **cup** water
4 slices turkey bacon	1/2 **cup** cider vinegar
1/2 **cup** chopped onions	2 1/2 **Tbsp** Splenda
2 **Tbsp** whole-wheat flour	1/16 **tsp** black pepper

Peel and dice the potatoes; place in boiling water. Cook until just soft. Fry bacon in a large skillet until crisp; remove and drain. Place the onions in the skillet and cook until tender. Slowly stir in flour; blend well. Add water and vinegar; cook, stirring, until bubbly and slightly thick. Stir in Splenda and pepper; simmer for 10 minutes. Crumble bacon. Carefully stir bacon and potatoes into hot mixture. Heat through, stirring gently to coat potato slices. Serve warm.

Exchanges/Choices

2 Starch

Basic Nutritional Values

Calories 160
 Calories from Fat 25
Total Fat . . . . 3.0 g
 Saturated Fat . . . . 0.8 g
 Trans Fat . . . . 0.0 g
Cholesterol . . . . 15 mg
Sodium . . . . 180 mg
Total Carbohydrate . . . 28 g
 Dietary Fiber . . . . 3 g
 Sugars . . . . 4 g
Protein . . . . 5 g

Turkey Divan
Serves 4   Serving size: 1/4 recipe

   2 **tsp** sodium-free chicken
     bouillon

1 1/2 **cups** water

   2 **Tbsp** Smart Balance
     margarine

   2 **Tbsp** whole-wheat flour

1/8 **tsp** ground nutmeg

   2 **Tbsp** reduced-fat Parmesan
     cheese

1/2 **cup** fat-free half and half

   12 **oz** frozen broccoli

3/4 **lb** turkey breast (trimmed
     of visible fat), cooked and
     cubed

1. Combine bouillon and water in a small bowl to form a broth; set aside.

2. Melt margarine in a saucepan over low heat. Stir in flour and nutmeg.
Cook, stirring constantly, until mixture is smooth and bubbly. Stir in broth
and heat to boiling, stirring constantly. Boil and stir 1 minute. Remove from
heat and stir in Parmesan cheese and half and half.

3. Arrange broccoli and turkey pieces in a shallow baking dish and cover
with the sauce. Sprinkle a little more Parmesan cheese over the top. Broil in
oven about 3–5 inches from heat until cheese is bubbly and slightly brown.

Exchanges/Choices

1/2 Fat-Free Milk
1 Vegetable
3 Lean Meat
1/2 Fat

Basic Nutritional Values

Calories 220
 Calories from Fat 65
Total Fat. . . . . 7.0 g
 Saturated Fat . . . . 2.1 g
 Trans Fat. . . . . 0.0 g
Cholesterol. . . . . 65 mg
Sodium. . . . . 210 mg
Total Carbohydrate . . . 14 g
 Dietary Fiber. . . . . 3 g
 Sugars . . . . 6 g
Protein . . . . 26 g

Broccoli Slaw
Serves 4   Serving size: 1/4 recipe

1/4 **cup** fat-free plain yogurt

1/4 **cup** canola mayonnaise

   3 **Tbsp** cider vinegar

   2 **tsp** Splenda

   1 **(8-oz)** can sliced water
     chestnuts, drained and
     rinsed, coarsely chopped

1/2 **cup** finely diced red onion

   2 **cups** broccoli, finely
     chopped

     Pepper, to taste

Whisk together yogurt, mayonnaise, vinegar, and Splenda in a large bowl.
Add water chestnuts, onion, and broccoli; toss to coat. Cover and refrigerate
for up to 2 days.

Exchanges/Choices

2 Vegetable
1 Fat

Basic Nutritional Values

Calories 100
 Calories from Fat 40
Total Fat. . . . . 4.5 g
 Saturated Fat . . . . 0.0 g
 Trans Fat. . . . . 0.0 g
Cholesterol. . . . . 0 mg
Sodium. . . . . 120 mg
Total Carbohydrate . . . 12 g
 Dietary Fiber. . . . . 3 g
 Sugars . . . . 5 g
Protein . . . . 2 g

Oatmeal and Apple Muffins
Serves 8   Serving size: 1 muffin

1/4 **cup** egg substitute

2/3 **cup** whole-wheat flour

2 **tsp** baking powder

2 **tsp** cinnamon

1 **tsp** nutmeg

1/2 **cup** nonfat milk

1 **cup** raisins

1 apple, peeled, cored, and chopped

1/4 **cup** natural unsweetened applesauce

2/3 **cup** rolled oats

4 **Tbsp** Splenda Brown Sugar Blend

Preheat oven to 400°F. Beat egg substitute. Sift together flour, baking powder, cinnamon, and nutmeg. Combine all ingredients, mixing just to moisten. Spoon batter into muffin cups until 3/4 full. Bake for 15–20 minutes.

Exchanges/Choices

3 Carbohydrate

Basic Nutritional Values

Calories 190
 Calories from Fat 10
Total Fat . . . . 1.0 g
 Saturated Fat . . . . 0.2 g
 Trans Fat . . . . 0.0 g
Cholesterol . . . . 0 mg
Sodium . . . . 120 mg
Total Carbohydrate . . . 44 g
 Dietary Fiber . . . . 3 g
 Sugars . . . . 28 g
Protein . . . . 4 g

Beef and Black Bean Chili
Serves 4   Serving size: 1/4 recipe

1 **lb** 96% lean ground beef

1 **(15-oz)** can no-added-salt black beans

1 **cup** no-added-salt chunky salsa

1 **(8-oz)** can no-added-salt tomato sauce

1 **Tbsp** chili seasoning mix

Cook meat in a large saucepan over medium-high heat until meat is browned, stirring until it crumbles. Drain away any fat. While meat cooks, drain and mash beans. Add mashed beans, salsa, tomato sauce, and seasoning mix to saucepan; stir well. Cook over medium heat 10 minutes or until thoroughly heated. Spoon into serving bowls.

Exchanges/Choices

1 Starch
1 Vegetable
4 Lean Meat

Basic Nutritional Values

Calories 280
 Calories from Fat 55
Total Fat . . . . 6.0 g
 Saturated Fat . . . . 2.7 g
 Trans Fat . . . . 0.1 g
Cholesterol . . . . 70 mg
Sodium . . . . 290 mg
Total Carbohydrate . . . 25 g
 Dietary Fiber . . . . 7 g
 Sugars . . . . 10 g
Protein . . . . 31 g

Peas and Cheese Salad

Serves 4   Serving size: 1/4 recipe

3 1/2 **Tbsp** canola mayonnaise

2 **tsp** prepared mustard

1/3 **tsp** basil leaves, crushed
Dash black pepper

2 **cups** frozen peas, thawed

2 **oz** fat-free cheddar cheese slices, diced

1 1/2 **oz** reduced-fat shredded sharp cheddar cheese

4 **oz** water chestnuts sliced, drained

5 **Tbsp** green onions, sliced

4 romaine lettuce leaves

In a large bowl, combine mayonnaise, mustard, basil, and pepper until blended. Stir in peas, cheese, water chestnuts, and green onions until well coated. Cover and chill at least 2 hours. To serve, spoon onto romaine leaves.

Exchanges/Choices

1 Starch
1 Lean Meat
1 Fat

Basic Nutritional Values

Calories 170
Calories from Fat 65
Total Fat . . . . 7.0 g
Saturated Fat . . . . 1.4 g
Trans Fat . . . . 0.0 g
Cholesterol . . . . 10 mg
Sodium . . . . 460 mg
Total Carbohydrate . . . . . 17 g
Dietary Fiber . . . . 6 g
Sugars . . . . 7 g
Protein . . . . 11 g

Scalloped Potatoes

Serves 4   Serving size: 1/4 recipe

1 medium onion, chopped

1 **tsp** Smart Balance Omega oil

1 **tsp** minced garlic

1 **tsp** minced thyme

1/4 **tsp** ground black pepper

2 **cups** russet potatoes, peeled and sliced 1/8-inch thick

1 **cup** nonfat milk

2 bay leaves

2 **Tbsp** cornstarch

1 **Tbsp** water

3 **Tbsp** fat-free cream cheese

2 **Tbsp** reduced-fat Parmesan cheese

Exchanges/Choices

1 Starch
1/2 Fat-Free Milk
1 Vegetable

Basic Nutritional Values

Calories 160
  Calories from Fat 20
Total Fat . . . . 2.0 g
  Saturated Fat . . . . 0.5 g
  Trans Fat . . . . 0.0 g
Cholesterol . . . . 5 mg
Sodium . . . . 185 mg
Total Carbohydrate . . . 29 g
  Dietary Fiber . . . . 2 g
  Sugars . . . . 6 g
Protein . . . . 6 g

1. Adjust an oven rack to the middle position and preheat the oven to 450°F. Combine the onion and oil in a large pot. Cover and cook over medium-low heat, stirring occasionally, until the onion is softened, 8–10 minutes. Stir in the garlic, thyme, and pepper; cook until fragrant, about 1 minute.

2. Add the potatoes, milk, and bay leaves and bring to a simmer. Cover, reduce heat to low, and simmer until partially tender, about 10 minutes. Discard the bay leaves. Whisk the cornstarch and water together and add to the pot; bring to a simmer. Remove from heat and stir in the cream cheese and 1 Tbsp Parmesan cheese, being careful not to break up the potatoes.

3. Transfer the mixture to an 8-inch square baking dish and sprinkle with the remaining Parmesan. Cover the dish with foil and bake for 20 minutes. Uncover and continue to bake until the potatoes are completely tender. Let cool for 10 minutes before serving.

Sautéed Zucchini and Red Peppers

Serves 4   Serving size: 1/4 recipe

2 medium red bell peppers, seeded and cut into 1/2-inch strips

2 medium zucchini, cut into 1/2-inch strips

1 clove garlic, minced

2 **Tbsp** Smart Balance Omega oil

Black pepper, to taste

2 **Tbsp** minced parsley

In a large skillet over medium heat, sauté peppers, zucchini, and garlic in oil until zucchini is golden. Season with pepper and parsley. Serve hot.

Exchanges/Choices

2 Vegetable
1 Fat

Basic Nutritional Values

Calories 95
 Calories from Fat 65
Total Fat. . . . . 7.0 g
 Saturated Fat . . . . 0.6 g
 Trans Fat. . . . . 0.0 g
Cholesterol . . . . 0 mg
Sodium. . . . . 15 mg
Total Carbohydrate . . . 8 g
 Dietary Fiber . . . . 3 g
 Sugars . . . . 5 g
Protein . . . . 2 g

Chocolate Zucchini Cake

Serves 12   Serving size: 1 slice

1/4 **cup** Smart Balance Light margarine

1/2 **cup** unsweetened applesauce

1 3/4 **cups** Splenda

3 egg whites

1 **tsp** pure vanilla extract

1/2 **cup** fat-free buttermilk

2 1/2 **cup** whole-wheat flour

1/2 **tsp** salt

4 **Tbsp** cocoa powder

1 **tsp** baking soda

1/2 **tsp** ground cinnamon

2 **cups** fresh zucchini grated with skin (about 1 medium)

Nonstick cooking spray

Exchanges/Choices

1 1/2 Carbohydrate
1/2 Fat

Basic Nutritional Values

Calories 140
 Calories from Fat 20
Total Fat. . . . . 2.5 g
 Saturated Fat . . . . 0.8 g
 Trans Fat. . . . . 0.0 g
Cholesterol . . . . 0 mg
Sodium. . . . . 175 mg
Total Carbohydrate . . . 25 g
 Dietary Fiber . . . . 4 g
 Sugars . . . . 5 g
Protein . . . . 6 g

1. Preheat oven 350°F.

2. Mix margarine, applesauce, and Splenda together. Add egg whites and beat well. Add vanilla and buttermilk. Blend well.

3. Sift together flour, salt, cocoa powder, baking soda, and cinnamon.

4. Blend together wet and dry ingredients. Fold in grated zucchini. Spray a 9 × 13-inch glass baking dish with nonstick cooking spray. Pour mixture into baking dish. Bake for 60 minutes.

Sloppy Joes

Serves 4   Serving size: 1 sandwich

- **1 lb** 96% lean ground beef
- **1/2 cup** chopped onions
- **6 Tbsp** diced celery
- **1/4 cup** green bell peppers, chopped
- **1 (8-oz)** can no-added-salt tomato sauce
- **1 Tbsp** Worcestershire sauce
- **1 tsp** black pepper

Brown ground beef and thoroughly drain. Add onions, celery, and green pepper. Cook over medium heat for 5 minutes; then add tomato sauce, Worcestershire sauce, and pepper. Turn heat to low and simmer for 10–15 minutes. Spoon onto buns to serve.

Exchanges/Choices

2 Vegetable
3 Lean Meat

Basic Nutritional Values

Calories	175
Calories from Fat	40
Total Fat	4.5 g
Saturated Fat	2.0 g
Trans Fat	0.3 g
Cholesterol	60 mg
Sodium	155 mg
Total Carbohydrate	8 g
Dietary Fiber	1 g
Sugars	5 g
Protein	25 g

Cinnamon Apple Yogurt

Serves 4   Serving size: 1/4 serving

- **2 cups** vanilla fat-free yogurt
- **1/2 cup** unsweetened applesauce
- **4 tsp** Splenda
- **2 tsp** ground cinnamon

Spoon 1/2 cup yogurt into each of four dessert dishes. Top each with 2 Tbsp applesauce, 1 tsp Splenda, and 1/2 tsp cinnamon.

Exchanges/Choices

1 Carbohydrate

Basic Nutritional Values

Calories	90
Calories from Fat	0
Total Fat	0.0 g
Saturated Fat	0.0 g
Trans Fat	0.0 g
Cholesterol	0 mg
Sodium	65 mg
Total Carbohydrate	18 g
Dietary Fiber	0 g
Sugars	14 g
Protein	4 g

Veal Parmesan Hoagie

Serves 4   Serving size: 1 hoagie

- **1 Tbsp** Smart Balance margarine
- **12 oz** veal round steak
- **2 Tbsp** reduced-fat Parmesan cheese
- **4** whole-wheat buns
- **1 cup** light red pasta sauce
- **2 Tbsp** shredded fat-free mozzarella cheese

Melt margarine in a shallow baking dish. Place veal in a baking dish and sprinkle with Parmesan cheese. Bake at 350°F for 20 minutes; turn meat over and bake another 20 minutes, until tender. Place the veal on the buns, pour pasta sauce over meat, and top with mozzarella cheese. Return to oven for 3–4 minutes to heat the sauce and melt the cheese.

This recipe is high in sodium.

Exchanges/Choices

2 Starch
1 Vegetable
3 Lean Meat
1/2 Fat

Basic Nutritional Values

Calories 340
 Calories from Fat 70
Total Fat . . . . 8.0 g
 Saturated Fat . . . . 2.3 g
 Trans Fat . . . . 0.0 g
Cholesterol . . . . 70 mg
Sodium . . . . 660 mg
Total Carbohydrate . . . 41 g
 Dietary Fiber . . . . 6 g
 Sugars . . . . 10 g
Protein . . . . 27 g

Southwest Tomato Salad

Serves 4   Serving size: 1/4 recipe

- **2 cups** diced tomatoes (about 4 medium tomatoes)
- **1/2 cup** diced green bell pepper
- **1/2 cup** chopped, peeled cucumber
- **1/2 cup** finely chopped red onion
- **1 Tbsp** minced jalapeño
- **1/2 cup** seasoned croutons
- **1/4 cup** light Italian salad dressing

In a large bowl, combine tomatoes, green bell pepper, cucumber, onion, and jalapeño. Add croutons and dressing; toss thoroughly to combine.

Exchanges/Choices

2 Vegetable
1/2 Fat

Basic Nutritional Values

Calories 70
 Calories from Fat 20
Total Fat . . . . 2.0 g
 Saturated Fat . . . . 0.4 g
 Trans Fat . . . . 0.0 g
Cholesterol . . . . 0 mg
Sodium . . . . 245 mg
Total Carbohydrate . . . 12 g
 Dietary Fiber . . . . 2 g
 Sugars . . . . 6 g
Protein . . . . 2 g

Baked Apples

Serves 4   Serving size: 1/4 recipe

4 medium tart baking apples (Jonathan, York, or Rome Beauty), peeled and cored

1/4 cup Splenda

2 1/2 Tbsp Smart Balance margarine

3 Tbsp sugar-free preserves (any kind)

1 tsp pumpkin pie spice

3 Tbsp raisins

3/4 cup water

1. Preheat oven to 350°F.

2. With the tip of a knife, make six 1/4-inch deep cuts in each apple, from top to halfway down. Place the apples in an 8 × 8 × 2-inch baking dish.

3. In a small bowl, combine the Splenda, margarine, fruit preserves, and spice. Stir in raisins.

4. Stuff each apple with one-fourth of the mixture. Pour water into the bottom of the baking dish; cover with foil and seal tightly. Bake for 50–60 minutes or until fork-tender. Remove foil and gently transfer apples to four small dessert bowls. Spoon a little of the juice from the bottom of the pan over each apple.

Exchanges/Choices

2 Fruit
1 Fat

Basic Nutritional Values

Calories	150
Calories from Fat	55
Total Fat	6.0 g
Saturated Fat	1.6 g
Trans Fat	0.0 g
Cholesterol	0 mg
Sodium	60 mg
Total Carbohydrate	28 g
Dietary Fiber	3 g
Sugars	23 g
Protein	0 g

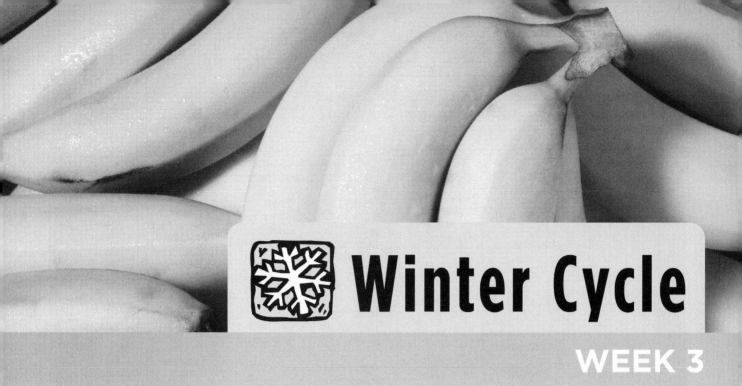

Winter Cycle

WEEK 3

Featured Recipes

Salisbury Steak

Baked Tomatoes and Squash

Ambrosia Salad

Gram's Gingerbread

Cranberry Ham Kabob

Sweet Potato Casserole

Red Lentil Soup

Jamaican Chicken

Vinegary Beets and Walnuts

Spicy Turkey Pitas

Carrot-Pineapple Coleslaw†

Stir-Fry Beef and Vegetables

Cauliflower Parmigiana

Broiled Haddock

Sauerkraut Salad

Banana Bran Muffin*

Dilled Cucumber Salad

Chicken with Artichoke Hearts

Green Bean Casserole

Whole-Wheat Blueberry Muffins

Macaroni and Cheese with Tomatoes

Tomato Asparagus Salad†

Baked Sweet Potato Fries

Asparagus Dijon

Peach and Apple Crisp

Whole-Wheat Pancakes or Waffles*

Beef and Barley Stew

Cinnamon Red Cabbage

Vegetable Lasagna

Fruit and Crème Parfait

*Indicates that the recipe has been used previously.

†This recipe is used as a snack, but its ingredients are in the shopping list.

	Sunday	Monday	Tuesday	Wednesday	Thursday	Friday	Saturday
Breakfast	3/4 cup multi-bran cereal 1 small orange 1 cup nonfat milk 1/4 cup egg substitute, scrambled	1 cup oatmeal 1/2 grapefruit 1 cup nonfat milk 1 oz reduced-fat cheese 2 Brazil nuts	1/2 whole-grain bagel 1 small banana 1 cup nonfat milk 1 Tbsp cashew butter	1/2 cup Kashi cereal 1 slice whole-grain bread 1 kiwi fruit 1 cup nonfat milk 2 egg whites, scrambled 2 tsp margarine	Banana Bran Muffin* 3/4 multigrain Cheerios 1 cup nonfat milk 6 almonds 1 tsp margarine	Whole-Wheat Blueberry Muffins 1 1/2 cups puffed cereal 1 cup cantaloupe 1 cup nonfat milk 1 oz turkey kielbasa (or other lean sausage) 2 1/4 tsp peanut butter (or cashew butter)	Whole-Wheat Pancakes or Waffles* 1/4 cup sugar-free maple syrup 3/4 cup fresh pineapple 1 cup nonfat milk 1/2 tsp margarine
Lunch	Salisbury Steak (1/2 serving) Baked Tomatoes and Squash Ambrosia Salad (1/8 recipe) Gram's Gingerbread	Red Lentil Soup 3 saltine crackers 1 small nectarine 1 cup spinach salad 1 tsp olive oil and vinegar (for dressing)	Spicy Turkey Pitas 1 cup oven-baked French fries 1 tangerine 8 black olives	Cauliflower Parmigiana 1 small dinner roll 1 1/2 cups mixed peas and corn 1 medium peach 1 oz lean turkey ham 1 oz reduced-fat provolone cheese 1/2 Tbsp salad dressing	Dilled Cucumber Salad 1 small dinner roll 2 oz baked tortilla chips 1/2 grapefruit 2 oz broiled fish 1 tsp tartar sauce	Macaroni and Cheese with Tomatoes 1/2 cup blackberries 1 cup leafy greens (for salad) 2 pecans	Beef and Barley Stew Cinnamon Red Cabbage 1 slice rye (or other) bread 1 tsp margarine
Snack A							
Snack B							
Dinner	Cranberry Ham Kabob Sweet Potato Casserole 2 Tbsp pine nuts	Jamaican Chicken Vinegary Beets and Walnuts 1/2 cup fruit cocktail 1/2 cup nonfat milk 1/2 Tbsp toasted pumpkin seeds	Stir-Fry Beef and Vegetables 1/2 cup red potatoes, boiled or roasted 1 slice multigrain bread 1/2 large pear 1 cup nonfat milk 1/2 tsp margarine	Broiled Haddock Sauerkraut Salad 2/3 cup brown rice 1 medium peach 1 cup nonfat milk	Chicken with Artichoke Hearts (1/2 serving) Green Bean Casserole 1 slice whole-wheat bread 3/4 cup berries (any kind) 1 cup nonfat milk 1 tsp margarine 2 Brazil nuts	Baked Sweet Potato Fries Asparagus Dijon Peach and Apple Crisp 1/2 cup unsweetened applesauce 1 cup nonfat milk 1/2 cup cooked kale 3 oz broiled pork chops	Vegetable Lasagna Fruit and Crème Parfait

*Indicates that the recipe has been used previously.

	Sunday	Monday	Tuesday	Wednesday	Thursday	Friday	Saturday
Breakfast	3/4 cup multi-bran cereal 1 small orange 1 cup nonfat milk 1/4 cup egg substitute, scrambled 10 peanuts	1 cup oatmeal 1/2 grapefruit 1 cup nonfat milk 1 oz reduced-fat cheese 2 Brazil nuts	1/2 whole-grain bagel 1 small banana 1 cup nonfat milk 1/4 cup low-fat cottage cheese 1 Tbsp cashew butter	1/2 cup Kashi cereal 1 slice whole-grain bread 1 kiwi fruit 1 cup nonfat milk 2 egg whites, scrambled 2 tsp margarine	Banana Bran Muffin* 3/4 multigrain Cheerios 1 cup nonfat milk 6 almonds 1 tsp margarine	Whole-Wheat Blueberry Muffins 1 1/2 cups puffed cereal 1 cup cantaloupe 1 cup nonfat milk 1 oz turkey kielbasa (or other lean sausage) 2 1/4 tsp peanut butter (or cashew butter)	Whole-Wheat Pancakes or Waffles* 1/4 cup sugar-free maple syrup 3/4 cup fresh pineapple 1 cup nonfat milk 1/2 tsp margarine
Lunch	Salisbury Steak (3/4 serving) Baked Tomatoes and Squash Ambrosia Salad (1/8 recipe) Gram's Gingerbread	Red Lentil Soup 3 saltine crackers 1 small nectarine 1 cup spinach salad 2 tsp olive oil and vinegar (for dressing) 1 oz reduced-fat cheese	Spicy Turkey Pitas 1 cup oven-baked French fries 1 tangerine 8 black olives 5 hazelnuts	Cauliflower Parmigiana 1 small dinner roll 1 1/2 cups mixed peas and corn 1 medium peach 1 oz lean turkey ham 1 oz reduced-fat provolone cheese 1/2 Tbsp salad dressing	Dilled Cucumber Salad 1 small dinner roll 2 oz baked tortilla chips 1/2 grapefruit 1 oz broiled fish 1 tsp tartar sauce 1 oz avocado	Macaroni and Cheese with Tomatoes 1/2 cup blackberries 1 cup leafy greens (for salad) 6 pecans	Beef and Barley Stew Cinnamon Red Cabbage 1 slice rye (or other) bread 2 tsp margarine
Snack A	2 Tbsp avocado 1 cup tomato soup	1 1/2 tsp peanut butter 1 small apple	16 pistachios 1/2 cup pineapple chunks	4 pecans 4 apricots	10 peanuts 3/4 mandarin oranges packed in juice	2 Brazil nuts 1 small orange	6 almonds 1/2 cup mango
Snack B	1 cup nonfat milk	1 cup nonfat milk	1 cup nonfat milk	1 cup nonfat milk	1 cup nonfat milk	1 cup nonfat milk	1 cup nonfat milk
Dinner	Cranberry Ham Kabob Sweet Potato Casserole 2 Tbsp pine nuts	Jamaican Chicken Vinegary Beets and Walnuts 1/2 cup fruit cocktail 1/2 cup nonfat milk 1/2 Tbsp toasted pumpkin seeds	Stir-Fry Beef and Vegetables 1/2 cup red potatoes, boiled or roasted 1 slice multigrain bread 1/2 large pear 1 cup nonfat milk 1/2 tsp margarine	Broiled Haddock Sauerkraut Salad 2/3 cup brown rice 1 medium peach 1 cup nonfat milk	Chicken with Artichoke Hearts Green Bean Casserole 1 slice whole-wheat bread 3/4 cup berries (any kind) 1 cup nonfat milk 1 tsp margarine 2 Brazil nuts	Baked Sweet Potato Fries Asparagus Dijon Peach and Apple Crisp 1/2 cup unsweetened applesauce 1 cup nonfat milk 1/2 cup cooked kale 4 oz broiled pork chops	Vegetable Lasagna Fruit and Crème Parfait

*Indicates that the recipe has been used previously.

2000 calorie MEAL PLAN WINTER WEEK 3

	Sunday	Monday	Tuesday	Wednesday	Thursday	Friday	Saturday
Breakfast	3/4 cup multi-bran cereal 1 small orange 1 cup nonfat milk 1/4 cup egg substitute, scrambled 10 peanuts	1 cup oatmeal 1/2 grapefruit 1 cup nonfat milk 1 oz reduced-fat cheese 2 Brazil nuts	1/2 whole-grain bagel 1 small banana 1 cup nonfat milk 1/4 cup low-fat cottage cheese 1 Tbsp cashew butter	1/2 cup Kashi cereal 1 slice whole-grain bread 1 kiwi fruit 1 cup nonfat milk 2 egg whites, scrambled 2 tsp margarine	Banana Bran Muffin* 3/4 multigrain Cheerios 1 cup nonfat milk 6 almonds 1 tsp margarine	**Whole-Wheat Blueberry Muffins** 1 1/2 cups puffed cereal 1 cup cantaloupe 1 cup nonfat milk 1 oz turkey kielbasa (or other lean sausage) 2 1/4 tsp peanut butter (or cashew butter)	**Whole-Wheat Pancakes or Waffles*** 1/4 cup sugar-free maple syrup 3/4 cup fresh pineapple 1 cup nonfat milk 1/2 tsp margarine
Lunch	**Salisbury Steak** (3/4 serving) **Baked Tomatoes and Squash** **Ambrosia Salad** (1/8 recipe) **Gram's Gingerbread**	**Red Lentil Soup** 3 saltine crackers 1 small nectarine 2 cups spinach salad 2 tsp olive oil and vinegar (for dressing) 1 oz reduced-fat cheese	**Spicy Turkey Pitas** 1 cup oven-baked French fries 3 tangerines 8 black olives 5 hazelnuts	**Cauliflower Parmigiana** 1 small dinner roll 1 1/2 cups mixed peas and corn 2 medium peaches 1 oz lean turkey ham 1 oz reduced-fat provolone cheese 1 1/2 Tbsp salad dressing	**Dilled Cucumber Salad** 1 small dinner roll 2 oz baked tortilla chips 1/2 grapefruit 1/2 cup cooked collard greens 1 oz broiled fish 1 tsp tartar sauce 1 oz avocado	**Macaroni and Cheese with Tomatoes** 1 1/2 cup blackberries 2 cups leafy greens (for salad) 6 pecans	**Beef and Barley Stew** **Cinnamon Red Cabbage** 1 slice rye (or other) bread 1/2 cup mixed fruit 2 tsp margarine
Snack A	1/2 cup nonstarchy vegetables (for soup) 2 Tbsp avocado 1 cup tomato soup	1 cup raw celery 1 1/2 tsp peanut butter 1 small apple	**Carrot-Pineapple Coleslaw**	1 cup raw zucchini 4 pecans 4 apricots	1 cup cucumber slices 10 peanuts 3/4 cup mandarin oranges packed in juice	**Tomato Asparagus Salad**	1 cup mixed raw vegetables 6 almonds 1/2 cup mango
Snack B	small unfrosted brownie 1 cup nonfat milk	2 small sandwich cookies 1 cup nonfat milk	5 vanilla wafers 1 cup nonfat milk	1 small muffin 1/2 tsp margarine 1 cup nonfat milk	1 half ear, corn on the cob 1 tsp margarine 1 cup nonfat milk	8 animal crackers 1 cup nonfat milk	1 waffle 1/2 Tbsp peanut butter 1 cup nonfat milk
Dinner	**Cranberry Ham Kabob** **Sweet Potato Casserole** 2 Tbsp pine nuts	**Jamaican Chicken** **Vinegary Beets and Walnuts** 1/2 cup fruit cocktail 1/2 cup nonfat milk 1/2 Tbsp toasted pumpkin seeds	**Stir-Fry Beef and Vegetables** 1/2 cup red potatoes, boiled or roasted 1 slice multigrain bread 1/2 large pear 1 cup nonfat milk 1/2 tsp margarine	**Broiled Haddock** **Sauerkraut Salad** 2/3 cup brown rice 1 medium peach 1 cup nonfat milk	**Chicken with Artichoke Hearts** **Green Bean Casserole** 1 slice whole-wheat bread 3/4 cup berries (any kind) 1 cup nonfat milk 1 tsp margarine 2 Brazil nuts	**Baked Sweet Potato Fries** **Asparagus Dijon** **Peach and Apple Crisp** 1/2 cup unsweetened applesauce 1 cup nonfat milk 1/2 cup cooked kale 4 oz broiled pork chops	**Vegetable Lasagna** **Fruit and Crème Parfait**

*Indicates that the recipe has been used previously.

	Sunday	Monday	Tuesday	Wednesday	Thursday	Friday	Saturday
Breakfast	3/4 cup multi-bran cereal 1 small orange 1 cup nonfat milk 1/2 cup egg substitute, scrambled 10 peanuts	1 cup oatmeal 1/2 grapefruit 1 cup nonfat milk 2 oz reduced-fat cheese 2 Brazil nuts	1/2 whole-grain bagel 1 small banana 1 cup nonfat milk 1/4 cup low-fat cottage cheese 1 Tbsp cashew butter	1/2 cup Kashi cereal 1 slice whole-grain bread 1 kiwi fruit 1 cup nonfat milk 4 egg whites, scrambled 2 tsp margarine	**Banana Bran Muffin*** 3/4 multigrain Cheerios 1 cup nonfat milk 1 oz lean sausage 6 almonds 1 tsp margarine	**Whole-Wheat Blueberry Muffins** 1 1/2 cups puffed cereal 1 cup cantaloupe 1 cup nonfat milk 2 oz turkey kielbasa (or other lean sausage) 2 1/4 tsp peanut butter (or cashew butter)	**Whole-Wheat Pancakes or Waffles*** 1/4 cup sugar-free maple syrup 3/4 cup fresh pineapple 1 cup nonfat milk 1 oz lean ham 1/2 tsp margarine
Lunch	**Salisbury Steak** (3/4 serving) **Baked Tomatoes and Squash** **Ambrosia Salad** (1/8 recipe) **Gram's Gingerbread**	**Red Lentil Soup** 3 saltine crackers 2 small nectarines 2 cups spinach salad 2 tsp olive oil and vinegar (for dressing) 1 oz reduced-fat cheese	**Spicy Turkey Pitas** 1 cup oven-baked French fries 3 tangerines 8 black olives 5 hazelnuts	**Cauliflower Parmigiana** 1 small dinner roll 1 1/2 cups mixed peas and corn 2 medium peaches 1 oz lean turkey ham 1 oz reduced-fat provolone cheese 1 1/2 Tbsp salad dressing	**Dilled Cucumber Salad** 1 small dinner roll 2 oz baked tortilla chips 1/2 grapefruit 1/2 cup cooked collard greens 1 oz broiled fish 1 tsp tartar sauce 1 oz avocado	**Macaroni and Cheese with Tomatoes** 1 1/2 cup blackberries 2 cup leafy greens (for salad) 6 pecans	**Beef and Barley Stew** **Cinnamon Red Cabbage** 1 slice rye (or other) bread 1/2 cup mixed fruit 2 tsp margarine
Snack A	1/2 cup nonstarchy vegetables (for soup) 2 Tbsp avocado 1 cup tomato soup	1 cup raw celery 1 1/2 tsp peanut butter 1 small apple	**Carrot-Pineapple Coleslaw**	1 cup raw zucchini 4 pecans 4 apricots	1 cup cucumber slices 10 peanuts 3/4 cup mandarin oranges packed in juice	**Tomato Asparagus Salad**	1 cup mixed raw vegetables 6 almonds 1/2 cup mango
Snack B	small unfrosted brownie 1 cup nonfat milk	2 small sandwich cookies 1 cup nonfat milk	5 vanilla wafers 1 cup nonfat milk	1 small muffin 1/2 tsp margarine 1 cup nonfat milk	1 half ear, corn on the cob 1 tsp margarine 1 cup nonfat milk	8 animal crackers 1 cup nonfat milk	1 waffle 1/2 Tbsp peanut butter 1 cup nonfat milk
Dinner	**Cranberry Ham Kabob** **Sweet Potato Casserole** 2 Tbsp pine nuts	**Jamaican Chicken** **Vinegary Beets and Walnuts** 1/2 cup fruit cocktail 1 cup nonfat milk 1/2 Tbsp toasted pumpkin seeds 1/2 whole-wheat crackers	**Stir-Fry Beef and Vegetables** 1 cup red potatoes, boiled or roasted 1 slice multigrain bread 1/2 large pear 1 cup nonfat milk 1/2 tsp margarine	**Broiled Haddock** **Sauerkraut Salad** 2/3 cup brown rice 1 medium peach 1 cup nonfat milk	**Chicken with Artichoke Hearts** **Green Bean Casserole** 1 slice whole-wheat bread 3/4 cup berries (any kind) 1 cup nonfat milk 1 tsp margarine 2 Brazil nuts	**Baked Sweet Potato Fries** **Asparagus Dijon** **Peach and Apple Crisp** 1 slice pumpernickel (or other) bread 1/2 cup unsweetened applesauce 1 cup nonfat milk 1/2 cup cooked kale 4 oz broiled pork chops 1 tsp margarine	**Vegetable Lasagna** **Fruit and Crème Parfait**

*Indicates that the recipe has been used previously.

SHOPPING LIST WINTER WEEK 3

VEGETABLES

_____ asparagus
_____ bean sprouts
_____ bell peppers, green and red
_____ cabbage, red
_____ cabbage, shredded
_____ carrots
_____ cauliflower
_____ celery
_____ collard greens
_____ cucumber
_____ eggplant
_____ garlic
_____ green beans, French-style
_____ green onions
_____ kale
_____ lettuce
_____ mushrooms
_____ onions, yellow or white
_____ red potatoes
_____ spinach (frozen and fresh)
_____ summer squash
_____ sweet potatoes
_____ tomatoes
_____ tomatoes, red grape
_____ zucchini

MEATS

_____ beef roast, chuck
       or boneless
_____ beef steak, sirloin
_____ boneless ham
_____ chicken breasts, boneless,
       skinless
_____ ground beef, 96% lean
_____ ground turkey, lean
_____ haddock fillets
_____ ham, lean
_____ pork chops
_____ sausage, turkey, smoked,
       lean
_____ turkey ham, lean

FRUITS

_____ apples
_____ avocado
_____ bananas
_____ blackberries
_____ blueberries
_____ cantaloupe
_____ grapefruit
_____ green grapes, seedless
_____ kiwi fruit
_____ lemon
_____ nectarines
_____ oranges
_____ peaches
_____ pears
_____ pineapple (chunks
       and crushed)
_____ raisins
_____ tangerines

DAIRY

_____ buttermilk, fat-free
_____ egg substitute
_____ egg whites
_____ milk, nonfat
_____ Smart Balance Light
       margarine
_____ sour cream, fat-free
_____ whipped topping, fat-free
_____ yogurt, plain, fat-free

CHEESE

_____ American, fat-free,
       shredded
_____ cheddar, sharp, reduced-fat
_____ cottage cheese, fat-free or
       reduced-fat
_____ feta, reduced-fat
_____ mozzarella, fat-free and
       reduced-fat
_____ Parmesan, reduced-fat
_____ provolone, reduced-fat

BREAD, GRAINS, & PASTA

_____ bagel, whole-grain
_____ barley
_____ bread crumbs
_____ bread, pumpernickel,
       rye, or multigrain
_____ bread, whole-grain,
       whole-wheat
_____ bulgur
_____ dinner rolls
_____ elbow macaroni,
       whole-wheat
_____ lasagna noodles
_____ pita pocket bread

BEANS

_____ red lentils

NUTS

_____ almonds
_____ Brazil nuts
_____ hazelnuts
_____ peanuts
_____ pecans
_____ pine nuts
_____ walnuts

CONDIMENTS

_____ canola mayonnaise
_____ catsup, no-salt
_____ Dijon mustard
_____ horseradish
_____ tartar sauce
_____ Worcestershire sauce,
　　　 reduced-sodium

SPICES & HERBS

_____ bay leaf
_____ black pepper
_____ cayenne pepper
_____ cinnamon, ground
_____ cloves, ground
_____ cumin, ground
_____ cumin seed
_____ curry powder
_____ dill weed
_____ dry mustard
_____ ginger, ground
_____ nutmeg, ground
_____ paprika
_____ parsley
_____ red pepper flakes
_____ rosemary
_____ tarragon
_____ thyme leaves
_____ turmeric, ground

OTHER

_____ artichoke hearts
_____ beets, sliced
_____ black olives
_____ cereal, bran
_____ cereal, granola, low-fat
_____ cereal, Kashi
_____ cereal, multi-bran
_____ cereal, multigrain Cheerios
_____ cereal, puffed
_____ cornflakes
_____ crackers, saltine
_____ crackers, whole-wheat
_____ cranberry sauce
_____ dark beer
_____ French fries
_____ fruit cocktail, in light syrup
_____ maple syrup, sugar-free
_____ molasses
_____ orange marmalade,
　　　 sugar-free
_____ peanut butter or cashew
　　　 butter
_____ pumpkin seeds
_____ rice, brown
_____ salad dressing, reduced-fat
　　　 or fat-free
_____ sauerkraut
_____ spaghetti sauce, light
_____ tomato paste,
　　　 no-added-salt
_____ tomatoes, crushed,
　　　 no-added-salt
_____ tortilla chips, baked
_____ unsweetened applesauce
_____ water chestnuts
_____ wine, red

STAPLES

_____ baking powder
_____ baking soda
_____ bouillon, beef, sodium-free
_____ bouillon, chicken,
　　　 sodium-free
_____ cornstarch
_____ honey
_____ lemon juice
_____ lime juice
_____ nonstick cooking spray
_____ old-fashioned oats, rolled
_____ olive oil
_____ sherry, dry cooking
_____ Smart Balance Omega oil
_____ Splenda
_____ Splenda Brown Sugar
　　　 Blend
_____ vinegar, balsamic
_____ vinegar, cider
_____ vinegar, red wine
_____ vinegar, white
_____ whole-wheat flour

Salisbury Steak

Serves 4   Serving size: 1/4 recipe

1 **lb** 96% lean ground beef

1/3 **cup** onion, finely chopped

1/4 **cup** saltine crackers, crumbled

1 egg white, slightly beaten

1 **Tbsp** horseradish

1/8 **tsp** pepper

1 **Tbsp** sodium-free beef bouillon

2 **Tbsp** whole-wheat flour

1/2 **cup** water

4 **oz** mushrooms, sliced

In a medium bowl, combine the beef, onion, crackers, egg white, horseradish, and pepper, mixing lightly but thoroughly; shape into four 1/2-inch thick patties. Heat a large nonstick skillet over medium heat. Place beef patties in skillet; cook 7–8 minutes or until no longer pink and juices run clear, turning once. Remove from skillet and keep warm. Mix the bouillon and flour with the water and mushrooms; heat until thickened. Serve sauce over Salisbury steaks.

Exchanges/Choices

1/2 Starch
4 Lean Meat

Basic Nutritional Values

Calories 195
 Calories from Fat 45
Total Fat. . . . . 5.0 g
 Saturated Fat . . . . 2.1 g
 Trans Fat . . . . 0.5 g
Cholesterol. . . . . 60 mg
Sodium. . . . . 160 mg
Total Carbohydrate . . . 10 g
 Dietary Fiber . . . . 1 g
 Sugars . . . . 2 g
Protein . . . . 27 g

Baked Tomatoes and Squash

Serves 4   Serving size: 1/4 recipe

2 medium summer squash (about 1/2 lb each)

1 (10-oz) pkg frozen spinach, cooked and drained

3 oz reduced-fat feta cheese, crumbled

1/4 cup dry whole-wheat bread crumbs

1/4 cup green onions, finely chopped

2 Tbsp minced parsley

1/2 tsp dill weed

2 medium tomatoes

4 tsp reduced-fat grated Parmesan cheese

Paprika, to taste

Exchanges/Choices

2 Vegetable
1 Lean Meat
1 Fat

Basic Nutritional Values

Calories 135
 Calories from Fat 40
Total Fat. . . . . 4.5 g
 Saturated Fat. . . . . . . 2.6 g
 Trans Fat . . . . 0.0 g
Cholesterol. . . . . 10 mg
Sodium. . . . . 415 mg
Total Carbohydrate . . . 16 g
 Dietary Fiber . . . . 5 g
 Sugars . . . . 5 g
Protein . . . . 11 g

1. Preheat oven to 375°F.

2. Cut squash in half lengthwise. Scoop out centers (leaving a 1/2-inch shell) and reserve pulp and seeds. In a large skillet over medium heat, bring 1 inch of water to a boil. Add squash shells, cover, and cook for 10 minutes or until fork-tender. Remove shells and drain well; then transfer to a baking dish.

3. In a medium bowl, combine squash pulp with spinach, feta cheese, bread crumbs, green onions, parsley, and dill weed. Mound 1/4 of the mixture into each squash shell, packing lightly. Bake for 10 minutes.

4. Remove stems from tomatoes and cut in half crosswise. Sprinkle top of each half with 1 tsp Parmesan cheese. Place tomatoes beside squash in baking dish. Bake 15–20 minutes longer or until spinach mixture is set and vegetables are heated through. Sprinkle spinach with paprika and serve.

Ambrosia Salad

Serves 4   Serving size: 1/4 recipe

1   **cup** diced fresh oranges

2   fresh bananas, sliced

1   **cup** seedless green grapes

1/2   **cup** raisins

2   **Tbsp** lemon juice

1/4   **cup** canola mayonnaise

2/3   **cup** fat-free whipped topping

6   **Tbsp** nonfat milk

4   small lettuce leaves

Combine the oranges, bananas, grapes, and raisins; sprinkle with lemon juice and chill. Stir in mayonnaise and mix with remaining ingredients. Serve on lettuce.

Exchanges/Choices

3 Fruit
1 Fat

Basic Nutritional Values

Calories 235
  Calories from Fat 45
Total Fat . . . . 5.0 g
  Saturated Fat . . . . 0.2 g
  Trans Fat . . . . 0.0 g
Cholesterol . . . . 0 mg
Sodium . . . . 115 mg
Total Carbohydrate . . . 47 g
  Dietary Fiber . . . . 4 g
  Sugars . . . . 33 g
Protein . . . . 3 g

Gram's Gingerbread

Serves 8   Serving size: 1 square

1/2   **cup** Splenda

1/2   **cup** molasses

1/4   **cup** unsweetened apple-sauce

1/2   **cup** egg substitute or egg whites, beaten

1 1/2   **cup** whole-wheat flour

1   **tsp** ginger, ground

1   **tsp** baking soda

1/2   **cup** boiling water

Mix together all ingredients (except water); then add water. Mix thoroughly. Bake at 350°F until a toothpick inserted into the center comes out clean.

Exchanges/Choices

2 Carbohydrate

Basic Nutritional Values

Calories 155
  Calories from Fat 0
Total Fat . . . . 0.0 g
  Saturated Fat . . . . 0.1 g
  Trans Fat . . . . 0.0 g
Cholesterol . . . . 0 mg
Sodium . . . . 195 mg
Total Carbohydrate . . . 35 g
  Dietary Fiber . . . . 3 g
  Sugars . . . . 14 g
Protein . . . . 5 g

Cranberry Ham Kabob

Serves 4   Serving size: 1/4 recipe

1 lb boneless ham, cut into
     16 1/2-inch cubes
     (trimmed of visible fat)

2 cups pineapple chunks
     (drained of syrup)

1 red pepper, cut into
     1-inch squares

1 green pepper, cut into
     1-inch squares

8 oz jellied cranberry sauce

1/8 tsp ground cloves

1 tsp dry mustard

1 Tbsp cider vinegar

Using 8 wooden or metal skewers, thread 2 ham chunks, 4 pineapple chunks, and red and green pepper pieces on each. Place in a single layer in a shallow baking pan. In a small bowl, mix cranberry sauce, cloves, mustard, and vinegar. Pour mixture over kabobs. Bake at 400°F for 15–20 minutes, basting often.

This recipe is high in sodium.

Exchanges/Choices

1 Fruit
1 1/2 Carbohydrate
1 Vegetable
2 Lean Meat

Basic Nutritional Values

Calories 250
  Calories from Fat 30
Total Fat . . . . 3.5 g
  Saturated Fat . . . . 1.1 g
  Trans Fat . . . . 0.0 g
Cholesterol . . . . 30 mg
Sodium . . . . 765 mg
Total Carbohydrate . . . 40 g
  Dietary Fiber . . . . 3 g
  Sugars . . . . 37 g
Protein . . . . 15 g

Sweet Potato Casserole

Serves 4   Serving size: 1/4 recipe

2 large sweet potatoes

1 cup mashed ripe bananas
     (about 2 medium)

1 tsp curry powder

1/3 cup fat-free sour cream

1/2 cup egg substitute

Cook sweet potatoes in the microwave for about 5 minutes. Scrape potato from the skins to get 1 cup mashed sweet potatoes. In large bowl, combine all ingredients. Beat with an electric mixer until mixed and very fluffy. Pour into a 1-quart casserole dish. Bake at 350°F for 20 minutes or until puffed and lightly browned.

Exchanges/Choices

1 Starch
1 Fruit

Basic Nutritional Values

Calories 170
  Calories from Fat 5
Total Fat . . . . 0.5 g
  Saturated Fat . . . . 0.1 g
  Trans Fat . . . . 0.0 g
Cholesterol . . . . 0 mg
Sodium . . . . 80 mg
Total Carbohydrate . . . 34 g
  Dietary Fiber . . . . 3 g
  Sugars . . . . 13 g
Protein . . . . 6 g

Red Lentil Soup

Serves 4   Serving size: 1/4 recipe

2 Tbsp Smart Balance Omega oil	**1/4 cup** bulgur
2 onions, chopped (1 1/2 cups)	**2 Tbsp** no-added-salt tomato paste
3 cloves garlic, minced	**1** bay leaf
1 Tbsp ground cumin	**1 tsp** paprika
2 Tbsp sodium-free chicken bouillon	**1 tsp** cayenne pepper
2 cups water	**3 Tbsp** lemon juice
1 cup red lentils	Freshly ground pepper, to taste

1. Heat 1 Tbsp oil in a soup pot or Dutch oven over medium-high heat. Add onions and cook, stirring, until softened, 3–5 minutes. Add garlic and cumin; cook for 1 minute. Add bouillon, water, lentils, bulgur, tomato paste, and bay leaf; bring to a simmer, stirring occasionally. Cover and cook over low heat until the lentils are very tender, 25–30 minutes. Discard the bay leaf. Add the paprika and cayenne pepper.

2. Ladle about 2 cups of the soup into a food processor and puree. Return the pureed soup to the soup pot and heat through. Stir in lemon juice and season with ground pepper. Just before serving, ladle into bowls.

Exchanges/Choices

2 1/2 Starch
1 Lean Meat
1 Fat

Basic Nutritional Values

Calories 290
  Calories from Fat 70
Total Fat . . . . 8.0 g
  Saturated Fat . . . . 0.6 g
  Trans Fat . . . . 0.0 g
Cholesterol . . . . 0 mg
Sodium . . . . 15 mg
Total Carbohydrate . . . 42 g
  Dietary Fiber . . . . 13 g
  Sugars . . . . 5 g
Protein . . . . 14 g

Jamaican Chicken

Serves 4   Serving size: 1/4 recipe

6 oz turkey smoked sausage

1 lb boneless, skinless chicken breast (trimmed of visible fat)

1/3 medium green pepper

1 lb tomatoes

2/3 cup chopped onion

2/3 cup whole-grain rice

1/3 cup no-salt catsup

1 cup water

Cut sausage into 1/2-inch-thick slices. Cut chicken into small pieces. Chop green pepper and tomatoes. Brown the sausage in a skillet and drain away fat. Add onion and chicken. Brown in 10 minutes, stirring occasionally; drain. Add green pepper, tomatoes, catsup, rice, and water; cover and bring to a boil. Reduce heat; cover and simmer for 25 minutes or until rice is tender. Uncover and simmer 5 more minutes.

Exchanges/Choices

2 Starch
2 Vegetable
3 Lean Meat
1/2 Fat

Basic Nutritional Values

Calories 370
  Calories from Fat 80
Total Fat . . . . 9.0 g
  Saturated Fat . . . . 2.5 g
  Trans Fat . . . . 0.0 g
Cholesterol . . . . 95 mg
Sodium . . . . 480 mg
Total Carbohydrate . . . 42 g
  Dietary Fiber . . . . 4 g
  Sugars . . . . 11 g
Protein . . . . 34 g

Vinegary Beets and Walnuts

Serves 4   Serving size: 1/4 recipe

1 **(15-oz) can** sliced beets, drained

1/2 **cup** balsamic vinegar

1 **Tbsp + 1 tsp** Splenda Brown Sugar Blend

Nonstick cooking spray

1/4 **cup** walnut halves, chopped

1/2 **tsp** ground cinnamon

1/2 **tsp** ground nutmeg

1. In a medium bowl, add the beets and a small amount of water. Microwave for 2–3 minutes or until the beets are warm through. Keep covered and set aside.

2. In a small saucepan, stir together vinegar and 1 Tbsp Splenda Brown Sugar Blend. Bring to a simmer, stirring constantly, until sugar is dissolved. Simmer for 6–8 minutes or until the mixture is reduced by half. Remove from heat and set aside.

3. Spray a skillet with nonstick cooking spray and put over medium heat. Add walnuts, cinnamon, and nutmeg, and dry roast for 2–3 minutes. Stir in the vinegar mixture and remaining Splenda Brown Sugar Blend; keep warm. Drain the beets and transfer to a serving dish. Pour the vinegar-walnut mixture over the beets.

Exchanges/Choices

1/2 Carbohydrate
1 Vegetable
1 Fat

Basic Nutritional Values

Calories 100
Calories from Fat 40
Total Fat . . . . 4.5 g
Saturated Fat . . . . 0.5 g
Trans Fat . . . . 0.0 g
Cholesterol . . . . 0 mg
Sodium . . . . 135 mg
Total Carbohydrate . . . 16 g
Dietary Fiber . . . . 2 g
Sugars . . . . 12 g
Protein . . . . 2 g

Spicy Turkey Pitas

Serves 4   Serving size: 1 pita sandwich

2 **tsp** Smart Balance Omega oil	**1/4** **cup** raisins
1 small red bell pepper, seeded and diced	**1/4** **cup** black olives, finely diced
1 small onion, diced	**1** **tsp** ground cumin
3 cloves garlic, minced	**1/2** **tsp** red pepper flakes
12 **oz** lean ground turkey	**2** pita pocket breads
1 **(15-oz)** can no-added-salt crushed tomatoes	

Add the oil to a medium skillet and coat the bottom of the pan. Put over heat and sauté pepper and onion for about 4 minutes. Stir in the garlic, reduce heat, and cook for another 4 minutes. Add the turkey, stir to break up the meat. Stir in remaining ingredients and increase heat until boiling. Lower heat and cook 10 minutes. Cut pita bread into halves and spoon an equal amount of the turkey mixture into each half.

Exchanges/Choices

1 Starch
1/2 Fruit
2 Vegetable
4 Lean Meat

Basic Nutritional Values

Calories 345	
Calories from Fat 80	
Total Fat. . . . . 9.0 g	
Saturated Fat . . . . 1.8 g	
Trans Fat . . . . 0.0 g	
Cholesterol. . . . . 65 mg	
Sodium. . . . . 290 mg	
Total Carbohydrate. . . 35 g	
Dietary Fiber . . . . 4 g	
Sugars . . . . 12 g	
Protein . . . . 31 g	

Carrot-Pineapple Coleslaw

Serves 4   Serving size: 1/4 recipe

2 **cups** shredded carrots	**1/4** **cup** plain fat-free yogurt
1 **cup** shredded cabbage	**1** **Tbsp** Splenda
2 **cups** crushed, canned pineapple, drained and juice reserved	**1** **Tbsp** cider vinegar
1/4 **cup** canola mayonnaise	**1/2** **tsp** ground black pepper

In large bowl, toss together carrots, cabbage, and pineapple. In a small bowl, stir together the reserved pineapple juice, mayonnaise, yogurt, Splenda, vinegar, and black pepper. Pour dressing over slaw; toss gently. Cover and refrigerate 2–24 hours.

Exchanges/Choices

1 Fruit
1 Vegetable
1 Fat

Basic Nutritional Values

Calories 140	
Calories from Fat 45	
Total Fat. . . . . 5.0 g	
Saturated Fat . . . . 0.0 g	
Trans Fat . . . . 0.0 g	
Cholesterol. . . . . 0 mg	
Sodium. . . . . 140 mg	
Total Carbohydrate. . . 23 g	
Dietary Fiber . . . . 3 g	
Sugars . . . . 19 g	
Protein 2g	

Stir-Fry Beef and Vegetables

Serves 4   Serving size: 1/4 recipe

- **1 lb** sirloin beef steak (trimmed of visible fat)
- **1** egg white
- **3 tsp** cornstarch
- **6 oz** bean sprouts, rinsed
- **1** celery stalk, thinly sliced
- **1** small tomato, cut into wedges
- **2/3** red or green bell pepper, quartered and cut into 1/2-inch pieces
- **6 Tbsp** water chestnuts, sliced
- **4** green onions, sliced into 1/2-inch pieces
- **3 Tbsp** reduced-sodium Worcestershire sauce
- **2 Tbsp** dry cooking sherry
- **2 Tbsp** Smart Balance Omega oil

Fresh ground pepper, to taste

Exchanges/Choices

2 Vegetable
3 Lean Meat
1 1/2 Fat

Basic Nutritional Values

Calories 260
　Calories from Fat 110
Total Fat. . . . . 12.0 g
　Saturated Fat . . . . 2.2 g
　Trans Fat. . . . . 0.1 g
Cholesterol. . . . . 40 mg
Sodium. . . . . 125 mg
Total Carbohydrate . . . 13 g
　Dietary Fiber . . . . 3 g
　Sugars . . . . 7 g
Protein. . . . . 26 g

1. Slice steak diagonally into 1/4-inch slices. In a small bowl, blend egg white and 2 tsp cornstarch. Add steak slices and cover with mixture; set aside.

2. Drain bean sprouts well. Combine celery, tomato wedges, and red or green pepper; set aside. Place water chestnuts and green onions in a small bowl; add Worcestershire sauce, remaining 1 tsp cornstarch, and dry cooking sherry.

3. Heat 1 Tbsp oil over high heat in a nonstick or heavy skillet. Add steak and stir-fry until it loses its pink color, stirring constantly. Remove and set aside. Add 1 Tbsp oil to skillet; add bean sprouts, celery, tomato wedges, and red or green pepper; stir-fry for 3–4 minutes or until crisp-tender. Add water chestnuts and onions with sauce mixture. Stir-fry for 1 minute; add steak and continue to stir-fry until heated through. Add pepper to taste.

Cauliflower Parmigiana

Serves 4   Serving size: 1/4 recipe

5	**cups** cauliflower	**1 1/2 cup** nonfat milk
1	**Tbsp** Smart Balance margarine	**1/4 cup** shredded reduced-fat Parmesan cheese
1/2	**tsp** ground cumin	Black pepper, to taste
2	**Tbsp** whole-wheat flour	

1. Cut cauliflower into 1 1/2-inch florets.

2. In a saucepan, melt the margarine over low heat; add the cumin and whole-wheat flour. Cook, stirring, for 3 minutes. Add the milk; bring to a boil, then simmer for 1 minute. Stir in Parmesan and pepper to taste. Cook the sauce over low heat, stirring, until cheese is melted. Remove pan from the heat and keep the sauce warm.

3. In a steamer set over boiling water, steam the cauliflower, covered, for 5 minutes or until just tender. Transfer to a 3-cup baking dish. Drizzle the cauliflower with the sauce and bake the gratin in the upper third of a preheated oven set at 400°F for 15 minutes or until it is golden and bubbly.

Exchanges/Choices

1/2 Fat-Free Milk
2 Vegetable
1/2 Fat

Basic Nutritional Values

Calories	130
Calories from Fat	35
Total Fat	4.0 g
Saturated Fat	1.4 g
Trans Fat	0.0 g
Cholesterol	10 mg
Sodium	230 mg
Total Carbohydrate	17 g
Dietary Fiber	4 g
Sugars	8 g
Protein	8 g

Broiled Haddock

Serves 4   Serving size: 1/4 recipe

	Nonstick cooking spray	**1 tsp** dry mustard
1/4	**cup** lemon juice	**2 Tbsp** Smart Balance Omega oil
1	**Tbsp** dried parsley	
1/2	**tsp** dried tarragon	**1 lb** haddock fillets

Lightly spray the oven broiler rack with nonstick cooking spray. Preheat broiler. In a small bowl, combine the lemon juice, parsley, tarragon, and mustard. Pour the oil into a small broiler-proof baking dish and place the fish in the dish. Pour the lemon juice mixture over the fish; broil for about 4 minutes. Check the fish, spoon juice over fish, and broil for another 4–6 minutes, until the fish flakes easily when tested with a fork.

Exchanges/Choices

3 Lean Meat
1/2 Fat

Basic Nutritional Values

Calories	165
Calories from Fat	70
Total Fat	8.0 g
Saturated Fat	0.7 g
Trans Fat	0.0 g
Cholesterol	65 mg
Sodium	80 mg
Total Carbohydrate	1 g
Dietary Fiber	0 g
Sugars	0 g
Protein	22 g

Sauerkraut Salad

Serves 4   Serving size: 1/4 recipe

1/3 **cup** vinegar

1/2 **cup** Splenda

1/2 **cup** diced celery

1/2 **cup** diced bell pepper

1/2 **cup** diced onion

1 1/2 **cups** sauerkraut, drained

Pour the vinegar over the Splenda in a saucepan and heat. Pour this mixture over the celery, peppers, and onion and then let cool. Add this mixture to the sauerkraut; toss together. Cover and chill for 3 hours before serving.

Exchanges/Choices

2 Vegetable

Basic Nutritional Values

Calories 40
  Calories from Fat . . . 0
Total Fat . . . . 0.0 g
  Saturated Fat . . . . 0.0 g
  Trans Fat . . . . 0.0 g
Cholesterol . . . . 0 mg
Sodium . . . . 365 mg
Total Carbohydrate . . . 10 g
  Dietary Fiber . . . . 3 g
  Sugars . . . . 5 g
Protein . . . . 1 g

Banana Bran Muffin

Serves 8   Serving size: 1 muffin

2/3 **cup** bran cereal	3/16 **tsp** ground nutmeg
2/3 **cup** plain fat-free yogurt	2 **cups** bananas, mashed
5/8 **cup** whole-wheat flour	1/4 **cup** unsweetened applesauce
5 **Tbsp** Splenda	1/2 **cup** egg substitute, beaten
1 **tsp** ground cinnamon	
1/2 **tsp** baking soda	

1. Preheat oven to 375°F. Place paper liners in muffin pan cups.

2. In a medium bowl, mix cereal and yogurt. Let stand for 5 minutes or until cereal is softened and breaks up.

3. Meanwhile, in a small bowl, combine the flour, Splenda, cinnamon, baking soda, and nutmeg; set aside.

4. Stir banana, applesauce, and egg substitute into cereal mixture. Stir in flour mixture until moistened. Fill muffin cups to about 2/3 full. Bake for 20–25 minutes or until muffins are lightly browned on top. Remove from pan and let cool on a wire rack before serving.

Exchanges/Choices

1 Starch
1 Fruit

Basic Nutritional Values

Calories 120
 Calories from Fat 5
Total Fat . . . . 0.5 g
 Saturated Fat . . . . 0.2 g
 Trans Fat . . . . 0.0 g
Cholesterol . . . . 0 mg
Sodium . . . . 135 mg
Total Carbohydrate . . . 27 g
 Dietary Fiber . . . . 5 g
 Sugars . . . . 11 g
Protein . . . . 5 g

Dilled Cucumber Salad

Serves 4   Serving size: 1/4 recipe

1/4 **cup** fat-free sour cream	1 1/2 **Tbsp** dill weed
1 **Tbsp** canola mayonnaise	Black pepper, to taste
1/4 **cup** plain fat-free yogurt	1 1/2 medium cucumber
1 1/2 **Tbsp** lime juice	

In a bowl, whisk together sour cream, mayonnaise, yogurt, lime juice, dill, and pepper. Peel the cucumbers and cut crosswise into 1/8-inch-thick slices. Stir them into the dressing. Serve chilled.

Exchanges/Choices

1 Vegetable

Basic Nutritional Values

Calories 40
 Calories from Fat 15
Total Fat . . . . 1.5 g
 Saturated Fat . . . . 0.0 g
 Trans Fat . . . . 0.0 g
Cholesterol . . . . 5 mg
Sodium . . . . 45 mg
Total Carbohydrate . . . 4 g
 Dietary Fiber . . . . 1 g
 Sugars . . . . 3 g
Protein . . . . 2 g

Chicken with Artichoke Hearts

Serves 4   Serving size: 1/4 recipe

- **1 lb** boneless, skinless chicken breasts (trimmed of visible fat)
- **2 Tbsp** Smart Balance margarine
- **2 Tbsp** whole-wheat flour
- **1 Tbsp** lemon juice
- **1 Tbsp** sodium-free chicken bouillon
- **1 cup** water
- **1 cup** fat-free sour cream
- **1 (14-oz)** can artichoke hearts, drained
- **2 cups** cooked brown rice

Brown chicken on both sides and then set aside. Melt margarine; add flour, lemon juice, bouillon, water, and sour cream. Mix well and stir over medium heat until sauce thickens. Put chicken and artichokes in a baking dish. Pour sauce over chicken and artichokes. Bake at 350°F for 1 hour. Serve with sauce over rice.

Exchanges/Choices

2 Starch
1 Vegetable
4 Lean Meat

Basic Nutritional Values

Calories	365
Calories from Fat	80
Total Fat	9.0 g
Saturated Fat	2.2 g
Trans Fat	0.0 g
Cholesterol	70 mg
Sodium	320 mg
Total Carbohydrate	33 g
Dietary Fiber	3 g
Sugars	4 g
Protein	33 g

Green Bean Casserole

Serves 4   Serving size: 1/4 recipe

- **2 Tbsp** Smart Balance Light margarine
- **2 Tbsp** whole-wheat flour
- **1/4 tsp** Splenda
- **1 tsp** grated onion
- **3/4 cup** fat-free sour cream
- **16 oz** frozen French-style green beans, cooked
- **1/2 cup** fat-free shredded cheddar cheese
- **1/4 cup** cornflake crumbs

Melt 1 Tbsp margarine in a skillet and add flour. Cook gently; remove from heat. Stir in Splenda, grated onion, and sour cream; then fold in the green beans. Place in a casserole dish, cover with cheese. Mix cornflake crumbs with the remaining 1 Tbsp margarine; add to casserole dish. Bake at 350°F until hot and bubbly.

Exchanges/Choices

1/2 Starch
2 Vegetable
1 Lean Meat

Basic Nutritional Values

Calories	140
Calories from Fat	25
Total Fat	3.0 g
Saturated Fat	0.8 g
Trans Fat	0.0 g
Cholesterol	5 mg
Sodium	255 mg
Total Carbohydrate	16 g
Dietary Fiber	4 g
Sugars	5 g
Protein	10 g

Whole-Wheat Blueberry Muffins
Serves 12   Serving size: 1 muffin

1   **cup** whole-wheat flour

5 1/2   **Tbsp** Splenda

1   **tsp** baking powder

6   **Tbsp** nonfat milk

3   **Tbsp** Smart Balance margarine

1/2   **cup** egg substitute

1/2   **cup** blueberries

Preheat oven to 400°F. In a medium bowl, combine flour, Splenda, and baking powder. In a small bowl, beat milk, margarine, and egg substitute; stir into dry ingredients until just moist. Fold in blueberries and spoon batter into 12 paper-lined muffin cups. Bake for 20–25 minutes or until golden brown. Serve immediately.

Exchanges/Choices

1/2 Starch
1/2 Fat

Basic Nutritional Values

Calories 70
 Calories from Fat 20
Total Fat. . . . . .2.5 g
 Saturated Fat . . . . .0.7 g
 Trans Fat. . . . . .0.0 g
Cholesterol. . . . . .0 mg
Sodium. . . . . .75 mg
Total Carbohydrate. . .9 g
 Dietary Fiber. . . . . .1 g
 Sugars . . . . .2 g
Protein. . . . . .3 g

Macaroni and Cheese with Tomatoes
Serves 4   Serving size: 1/4 recipe

8   **oz** whole-wheat elbow macaroni, uncooked

2   tomatoes, sliced

1/2   **cup** bread crumbs

2   **Tbsp** Smart Balance Light margarine

1   **Tbsp** whole-wheat flour

1/4   **tsp** dry mustard

2   **cups** nonfat milk

2   **oz** shredded fat-free American cheese

2   **oz** reduced-fat sharp cheddar cheese

Prepare pasta according to package directions and drain. Preheat oven to 375°F. Slice the tomatoes into 1/2-inch-thick slices. Set aside on a small plate. Crumble the bread crumbs with your fingertips; set aside on a small plate. In a 2-quart saucepan over medium heat, melt the margarine. Add the flour and dry mustard; then cook for 2–3 minutes. Add the milk little by little and continue stirring until mixture thickens. Add cheese and stir until melted. Place 1/3 of the tomato slices in the bottom of a baking dish; add half the pasta. Place another 1/3 of the tomato slices on top and then add the rest of the pasta. Pour the sauce over the dish. Arrange the last 1/3 of the tomato slices on top and sprinkle with bread crumbs. Bake for 20 minutes.

Exchanges/Choices

3 Starch
1/2 Fat-Free Milk
1 Lean Meat
1/2 Fat

Basic Nutritional Values

Calories 355
 Calories from Fat 65
Total Fat. . . . . .7.0 g
 Saturated Fat . . . . .2.8 g
 Trans Fat. . . . . .0.0 g
Cholesterol. . . . . .15 mg
Sodium. . . . . .450 mg
Total Carbohydrate. . .56 g
 Dietary Fiber. . . . . .6 g
 Sugars . . . . .10 g
Protein. . . . . .21 g

Tomato Asparagus Salad
Serves 4   Serving size: 1/4 recipe

1 lb asparagus

1 pint red grape tomatoes,
       cut in half lengthwise

2 Tbsp Smart Balance
       Omega oil

1 medium lemon, juiced
       Pepper, to taste

Blanch the asparagus in a large pot of boiling water until just tender, about 1–2 minutes for very thin spears and 4–5 minutes for thicker spears. Drain and place in an ice water bath until completely chilled. Cut the asparagus into 1-inch pieces. Toss the asparagus with the remaining ingredients; divide among four chilled salad plates to serve.

Exchanges/Choices
2 Vegetable
1 1/2 Fat

Basic Nutritional Values
Calories 100
  Calories from Fat 70
Total Fat . . . . 8.0 g
  Saturated Fat . . . . 0.5 g
  Trans Fat . . . . 0.0 g
Cholesterol . . . . 0 mg
Sodium . . . . 20 mg
Total Carbohydrate . . . 8 g
  Dietary Fiber . . . . 3 g
  Sugars . . . . 4 g
Protein . . . . 3 g

Baked Sweet Potato Fries
Serves 4   Serving size: 1/4 recipe

2 medium sweet potatoes

1 1/2 Tbsp Smart Balance
       Omega oil

1 tsp curry powder

1/4 tsp ground turmeric

1/4 tsp cumin seed

1/4 tsp ground ginger

Preheat oven to 400°F. Wash and scrub sweet potatoes, leaving the skins on. Cut them into sticks about 1/4–1/2 inch wide and 2–4 inches long; set aside. In a 2-quart mixing bowl, mix together the oil and spices. Add potato sticks to bowl; stir to coat. Arrange sticks on a baking sheet; bake for 30–40 minutes or until fries are tender on the inside and slightly golden on the outside. Halfway through baking, stir with spatula to prevent fries from sticking.

Exchanges/Choices
1 Starch
1 Fat

Basic Nutritional Values
Calories 115
  Calories from Fat 45
Total Fat . . . . 5.0 g
  Saturated Fat . . . . 0.4 g
  Trans Fat . . . . 0.0 g
Cholesterol . . . . 0 mg
Sodium . . . . 25 mg
Total Carbohydrate . . . 16 g
  Dietary Fiber . . . . 3 g
  Sugars . . . . 5 g
Protein . . . . 2 g

Asparagus Dijon
Serves 4   Serving size: 1/4 recipe

1 **lb** trimmed asparagus

1/4 **cup** Dijon mustard

1/4 **cup** dark beer

3 **Tbsp** honey

1/2 **tsp** minced garlic

1/4 **tsp** crushed dried thyme leaves

Add asparagus to boiling water and cook uncovered, about 2 minutes or until barely tender. Drain. In a separate bowl, combine mustard, beer, honey, garlic, and thyme; mix well. Pour over cooked asparagus.

Exchanges/Choices

1 Carbohydrate
1 Vegetable

Basic Nutritional Values

Calories	95
Calories from Fat	10
Total Fat	1.0 g
Saturated Fat	0.0 g
Trans Fat	0.0 g
Cholesterol	0 mg
Sodium	375 mg
Total Carbohydrate	21 g
Dietary Fiber	2 g
Sugars	15 g
Protein	3 g

Peach and Apple Crisp
Serves 4   Serving size: 1/4 recipe

2 **cups** sliced peaches (fresh, frozen, or canned light)

1 1/2 **cups** apples, peeled and sliced

3 1/2 **Tbsp** Splenda

2 **Tbsp** + 2 **tsp** whole-wheat flour

1 **tsp** ground cinnamon

1 **tsp** ground nutmeg

3 **Tbsp** old-fashioned oats

2 **Tbsp** Smart Balance Light margarine, melted

Preheat oven to 400°F. Place peaches and apples in a large bowl. In a small bowl, mix 2 Tbsp Splenda, 2 tsp flour, 1/2 tsp cinnamon, and 1/2 tsp nutmeg. Sprinkle over fruit and toss until fruit is evenly coated; mound mixture in a 1-quart casserole. In a small bowl, mix oats, 2 Tbsp flour, 1 1/2 Tbsp Splenda, 1/2 tsp cinnamon, and 1/2 tsp nutmeg. Stir in margarine until mixture is evenly moistened. Spoon over fruit. Bake in lower third of the oven for 30 minutes or until juices are bubbly and topping is browned. Serve warm.

Exchanges/Choices

1 1/2 Carbohydrate
1/2 Fat

Basic Nutritional Values

Calories	130
Calories from Fat	40
Total Fat	4.5 g
Saturated Fat	1.3 g
Trans Fat	0.0 g
Cholesterol	0 mg
Sodium	40 mg
Total Carbohydrate	22 g
Dietary Fiber	3 g
Sugars	14 g
Protein	2 g

Whole-Wheat Pancakes or Waffles

Serves 4   Serving size: 2 pancakes or waffles

1/2 **cup** rolled oats

1/2 **cup** whole-wheat flour, sifted

2 **tsp** baking powder

2 **Tbsp** Splenda

1/2 **cup** egg substitute, beaten well

3/4 **cup** nonfat milk

2 **Tbsp** Smart Balance Omega oil

Nonstick cooking spray

Stir together dry ingredients. Combine egg substitute, milk, and oil; stir into flour mixture. Cook on a griddle lightly coated with nonstick spray until golden brown, then turn. Can also be made in a waffle iron.

Exchanges/Choices

1 1/2 Starch
1 1/2 Fat

Basic Nutritional Values

Calories 185
  Calories from Fat 70
Total Fat . . . . 8.0 g
  Saturated Fat . . . . 0.7 g
  Trans Fat . . . . 0.0 g
Cholesterol . . . . 0 mg
Sodium . . . . 265 mg
Total Carbohydrate . . . 22 g
  Dietary Fiber . . . . 3 g
  Sugars . . . . 3 g
Protein . . . . 8 g

Beef and Barley Stew

Serves 4   Serving size: 1/4 recipe

24 **oz** chuck roast or boneless beef (trimmed of visible fat)

1/2 **cup** barley, uncooked

1/4 **tsp** pepper

3/4 **tsp** dried rosemary, crushed

2 **cups** water

4 medium carrots, sliced

2 medium onions, sliced

Place meat and barley in a large baking pot or Dutch oven. Season with pepper and rosemary. Add water, carrots, and onions. Heat to boiling; then lower heat. Cover and simmer until beef is tender, about 2–3 hours.

Exchanges/Choices

2 Starch
2 Vegetable
3 Lean Meat

Basic Nutritional Values

Calories 355
  Calories from Fat 65
Total Fat . . . . 7.0 g
  Saturated Fat . . . . 2.2 g
  Trans Fat . . . . 0.0 g
Cholesterol . . . . 85 mg
Sodium . . . . 135 mg
Total Carbohydrate . . . 43 g
  Dietary Fiber . . . . 8 g
  Sugars . . . . 8 g
Protein . . . . 30 g

Cinnamon Red Cabbage

Serves 4   Serving size: 1/4 recipe

- **4 cups** red cabbage
- **1** medium Granny Smith apple
- **1** medium pear
- **1/4 cup** sugar-free orange marmalade
- **1 tsp** cinnamon
- **1 tsp** ground cloves
- **3 Tbsp** red wine vinegar
- **3 Tbsp** red table wine

Thinly slice the cabbage. Peel and slice the apple. Peel and chop the pear. In a large pot, combine the cabbage, apple, pear, marmalade, cinnamon, cloves, vinegar, wine, and 1 cup water. Bring to a boil and cook the mixture, covered, over moderately low heat, stirring occasionally, for 3 hours. Serve the cabbage chilled as an accompaniment to cold sliced meats.

Exchanges/Choices

1 Fruit
1 Vegetable

Basic Nutritional Values

Calories 80
  Calories from Fat 0
Total Fat. . . . . 0.0 g
  Saturated Fat . . . . 0.1 g
  Trans Fat. . . . . 0.0 g
Cholesterol. . . . . 0 mg
Sodium. . . . . 15 mg
Total Carbohydrate. . . 22 g
  Dietary Fiber. . . . . 4 g
  Sugars . . . . 14 g
Protein. . . . . 1 g

Vegetable Lasagna

Serves 4   Serving size: 1/4 recipe

8 **oz** lasagna noodles

1/4 **cup** Smart Balance
Omega oil

1/2 medium eggplant, diced

1/4 **cup** onion, chopped

1 medium garlic clove, minced

1 **cup** zucchini, sliced

2 **cups** light spaghetti sauce

1 **cup** fat-free cottage cheese

1/2 **cup** reduced-fat cottage
cheese

1/2 **cup** fat-free buttermilk

1/4 **cup** egg substitute

1 **tsp** pepper

1 **oz** fat-free shredded
mozzarella cheese

1 **oz** reduced-fat shredded
mozzarella cheese

2 **Tbsp** reduced-fat grated
Parmesan cheese

Exchanges/Choices

3 Starch
1/2 Fat-Free Milk
4 Vegetable
2 Lean Meat
2 Fat

Basic Nutritional Values

Calories 550
 Calories from Fat 160
Total Fat. . . . . 18.0 g
 Saturated Fat . . . . 2.6 g
 Trans Fat. . . . . 0.0 g
Cholesterol. . . . . 15 mg
Sodium. . . . . 925 mg
Total Carbohydrate. . . 71 g
 Dietary Fiber. . . . . 6 g
 Sugars . . . . 19 g
Protein. . . . . 29 g

1. Cook and drain lasagna noodles according to package directions.

2. In 10-inch skillet over medium heat, heat the oil. Add eggplant, onion, and garlic; cook for 10 minutes, stirring often. Add zucchini; cook 5 minutes or until vegetables are crisp-tender. Stir in spaghetti sauce; heat through.

3. In a medium bowl, stir together cottage cheese, buttermilk, egg substitute, and pepper until blended. In a baking dish, layer 1/3 of the noodles and top with 1/2 of the vegetable mixture, 1/2 of the cottage cheese, and 1/2 of the mozzarella. Top with 1/3 of the noodles. Layer on the remaining vegetable mixture, cottage cheese, and mozzarella (reserve a small portion of the mozzarella). Top with last 1/3 of noodles; cover with foil. Bake at 350°F for 30 minutes. Uncover, sprinkle with Parmesan and reserved mozzarella. Bake 10 minutes more, until hot and bubbly. Let stand 10 minutes before serving.

This recipe is high in sodium.

Fruit and Crème Parfait

Serves 4   Serving size: 1/4 recipe

1 **cup** fat-free whipped topping

1 **cup** fat-free plain yogurt

1/4 **cup** Splenda

2 **cup** berries

1 **cup** low-fat granola cereal

Place whipped topping, yogurt, and Splenda in a medium bowl. Stir until thoroughly blended into a crème. To make each parfait, place a layer of each of the following amounts in a parfait glass in the order listed: 1/4 cup crème, 1/4 cup berries, 3 Tbsp granola, 3 Tbsp crème, 1/4 cup berries, 1 Tbsp crème, and finish with 1 Tbsp granola. Serve immediately or place in the refrigerator up to 2 hours before serving.

Exchanges/Choices
2 1/2 Carbohydrate

Basic Nutritional Values
Calories 185
  Calories from Fat 15
Total Fat . . . . 1.5 g
  Saturated Fat . . . . 0.4 g
  Trans Fat . . . . 0.0 g
Cholesterol . . . . 5 mg
Sodium . . . . 105 mg
Total Carbohydrate . . . 38 g
  Dietary Fiber . . . . 3 g
  Sugars . . . . 19 g
Protein . . . . 5 g

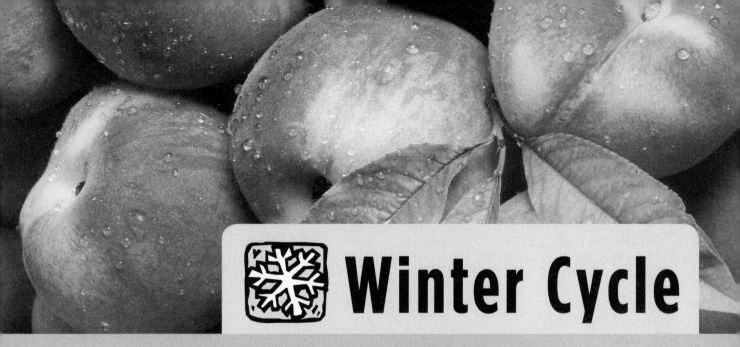

Winter Cycle

Featured Recipes

Cashew Pork

Hash Brown Potatoes

Scallops Coquille

Seasoned Chilled Vegetables*

Pita with Veggies

Chicken Eggplant Stir-Fry

Peach Cobbler

Zucchini Carrot Muffins*

New Orleans Chilled Rice

Raspberry Smoothie

Sweet Apple Pork Chops

Fruit Salad Medley

Fruit Medley

Veggie Melts

Whole-Wheat Pasta Salad

Baked Chicken Baja

Oatmeal and Apple Muffins*

Asian Chicken Pitas

Poppy Seed Fruit Salad

Cod Teriyaki

Carrot Slaw

Low-Fat Corn Bread

Whole-Grain Muffins*

Roast Beef and Swiss Roll-Up

Spinach-Orange Salad

Potato Salad

Zesty Orange Oats Peach Crisp

Fried Bananas*

Barbecued Pork Sandwich*

Oven-Roasted Tomatoes*

Skewered Chicken and Shrimp*

Cold Pasta Salad*

Carrots in Sherry Wine*

*Indicates that the recipe has been used previously.

1500 calorie MEAL PLAN WINTER WEEK 4

	Sunday	Monday	Tuesday	Wednesday	Thursday	Friday	Saturday
Breakfast	2 whole-grain waffles or pancakes 2 Tbsp sugar-free maple syrup 1 small orange 1 cup nonfat milk	1 whole-wheat English muffin 1/2 grapefruit 1 cup nonfat milk 1 oz lean turkey sausage 2 tsp margarine	**Zucchini Carrot Muffins*** 1 cup nonfat milk 1 oz Canadian bacon 1/2 tsp margarine	**Fruit Medley** 1/2 cup oatmeal 1 cup nonfat milk 1/4 cup egg substitute, scrambled 6 almonds	**Oatmeal and Apple Muffins*** 1 cup nonfat milk 1 egg, cooked as desired 1 tsp margarine	**Whole-Grain Muffins** (2)* 1 1/2 Tbsp fruit spread 1 cup nonfat milk 1 oz lean turkey sausage	**Fried Bananas*** 1/2 nonfat milk
Lunch	**Cashew Pork** **Hash Brown Potatoes** 1 dinner roll 1/2 cup peas 1/2 cup unsweetened applesauce	**Pita with Veggies** 2 oz baked tortilla chips 1 medium peach 1 oz reduced-fat cheese	**New Orleans Chilled Rice** **Raspberry Smoothie** 2 oz chicken breast	**Veggie Melts** **Whole-Wheat Pasta Salad** 1/2 cup cooked mustard greens	**Asian Chicken Pitas** **Poppy Seed Fruit Salad** 3/4 cup cooked corn and peas 10 peanuts	**Roast Beef and Swiss Roll-Up** (2) 3/4 oz pretzels 1 cup cantaloupe	**Barbecued Pork Sandwich*** **Oven-Roasted Tomatoes*** 1/2 ear corn on the cob 1/2 cup unsweetened plums 1/2 tsp margarine
Snack A							
Snack B							
Dinner	**Scallops Coquille** **Seasoned Chilled Vegetables*** 1/2 cup roasted red potatoes 1 slice whole-wheat bread 17 grapes 1 cup nonfat milk 1/2 cup green beans 1/2 tsp margarine	**Chicken Eggplant Stir-Fry** **Peach Cobbler** 12 cherries 1/2 cup nonfat milk 3 cashews	**Sweet Apple Pork Chops** **Fruit Salad Medley** 1/2 cup baked tater tots 1 cup steamed Brussels sprouts	**Baked Chicken Baja** 3 oz baked potato 1 slice multigrain bread 3/4 cup blackberries 1 cup nonfat milk 2 cups mixed salad vegetables 1/2 tsp olive oil and vinegar dressing	**Cod Teriyaki** **Carrot Slaw** **Low-Fat Corn Bread** 1/2 cup cooked green beans 1 tsp margarine	**Spinach-Orange Salad** **Potato Salad** **Zesty Orange Oats** **Peach Crisp** 1/2 cup nonfat milk 1/2 cup cooked squash 2 oz broiled beef	**Skewered Chicken and Shrimp*** **Cold Pasta Salad*** **Carrots in Sherry Wine*** 6 mixed nuts

*Indicates that the recipe has been used previously.

	Sunday	Monday	Tuesday	Wednesday	Thursday	Friday	Saturday
Breakfast	2 whole-grain waffles 2 Tbsp sugar-free maple syrup 1 small orange 1 cup nonfat milk 1/4 cup egg substitute, scrambled 1 1/2 tsp margarine	1 whole-wheat English muffin 1/2 grapefruit 1 cup nonfat milk 1 oz lean turkey sausage 2 tsp margarine	Zucchini Carrot Muffins* 1 cup nonfat milk 1 oz Canadian bacon 1/2 tsp margarine	Fruit Medley 1/2 cup oatmeal 1 cup nonfat milk 1/4 cup egg substitute, scrambled 6 almonds	Oatmeal and Apple Muffins* 1 cup nonfat milk 1 egg, cooked as desired 1 tsp margarine	Whole-Grain Muffins (2)* 1 1/2 Tbsp fruit spread 1 cup nonfat milk 1 oz lean turkey sausage	Fried Bananas* 1/2 nonfat milk
Lunch	Cashew Pork Hash Brown Potatoes 1 dinner roll 1/2 cup peas 1/2 cup unsweetened applesauce	Pita with Veggies 2 oz baked tortilla chips 1 medium peach 1 oz reduced-fat cheese 1 Tbsp sunflower seeds	New Orleans Chilled Rice Raspberry Smoothie 2 oz chicken breast 10 peanuts	Veggie Melts Whole-Wheat Pasta Salad 1/2 cup cooked mustard greens 1 oz reduced-fat cheese	Asian Chicken Pitas Poppy Seed Fruit Salad 3/4 cup cooked corn and peas 20 peanuts	Roast Beef and Swiss Roll-Up (2) 3/4 oz pretzels 1 cup cantaloupe 2 Brazil nuts	Barbecued Pork Sandwich* Oven-Roasted Tomatoes* 1/2 ear corn on the cob 1/2 cup unsweetened plums 1 1/2 tsp margarine
Snack A	1/2 cup light ice cream	5 hazelnuts 3/4 cup blueberries	16 pistachios 1 medium peach	4 walnuts 1 small apple	4 pecans 4 apricots	6 almonds 4 dried apple rings	6 almonds 3/4 cup blueberries
Snack B	1 cup nonfat milk	1 cup nonfat milk	1 cup nonfat milk	1 cup nonfat milk	1 cup nonfat milk	1 cup nonfat milk	1 cup fat-free yogurt
Dinner	Scallops Coquille Seasoned Chilled Vegetables* 1/2 cup roasted red potatoes 1 slice whole-wheat bread 17 grapes 1 cup nonfat milk 1/2 cup green beans 1/2 tsp margarine	Chicken Eggplant Stir-Fry Peach Cobbler 12 cherries 1 oz reduced-fat cheese 1/2 cup nonfat milk 3 cashews	Sweet Apple Pork Chops Fruit Salad Medley 1/2 cup baked tater tots 1 cup steamed Brussels sprouts 1 oz reduced-fat cheese	Baked Chicken Baja 3 oz baked potato 1 slice multigrain bread 3/4 cup blackberries 1 cup nonfat milk 2 cups mixed salad vegetables 1/2 tsp olive oil and vinegar dressing	Cod Teriyaki Carrot Slaw Low-Fat Corn Bread 1/2 cup cooked green beans 1 tsp margarine	Spinach-Orange Salad Potato Salad Zesty Orange Oats Peach Crisp 1/2 cup nonfat milk 1/2 cup cooked squash 3 oz broiled beef	Skewered Chicken and Shrimp* Cold Pasta Salad* Carrots in Sherry Wine* 6 mixed nuts

*Indicates that the recipe has been used previously.

2000 calorie MEAL PLAN WINTER WEEK 4

	Sunday	Monday	Tuesday	Wednesday	Thursday	Friday	Saturday
Breakfast	2 whole-grain waffles 2 Tbsp sugar-free maple syrup 1 small orange 1 cup nonfat milk 1/4 egg substitute, scrambled 1 1/2 tsp margarine	1 whole-wheat English muffin 1/2 grapefruit 1 cup nonfat milk 1 oz lean turkey sausage 2 tsp margarine	**Zucchini Carrot Muffins*** 1 cup nonfat milk 1 oz Canadian bacon 1/2 tsp margarine	**Fruit Medley** 1/2 cup oatmeal 1 cup nonfat milk 1/4 cup egg substitute, scrambled 6 almonds	**Oatmeal and Apple Muffins*** 1 cup nonfat milk 1 egg, cooked as desired 1 tsp margarine	**Whole-Grain Muffins** (2)* 1 1/2 Tbsp fruit spread 1 cup nonfat milk 1 oz lean turkey sausage	**Fried Bananas*** 1/2 nonfat milk
Lunch	**Cashew Pork Hash Brown Potatoes** 1 dinner roll 1/2 cup peas 1/2 cup unsweetened applesauce	**Pita with Veggies** 2 oz baked tortilla chips 2 medium peaches 1/2 cup steamed broccoli and/or cauliflower 1 oz reduced-fat cheese 1 Tbsp sunflower seeds	**New Orleans Chilled Rice** **Raspberry Smoothie** 2 oz chicken breast 10 peanuts	**Veggie Melts** **Whole-Wheat Pasta Salad** 1 kiwi fruit 1/2 cup cooked mustard greens 1 oz reduced-fat cheese	**Asian Chicken Pitas** **Poppy Seed Fruit Salad** 3/4 cup cooked corn and peas 1 1/4 cups strawberries 1/2 cup cooked broccoli florets 20 peanuts	**Roast Beef and Swiss Roll-Up** (2) 3/4 oz pretzels 1 cup cantaloupe 1 cup mixed salad greens 1 tsp olive oil and vinegar dressing	**Barbecued Pork Sandwich*** **Oven-Roasted Tomatoes*** 1/2 ear corn on the cob 1 cup unsweetened plums 1 cup raw vegetable sticks 1 1/2 tsp margarine
Snack A	1 cup nonstarchy vegetables 1/2 cup light ice cream	1 cup raw vegetable sticks 5 hazelnuts 3/4 cup blueberries	1 cup mixed vegetable sticks 16 pistachios 1 medium peach	1 cup celery 4 walnuts 1 small apple	1 cup mixed vegetable sticks 4 pecans 4 apricots	1 cup green pepper slices 6 almonds 4 dried apple rings	1 cup raw carrots 6 almonds 3/4 cup blueberries
Snack B	1/2 oz breadsticks 1/2 Tbsp peanut butter 1 cup nonfat milk	3/4 oz sugar-free cookies 1 cup nonfat milk	3 small graham cracker squares 1 1/2 tsp almond butter 1 cup nonfat milk	3/4 oz pretzels 1 cup nonfat milk	3 graham cracker squares 1 cup nonfat milk	3 cup popcorn 1 tsp margarine 1 cup nonfat milk	3/4 cup shredded wheat 3 macadamia nuts 1 cup fat-free yogurt
Dinner	**Scallops Coquille** **Seasoned Chilled Vegetables*** 1/2 cup roasted red potatoes 1 slice whole-wheat bread 17 grapes 1 cup nonfat milk 1/2 cup green beans 1/2 tsp margarine	**Chicken Eggplant Stir-Fry** **Peach Cobbler** 12 cherries 1/2 cup nonfat milk 1 oz reduced-fat cheese 3 cashews	**Sweet Apple Pork Chops** **Fruit Salad Medley** 1/2 cup baked tater tots 1 cup steamed Brussels sprouts 1 oz reduced-fat cheese	**Baked Chicken Baja** 3 oz baked potato 1 slice multigrain bread 3/4 cup blackberries 1 cup nonfat milk 2 cups mixed salad vegetables 1/2 tsp olive oil and vinegar dressing	**Cod Teriyaki** **Carrot Slaw** **Low-Fat Corn Bread** 1/2 cup cooked green beans 1 tsp margarine	**Spinach-Orange Salad** **Potato Salad** **Zesty Orange Oats Peach Crisp** 1/2 cup nonfat milk 1/2 cup cooked squash 3 oz broiled beef	**Skewered Chicken and Shrimp*** **Cold Pasta Salad*** **Carrots in Sherry Wine*** 6 mixed nuts

*Indicates that the recipe has been used previously.

86   Week 4 ▨ WINTER

	Sunday	Monday	Tuesday	Wednesday	Thursday	Friday	Saturday
Breakfast	2 whole-grain waffles 2 Tbsp sugar-free maple syrup 1 small orange 1 cup nonfat milk 1/2 cup egg substitute, scrambled 1 1/2 tsp margarine	1 whole-wheat English muffin 1/2 grapefruit 1 cup nonfat milk 2 oz lean turkey sausage 2 tsp margarine	Zucchini Carrot Muffins* 1 cup nonfat milk 2 oz Canadian bacon 1/2 tsp margarine	Fruit Medley 1/2 cup oatmeal 1 cup nonfat milk 1/2 cup egg substitute, scrambled 6 almonds	Oatmeal and Apple Muffins* 1 cup nonfat milk 1 egg, cooked as desired 1 oz reduced-fat cheese 1 tsp margarine	Whole-Grain Muffins (2)* 1 1/2 Tbsp fruit spread 1 cup nonfat milk 2 oz lean turkey sausage	Fried Bananas* 1/2 nonfat milk 1 oz lean sausage
Lunch	Cashew Pork Hash Brown Potatoes 1 dinner roll 1/2 cup peas 1/2 cup unsweetened applesauce	Pita with Veggies 2 oz baked tortilla chips 2 medium peaches 1/2 cup steamed broccoli and/or cauliflower 1 oz reduced-fat cheese 1 Tbsp sunflower seeds	New Orleans Chilled Rice Raspberry Smoothie 2 oz chicken breast 10 peanuts	Veggie Melts Whole-Wheat Pasta Salad 1 kiwi fruit 1 cup cooked mustard greens 1 oz reduced-fat cheese	Asian Chicken Pitas Poppy Seed Fruit Salad 3/4 cup cooked corn and peas 1 1/4 cup strawberries 1/2 cup cooked broccoli florets 20 peanuts	Roast Beef and Swiss Roll-Up (2) 3/4 oz pretzels 1 cup cantaloupe 1 cup mixed salad greens 1 tsp olive oil and vinegar dressing	Barbecued Pork Sandwich* Oven-Roasted Tomatoes* 1/2 ear corn on the cob 1 cup unsweetened plums 1 cup raw vegetable sticks 1 1/2 tsp margarine
Snack A	1 cup nonstarchy vegetables 1/2 cup light ice cream	1 cup raw vegetable sticks 5 hazelnuts 3/4 cup blueberries	1 cup mixed vegetable sticks 16 pistachios 1 medium peach	1 cup celery 4 walnuts 1 small apple	1 cup mixed vegetable sticks 4 pecans 4 apricots	1 cup green pepper slices 6 almonds 4 dried apple rings	1 cup raw carrots 6 almonds 3/4 cup blueberries
Snack B	1/2 oz breadsticks 1/2 Tbsp peanut butter 1 cup nonfat milk	3/4 oz sugar-free cookies 1 cup nonfat milk	3 small graham cracker squares 1 1/2 tsp almond butter 1 cup nonfat milk	3/4 oz pretzels 1 cup nonfat milk	3 graham cracker squares 1 cup nonfat milk	3 cup popcorn 1 tsp margarine 1 cup nonfat milk	3/4 cup shredded wheat 3 macadamia nuts 1 cup fat-free yogurt
Dinner	Scallops Coquille Seasoned Chilled Vegetables* 1 cup roasted red potatoes 1 slice whole-wheat bread 17 grapes 1 cup nonfat milk 1/2 cup green beans 1/2 tsp margarine	Chicken Eggplant Stir-Fry Peach Cobbler 12 cherries 1/2 cup nonfat milk 1 oz reduced-fat cheese 3 cashews	Sweet Apple Pork Chops Fruit Salad Medley 1/2 cup baked tater tots 1 cup steamed Brussels sprouts 1 oz reduced-fat cheese	Baked Chicken Baja 6 oz baked potato 1 slice multigrain bread 3/4 cup blackberries 1 cup nonfat milk 2 cups mixed salad vegetables 1/2 tsp olive oil and vinegar dressing	Cod Teriyaki Carrot Slaw Low-Fat Corn Bread 1/2 cup unsweetened peaches 1/2 cup cooked green beans 1 tsp margarine	Spinach-Orange Salad Potato Salad Zesty Orange Oats Peach Crisp 1 Tbsp raisins 1 cup nonfat milk 1/2 cup cooked squash 3 oz broiled beef	Skewered Chicken and Shrimp* Cold Pasta Salad* Carrots in Sherry Wine* 1 cup nonfat milk 6 mixed nuts

*Indicates that the recipe has been used previously.

VEGETABLES

_____ bean sprouts
_____ bell peppers, red and yellow
_____ broccoli
_____ Brussels sprouts
_____ carrot sticks or baby carrots
_____ carrots
_____ cauliflower
_____ celery
_____ corn on the cob
_____ cucumber
_____ eggplant
_____ garlic
_____ green beans
_____ lettuce, romaine
_____ mushrooms
_____ mustard greens
_____ onions, green
_____ onions, red
_____ onions, yellow or white
_____ peaches
_____ peas
_____ potatoes
_____ potatoes, red
_____ shallots
_____ spinach
_____ squash, any kind with a crooked neck
_____ tomatoes
_____ zucchini

MEATS

_____ bacon, Canadian
_____ beef, lean cut (for broiling on Friday)
_____ chicken breasts, boneless, skinless
_____ cod, fresh or frozen
_____ pork chops, boneless, sirloin
_____ pork tenderloin
_____ roast beef, deli-style
_____ sausage, turkey, lean
_____ scallops
_____ shrimp

FRUITS

_____ apples
_____ bananas
_____ blackberries
_____ blueberries
_____ cantaloupe
_____ cherries
_____ grapefruit
_____ grapes, seedless
_____ kiwi fruit
_____ oranges
_____ pineapple, chunks and crushed, no-added-sugar
_____ plums
_____ raisins
_____ raspberries
_____ strawberries

DAIRY

_____ egg substitute
_____ eggs
_____ half and half, fat-free
_____ milk, nonfat
_____ Smart Balance Light Spread
_____ Smart Balance margarine
_____ sour cream, fat-free
_____ whipped topping, fat-free
_____ yogurt, lemon, fat-free
_____ yogurt, plain, fat-free

CHEESE

_____ any kind, reduced-fat
_____ cheddar, sharp, reduced-fat
_____ mozzarella, fat-free
_____ Swiss, reduced-fat

BREAD, GRAINS, & PASTA

_____ bread, whole-grain, whole-wheat
_____ dinner rolls, whole-wheat
_____ English muffins, whole-wheat
_____ hamburger buns, whole-wheat
_____ pasta, shells or elbows, whole-wheat
_____ pita breads, whole-grain, 6-inch
_____ rice, whole-grain

NUTS

____ almonds
____ cashews
____ peanuts, dry roasted
____ sunflower seeds
____ walnuts

CONDIMENTS

____ canola mayonnaise
____ horseradish
____ mustard, Dijon
____ mustard, prepared
____ soy sauce, light
____ Worcestershire sauce

SPICES & HERBS

____ allspice
____ basil
____ cilantro
____ cinnamon, ground
____ dill seeds
____ dill weed
____ garlic powder
____ ginger, ground
____ gingerroot
____ lemon juice
____ marjoram
____ mint
____ mustard, dry
____ nutmeg, ground
____ paprika
____ parsley
____ pepper
____ red pepper flakes
____ rosemary
____ thyme

OTHER

____ apple cider
____ applesauce, unsweetened
____ biscuit mix
____ dill pickle
____ fruit spread
____ maple syrup, sugar-free
____ orange juice
____ poppy seeds
____ pretzels
____ salad dressing, Italian, light
____ tater tots, baked
____ tomato sauce, no-added-salt
____ tortilla chips, baked
____ tortillas, corn, 6-inch
____ waffles, whole-grain
____ water chestnuts

STAPLES

____ baking powder
____ bouillon, beef, sodium-free
____ bouillon, chicken, sodium-free
____ cornmeal
____ cornstarch
____ honey
____ lime juice
____ nonstick cooking spray
____ oats, old-fashioned
____ olive oil
____ sesame oil
____ sherry, dry cooking
____ Smart Balance Omega oil
____ Splenda
____ Splenda Brown Sugar Blend
____ vanilla extract
____ vinegar, apple cider
____ vinegar, malt
____ vinegar, rice
____ vinegar, rice wine
____ vinegar, tarragon
____ vinegar, white
____ white wine
____ whole-wheat flour

Cashew Pork

Serves 4   Serving size: 1/4 recipe

2 **tsp** Smart Balance Omega oil

3/4 **lb** boneless sirloin pork chops (trimmed of visible fat)

1/4 **cup** cashews, unsalted

1 garlic clove, minced

1/2 **tsp** grated gingerroot

1/2 **cup** red pepper, diced

1 **Tbsp** sodium-free chicken bouillon

1 **cup** water

1 **Tbsp** snipped parsley

Heat 1 tsp oil in a skillet. Over medium heat, cook pork chops for 6 minutes. Turn over and cook 7–9 minutes more or until desired doneness (slightly pink in center). Remove meat from skillet; keep warm. Using a food processor or blender, process or blend cashews until coarsely ground; set aside. Add remaining oil to hot skillet. Add garlic, ginger root, and red pepper. Cook and stir, about 15 seconds; stir in ground cashews. In a separate bowl, mix together bouillon and water to form a broth; slowly add to skillet, stirring until well blended. Stir in parsley. Serve sauce over pork. Sprinkle remaining cashews on each serving.

Exchanges/Choices
2 Lean Meat
1 1/2 Fat

Basic Nutritional Values
Calories 160
  Calories from Fat 70
Total Fat. . . . . 8.0 g
  Saturated Fat . . . . 1.3 g
  Trans Fat. . . . . 0.0 g
Cholesterol. . . . . 40 mg
Sodium. . . . . 210 mg
Total Carbohydrate . . . 5 g
  Dietary Fiber . . . . 0 g
  Sugars . . . . 1 g
Protein . . . . 16 g

Hash Brown Potatoes

Serves 4   Serving size: 1/4 recipe

1 **lb** baking potato, peeled and quartered

2 medium onions

2 **Tbsp** Smart Balance margarine

Pepper, to taste

In a medium saucepan over medium heat, boil potatoes in boiling water until tender. While the potatoes are cooking, brown the onions in a frying pan with half the margarine. Chop potatoes until almost mashed. Place potatoes with the onions in the frying pan. Pat down top evenly; dot with remaining margarine and sprinkle with pepper to taste. Cover; cook over low heat until bottom is browned. Move potatoes frequently to keep them from burning.

Exchanges/Choices
1 Starch
2 Vegetable
1/2 Fat

Basic Nutritional Values
Calories 145
  Calories from Fat 40
Total Fat. . . . . 4.5 g
  Saturated Fat . . . . 1.3 g
  Trans Fat. . . . . 0.0 g
Cholesterol. . . . . 0 mg
Sodium. . . . . 50 mg
Total Carbohydrate . . . 25 g
  Dietary Fiber . . . . 3 g
  Sugars . . . . 5 g
Protein . . . . 2 g

Scallops Coquille

Serves 4   Serving size: 1/4 recipe

2 **tsp** Smart Balance margarine

1 **Tbsp** chopped onion

1 **lb** scallops

1 **cup** sliced mushrooms

1/3 **cup** white wine

1 1/2 **tsp** lemon juice

Dash dried marjoram

Dash paprika

1 1/2 **Tbsp** Smart Balance Light Spread

2 **Tbsp** whole-wheat flour

1/2 **cup** fat-free half and half

1 **Tbsp** snipped parsley

Exchanges/Choices

1/2 Carbohydrate
3 Lean Meat

Basic Nutritional Values

Calories 170
　Calories from Fat 45
Total Fat. . . . . .5.0 g
　Saturated Fat . . . . .1.4 g
　Trans Fat. . . . . .0.0 g
Cholesterol. . . . . .45 mg
Sodium. . . . . .305 mg
Total Carbohydrate. . .7 g
　Dietary Fiber . . . . .1 g
　Sugars . . . . .2 g
Protein. . . . . .22 g

1. Combine margarine and onion in a 1 1/2-quart casserole. Microwave at high power for 1 minute.

2. Drain scallops and reserve liquid. Stir the following into the margarine and onions: scallops, mushrooms, wine, lemon juice, marjoram, and paprika. Microwave, covered, at high for 3 minutes. Drain and reserve liquid.

3. Place Smart Balance Light Spread in a small bowl. Microwave at high power until melted, about 30–60 seconds. Blend in whole-wheat flour. Stir in 1/2 cup reserved scallop liquid, half and half, and parsley. Microwave at medium-high (70%) until thickened, 3–5 minutes, stirring once. Stir sauce into scallops. Spoon scallop mixture into 4 small bowls. Microwave at medium-high until heated through, 2–3 minutes.

Seasoned Chilled Vegetables

Serves 4   Serving size: 1/4 recipe

1/2 **cup** carrots, thinly sliced

1/2 **cup** cauliflower florets

1/2 **cup** zucchini, quartered and thickly sliced

1 **Tbsp** sodium-free chicken bouillon

1/2 **cup** water

1/4 **cup** sliced celery

1/4 **cup** white vinegar

2 **Tbsp** red onions, coarsely chopped

2 **Tbsp** Smart Balance Omega oil

1 **tsp** Splenda

1 **tsp** prepared mustard

1/2 **tsp** dill seeds

1/2 **tsp** dried rosemary, crushed

1/2 **tsp** dried thyme, crushed

1/2 **tsp** black pepper

Exchanges/Choices

1 Vegetable
1 1/2 Fat

Basic Nutritional Values

Calories 85
  Calories from Fat 65
Total Fat . . . . 7.0 g
  Saturated Fat . . . . 0.5 g
  Trans Fat . . . . 0.0 g
Cholesterol . . . . 0 mg
Sodium . . . . 40 mg
Total Carbohydrate . . . 6 g
  Dietary Fiber . . . . 1 g
  Sugars . . . . 3 g
Protein . . . . 1 g

Place all ingredients in a 3-quart saucepan. Bring to a boil; reduce heat to low, cover, and simmer for 10 minutes or until vegetables are crisp-tender. Pour into a bowl and chill for 2 hours or until cold. Serve.

Pita with Veggies

Serves 4   Serving size: 1 sandwich

2 oz shredded fat-free
   mozzarella cheese

1 1/2 oz shredded reduced-fat
   sharp cheddar cheese

1/2 cup thinly sliced cauliflower

1/4 cup canola mayonnaise
   or low-fat salad dressing

1 tsp snipped dill weed
   (or 1/2 tsp dried)

1 medium tomato, chopped

1 small zucchini or carrot,
   shredded

2 (6-inch) pita breads,
   cut into halves

2 cups salad greens

Exchanges/Choices

1 Starch
1 Vegetable
1 Lean Meat
1 Fat

Basic Nutritional Values

Calories 195
   Calories from Fat 65
Total Fat . . . . 7.0 g
   Saturated Fat . . . . 1.4 g
   Trans Fat . . . . 0.0 g
Cholesterol . . . . 10 mg
Sodium . . . . 520 mg
Total Carbohydrate . . . 22 g
   Dietary Fiber . . . . 2 g
   Sugars . . . . 3 g
Protein . . . . 11 g

Mix all ingredients except pita breads and salad greens. Separate pita breads
along cut sides to form pockets. Arrange salad greens and vegetable mixture
in pockets.

Chicken Eggplant Stir-Fry

Serves 4　　　Serving size: 1/4 recipe

1/4 **cup** basil, coarsely chopped

2 **Tbsp** mint, chopped

3 green onions, coarsely chopped

2 cloves garlic, crushed

1 **tsp** ginger, ground

1/2 **cup** water

1 **Tbsp** sodium-free chicken bouillon

2 **Tbsp** Smart Balance Omega oil

1 small eggplant, pared (if desired)

1 yellow onion, coarsely chopped

1 red bell pepper, seeded and sliced

1 yellow bell pepper, seeded and sliced

3/4 **lb** boneless, skinless chicken breast, cut into 1/2-inch wide strips

Exchanges/Choices

4 Vegetable
2 Lean Meat
1 Fat

Basic Nutritional Values

Calories 240
　Calories from Fat 90
Total Fat. . . . . 10.0 g
　Saturated Fat . . . . 1.2 g
　Trans Fat. . . . . 0.0 g
Cholesterol. . . . . 50 mg
Sodium. . . . . 50 mg
Total Carbohydrate. . . 20 g
　Dietary Fiber. . . . . 5 g
　Sugars . . . . 8 g
Protein. . . . . 20 g

1. In a blender, blend the basil, mint, green onions, garlic, ginger, water, and chicken bouillon until minced but not pureed.

2. Place a nonstick frying pan over medium heat and add 1 Tbsp oil. Add the eggplant, onion, and bell peppers; sauté until vegetables are just tender, about 8 minutes. Remove the vegetables.

3. Add the remaining 1 Tbsp oil to the pan. Sauté chicken, about 3 minutes or until thoroughly cooked. Return the vegetables to the pan and stir until heated through, about 3 more minutes.

Peach Cobbler

Serves 4   Serving size: 1/4 recipe

Nonstick cooking spray

1/2 **cup** Splenda

1 **Tbsp** cornstarch

2 **cups** sliced peaches

2 **Tbsp** water

1 **cup** biscuit mix

1/4 **cup** nonfat milk

Exchanges/Choices

2 1/2 Carbohydrate
1/2 Fat

Basic Nutritional Values

Calories 200
 Calories from Fat 35
Total Fat. . . . . .4.0 g
 Saturated Fat . . . . .1.2 g
 Trans Fat. . . . . .1.2 g
Cholesterol. . . . . .0 mg
Sodium. . . . . .410 mg
Total Carbohydrate. . .35 g
 Dietary Fiber. . . . . .2 g
 Sugars . . . . .12 g
Protein. . . . . .5 g

Preheat oven to 425°F. Spray a round casserole dish with nonstick cooking spray. Mix 1/2 cup Splenda and cornstarch in a saucepan; stir in peaches and water. Heat to boiling, stirring constantly. Boil and stir 1 minute. Pour mixture into casserole dish. Mix biscuit mix according to package directions and drop dough by spoonfuls onto the hot peach mixture. Bake until golden brown, about 20 minutes. Serve with nonfat milk.

Zucchini Carrot Muffins

Serves 8   Serving size: 1 muffin

3/4 **cup** rolled oats	2 **tsp** ground nutmeg
2 1/2 **cups** whole-wheat flour	3 **Tbsp** Smart Balance Omega oil
2/3 **cup** nonfat milk	3 egg whites, beaten
1/2 **cup** wheat germ, toasted	1 **cup** carrots, finely shredded
3 **tsp** baking powder	1/2 **cup** zucchini, stemmed and grated
3/4 **cup** Splenda	
1 **Tbsp** ground cinnamon	

Preheat oven to 350°F. Combine all ingredients and mix well; pour into muffin liners in muffin pans. Bake for about 1 hour. Let cool for about 30 minutes before removing.

Exchanges/Choices

2 1/2 Carbohydrate
1 1/2 Fat

Basic Nutritional Values

Calories 260
 Calories from Fat 65
Total Fat . . . . 7.0 g
 Saturated Fat . . . . 0.9 g
 Trans Fat . . . . 0.0 g
Cholesterol . . . . 0 mg
Sodium . . . . 180 mg
Total Carbohydrate . . . 42 g
 Dietary Fiber . . . . 7 g
 Sugars . . . . 5 g
Protein . . . . 11 g

New Orleans Chilled Rice

Serves 4   Serving size: 1/4 recipe

3/4 **cups** whole-grain rice	1/2 **cup** shallots, chopped
1 **Tbsp** Smart Balance Omega oil	1/2 medium red pepper, chopped
1/2 **cup** chopped dill pickle	1/4 **cup** canola mayonnaise
1/2 **cup** celery, diced	1/4 **cup** fat-free plain yogurt
1/2 **cup** onion	1/2 **Tbsp** vinegar

Cook rice according to package directions. In a large bowl, combine all other ingredients with the cooked rice; chill before serving.

Exchanges/Choices

2 Starch
2 Vegetable
1 Fat

Basic Nutritional Values

Calories 255
 Calories from Fat 70
Total Fat . . . . 8.0 g
 Saturated Fat . . . . 0.4 g
 Trans Fat . . . . 0.0 g
Cholesterol . . . . 0 mg
Sodium . . . . 345 mg
Total Carbohydrate . . . 39 g
 Dietary Fiber . . . . 2 g
 Sugars . . . . 5 g
Protein . . . . 5 g

Raspberry Smoothie
Serves 4   Serving size: 1/4 recipe

8	**oz** fat-free lemon yogurt	**2**	**cups** raspberries
1	**cups** fat-free whipped topping	**4**	ice cubes

Combine ingredients in a blender; cover and process until smooth.

Exchanges/Choices
1 Carbohydrate

Basic Nutritional Values
Calories 85
  Calories from Fat 0
Total Fat . . . . 0.0 g
  Saturated Fat . . . . 0.0 g
  Trans Fat . . . . 0.0 g
Cholesterol . . . . 0 mg
Sodium . . . . 30 mg
Total Carbohydrate . . . 18 g
  Dietary Fiber . . . . 4 g
  Sugars . . . . 9 g
Protein . . . . 2 g

Sweet Apple Pork Chops
Serves 4   Serving size: 1/4 recipe

1 1/2	**cups** apple cider	**1/4**	**tsp** pepper
1/4	**cup** lemon juice	**1**	**tsp** cinnamon
2	**Tbsp** light soy sauce	**3/4**	**lb** boneless sirloin pork chops (trimmed of visible fat)
2	**Tbsp** honey		
1	clove garlic, minced		

1. Combine all ingredients except pork; mix well. Place pork in shallow dish; pour marinade over pork. Cover and refrigerate 6–24 hours.

2. Prepare a covered grill with drip pan in the center, banked by medium-hot coals. Grill chops for 20–25 minutes, turning once and basting occasionally with marinade.

Exchanges/Choices
1 Carbohydrate
2 Lean Meat

Basic Nutritional Values
Calories 150
  Calories from Fat 20
Total Fat . . . . 2.0 g
  Saturated Fat . . . . 0.3 g
  Trans Fat . . . . 0.0 g
Cholesterol . . . . 40 mg
Sodium . . . . 420 mg
Total Carbohydrate . . . 17 g
  Dietary Fiber . . . . 0 g
  Sugars . . . . 15 g
Protein . . . . 15 g

Fruit Salad Medley

Serves 4   Serving size: 1/4 recipe

1/2 **cup** strawberries, sliced

1/4 **cup** Splenda

1/2 **cup** blueberries
(or canned light)

1 banana, sliced

3 **tsp** lemon juice

2 oranges, peeled and sliced
crosswise

1/2 **cup** blackberries
(or canned light)

1/2 **cup** pineapple (fresh, frozen,
or canned light chunks)

1/2 **cup** orange juice
Sprig mint leaves

Exchanges/Choices

2 Fruit

Basic Nutritional Values

Calories 120
   Calories from Fat 5
Total Fat . . . . 0.5 g
   Saturated Fat . . . . 0.1 g
   Trans Fat . . . . 0.0 g
Cholesterol . . . . 0 mg
Sodium . . . . 0 mg
Total Carbohydrate . . . 29 g
   Dietary Fiber . . . . 5 g
   Sugars . . . . 21 g
Protein . . . . 2 g

In a medium bowl, stir together half of the strawberries and half of the Splenda; set aside. In a 2-quart serving bowl, add blueberries and layer bananas on top; sprinkle with lemon juice. Add a layer of strawberries with remaining Splenda, then oranges and blackberries. Arrange pineapple tidbits around outer edge. Layer remaining strawberry slices around pineapple tidbits. Pour orange juice over all the fruit. Cover and chill for 1 hour. Just before serving, top with mint leaves.

Fruit Medley

Serves 4   Serving size: 1/4 recipe

1 medium banana

1 **cup** seedless grapes

1 orange, peeled and sectioned

1 grapefruit, peeled and sectioned

1 **cup** canned light pineapple, juice reserved

Combine all ingredients and chill 30 minutes before serving. Be sure to cover the banana with the pineapple juice to keep it fresh.

Exchanges/Choices

2 Fruit

Basic Nutritional Values

Calories	130
Calories from Fat	5
Total Fat	0.5 g
Saturated Fat	0.1 g
Trans Fat	0.0 g
Cholesterol	0 mg
Sodium	0 mg
Total Carbohydrate	33 g
Dietary Fiber	3 g
Sugars	25 g
Protein	2 g

Veggie Melts

Serves 4   Serving size: 1 melt

1/4 **cup** cucumber, thinly sliced

1/2 **cup** shredded carrot

2 **Tbsp** green onions, sliced

2 **Tbsp** light Italian dressing

1/2 **cup** fat-free shredded mozzarella cheese

2 English muffins, split and toasted

Preheat broiler. Combine cucumber, carrot, green onions, and dressing; set aside. Sprinkle cheese evenly over muffin halves. Broil 1 minute or until cheese melts. Top muffin halves evenly with cucumber mixture. Serve immediately.

Exchanges/Choices

1 Starch
1 Lean Meat

Basic Nutritional Values

Calories	105
Calories from Fat	10
Total Fat	1.0 g
Saturated Fat	0.1 g
Trans Fat	0.0 g
Cholesterol	5 mg
Sodium	400 mg
Total Carbohydrate	17 g
Dietary Fiber	1 g
Sugars	3 g
Protein	7 g

Whole-Wheat Pasta Salad

Serves 4   Serving size: 1/4 recipe

8 oz whole-wheat pasta, shells or elbows

1/2 cup canola mayonnaise

1/2 cup celery, diced

1/2 cup onion, diced

2 Tbsp Dijon mustard

1 tsp dill weed

1/2 tsp marjoram

1/4 tsp black pepper

Cook pasta according to package directions. Drain. In a medium bowl, stir together all of the remaining ingredients until well blended. Stir in cooked pasta; gently toss until well coated. Cover and chill at least 2 hours before serving.

Exchanges/Choices

3 Starch
1 1/2 Fat

Basic Nutritional Values

Calories 305
  Calories from Fat 90
Total Fat. . . . . 10.0 g
  Saturated Fat . . . . 0.2 g
  Trans Fat. . . . . 0.0 g
Cholesterol. . . . . 0 mg
Sodium. . . . . 380 mg
Total Carbohydrate. . . 46 g
  Dietary Fiber . . . . 5 g
  Sugars . . . . 4 g
Protein. . . . . 9 g

Baked Chicken Baja

Serves 4   Serving size: 1/4 recipe

1 lb boneless, skinless chicken breast halves

1/4 tsp pepper

2 garlic cloves, minced

2 Tbsp Smart Balance Omega oil

4 Tbsp tarragon vinegar

3/4 cup dry sherry

Sprinkle chicken with pepper. In large frying pan over medium heat, crush garlic into oil. Stir in vinegar; add chicken and sauté, turning frequently, until golden brown, about 10 minutes. Remove chicken to baking dish; add sherry and place in 350°F oven for 10 minutes.

Exchanges/Choices

3 Lean Meat
1 1/2 Fat

Basic Nutritional Values

Calories 220
  Calories from Fat 90
Total Fat. . . . . 10.0 g
  Saturated Fat . . . . 1.3 g
  Trans Fat. . . . . 0.0 g
Cholesterol. . . . . 65 mg
Sodium. . . . . 60 mg
Total Carbohydrate. . . 4 g
  Dietary Fiber . . . . 0 g
  Sugars . . . . 2 g
Protein. . . . . 24 g

Oatmeal and Apple Muffins
Serves 8   Serving size: 1 muffin

1/4 **cup** egg substitute

2/3 **cup** whole-wheat flour

2 **tsp** baking powder

2 **tsp** cinnamon

1 **tsp** nutmeg

1/2 **cup** nonfat milk

1 **cup** raisins

1 apple, peeled, cored, and chopped

1/4 **cup** natural unsweetened applesauce

2/3 **cup** rolled oats

4 **Tbsp** Splenda Brown Sugar Blend

Preheat oven to 400°F. Beat egg substitute. Sift together flour, baking powder, cinnamon, and nutmeg. Combine all ingredients, mixing just to moisten. Spoon batter into muffin cups until 3/4 full. Bake for 15–20 minutes.

Exchanges/Choices

3 Carbohydrate

Basic Nutritional Values

Calories	190
Calories from Fat	10
Total Fat	1.0 g
Saturated Fat	0.2 g
Trans Fat	0.0 g
Cholesterol	0 mg
Sodium	120 mg
Total Carbohydrate	44 g
Dietary Fiber	3 g
Sugars	28 g
Protein	4 g

Asian Chicken Pitas
Serves 4   Serving size: 1 pita

1/2 **lb** boneless, skinless chicken breasts

1/2 **cup** bean sprouts

1/4 **cup** diced water chestnuts

1/4 **cup** sliced green onions

1 **Tbsp** rice vinegar

1 **Tbsp** light soy sauce

1 **tsp** sesame oil

2 (6- or 7-inch) whole-wheat pitas, cut in half crosswise

2 lettuce leaves

1. Place chicken in a medium saucepan; add water until the chicken in covered. Bring to a boil. Reduce heat to medium and cook, uncovered, for 15 minutes or until chicken is done. Drain. Let sit until chicken is cool to the touch. Chop chicken into bite-size pieces. Combine chicken, bean sprouts, water chestnuts, and green onions.

2. In a separate bowl, combine the vinegar, soy sauce, and oil; pour over chicken, tossing gently. Line each pita with half a lettuce leaf; spoon chicken mixture evenly into pita halves.

Exchanges/Choices

1 Starch
1 Vegetable
2 Lean Meat

Basic Nutritional Values

Calories	180
Calories from Fat	30
Total Fat	3.5 g
Saturated Fat	0.7 g
Trans Fat	0.0 g
Cholesterol	35 mg
Sodium	345 mg
Total Carbohydrate	22 g
Dietary Fiber	3 g
Sugars	2 g
Protein	16 g

Poppy Seed Fruit Salad

Serves 4   Serving size: 1/4 recipe

2 large oranges

1 1/2 **cup** cantaloupe cubes

1 **cup** fat-free yogurt
(any flavor)

1/2 **tsp** poppy seeds

4 mint sprigs (for garnish)

Cut each orange in half; then remove the flesh of the orange from each of the halves, taking care not to damage them. Dice the orange pulp. Retain the empty orange peels (they should look like little bowls). Remove the skin and seeds from the cantaloupe; dice into very small pieces. Place diced oranges and cantaloupe into the orange peel bowls, letting any extra spill over onto the plate. In a small bowl, whisk together the yogurt and poppy seeds; then pour over the fruit. Top each orange peel bowl with a sprig of mint.

Exchanges/Choices

1 Fruit
1/2 Fat-Free Milk

Basic Nutritional Values

Calories 105
  Calories from Fat 0
Total Fat . . . . 0.0 g
  Saturated Fat . . . . 0.1 g
  Trans Fat . . . . 0.0 g
Cholesterol . . . . 0 mg
Sodium . . . . 35 mg
Total Carbohydrate . . . 23 g
  Dietary Fiber . . . . 3 g
  Sugars . . . . 18 g
Protein . . . . 3 g

Cod Teriyaki

Serves 4   Serving size: 1/4 recipe

2 **Tbsp** light soy sauce

1/4 **cup** dry cooking sherry

2 **Tbsp** Splenda

1/2 **Tbsp** ginger, ground

1/8 **tsp** garlic powder

1/2 **cup** water

1 **lb** cod, fresh or frozen

Combine all ingredients, except fish, in an 8 × 8-inch baking dish. Stir until blended. Add fish, coating both sides. Cover; refrigerate 1 hour. Place fish fillets on a roasting rack. Microwave at high power (100%) until fish flakes easily in the center with a fork, 5–7 minutes. Rotate baking dish a half-turn after half the cooking time.

Exchanges/Choices

3 Lean Meat

Basic Nutritional Values

Calories 105
  Calories from Fat 10
Total Fat . . . . 1.0 g
  Saturated Fat . . . . 0.2 g
  Trans Fat . . . . 0.0 g
Cholesterol . . . . 50 mg
Sodium . . . . 205 mg
Total Carbohydrate . . . 1 g
  Dietary Fiber . . . . 0 g
  Sugars . . . . 1 g
Protein . . . . 20 g

Carrot Slaw

Serves 4   Serving size: 1/4 recipe

1/2 **cup** crushed pineapple
(or can of no-added-sugar
crushed pineapple)

1 **tsp** honey

1 **tsp** lemon juice

1/4 **tsp** nutmeg

1/2 **cup** fat-free sour cream

2 cups carrot, grated

Exchanges/Choices

1/2 Carbohydrate
1 Vegetable

Basic Nutritional Values

Calories 65
  Calories from Fat 0
Total Fat . . . . 0.0 g
  Saturated Fat . . . . 0.1 g
  Trans Fat . . . . 0.0 g
Cholesterol . . . . 5 mg
Sodium . . . . 55 mg
Total Carbohydrate . . . 11 g
  Dietary Fiber . . . . 2 g
  Sugars . . . . 8 g
Protein . . . . 3 g

Drain pineapple. In a medium bowl, mix honey, lemon juice, and nutmeg. Blend in sour cream. Add carrots and pineapple. Serve chilled.

Low-Fat Corn Bread

Serves 8   Serving size: 1/8 recipe

1/2 **cup** egg substitute

1/2 **cup** Splenda

3/4 **cup** nonfat milk

1/2 **cup** unsweetened applesauce

1 1/2 **cup** whole-wheat flour

2/3 **cup** cornmeal

1 **Tbsp** baking powder

Nonstick cooking spray

Exchanges/Choices

2 Starch

Basic Nutritional Values

Calories 150
  Calories from Fat 5
Total Fat . . . . 0.5 g
  Saturated Fat . . . . 0.1 g
  Trans Fat . . . . 0.0 g
Cholesterol . . . . 0 mg
Sodium . . . . 180 mg
Total Carbohydrate . . . 30 g
  Dietary Fiber . . . . 4 g
  Sugars . . . . 4 g
Protein . . . . 6 g

Beat together the egg substitute, Splenda, milk, and applesauce; set aside. In a separate bowl, sift and combine flour, cornmeal, and baking powder. Stir into egg mixture using as few strokes as possible. Spray an 8 × 8-inch baking pan with nonstick cooking spray. Bake at 400°F for 25–30 minutes or until a toothpick inserted near the middle comes out clean.

Whole-Grain Muffins
Serves 8   Serving size: 1 muffin

Nonstick cooking spray

3/4 **cup** whole-wheat flour

2 **tsp** baking powder

1 1/2 **Tbsp** Splenda

2/3 **cup** rolled oats cereal

1 **cup** nonfat milk

1/4 **cup** egg substitute

1/4 **cup** unsweetened applesauce

1. Lightly spray muffin pan cups with nonstick cooking spray; set aside.

2. Stir together the flour, baking powder, and Splenda; set aside.

3. Combine rolled oats and milk in a large mixing bowl; let stand until oats are softened, about 1–2 minutes. Add egg substitute and applesauce; beat well. Add whole-wheat flour mixture; gently stir to combine. Divide batter evenly among prepared muffin cups. Bake at 400°F for 25 minutes or until lightly browned.

Exchanges/Choices

1 Carbohydrate

Basic Nutritional Values

Calories 85
  Calories from Fat 5
Total Fat. . . . . 0.5 g
  Saturated Fat . . . . 0.1 g
  Trans Fat. . . . . 0.0 g
Cholesterol. . . . . 0 mg
Sodium. . . . . 120 mg
Total Carbohydrate. . . 16 g
  Dietary Fiber. . . . . 2 g
  Sugars . . . . 3 g
Protein. . . . . 5 g

Roast Beef and Swiss Roll-Up
Serves 4   Serving size: 3 roll-ups

1/2 **lb** deli-style roast beef

3 slices reduced-fat Swiss cheese

12 romaine lettuce leaves

2 small tomatoes, diced

12 (6-inch) corn tortillas

4 **Tbsp** horseradish (optional)

Place the tortillas on a flat surface and divide the roast beef evenly between the 12 tortillas. Cut the cheese into 12 slices and place one on each tortilla, followed by a lettuce leaf and some tomato. If desired, add horseradish. Roll up the tortillas and serve. If desired, warm roll-ups in the oven before serving.

Exchanges/Choices

2 Starch
1 Vegetable
2 Lean Meat
1/2 Fat

Basic Nutritional Values

Calories 305
  Calories from Fat 55
Total Fat. . . . . 6.0 g
  Saturated Fat . . . . 2.3 g
  Trans Fat. . . . . 0.0 g
Cholesterol. . . . . 40 mg
Sodium. . . . . 325 mg
Total Carbohydrate. . . 39 g
  Dietary Fiber. . . . . 5 g
  Sugars . . . . 4 g
Protein. . . . . 23 g

Spinach-Orange Salad

Serves 4   Serving size: 1/4 recipe

- 4 **cups** spinach, torn into pieces
- 2 medium oranges, peeled and sectioned, juice reserved (about 1/4 cup)
- 2/3 **cup** mushrooms, sliced
- 1/2 **cup** red onion, sliced
- 2 **Tbsp** Smart Balance Omega oil
- 2 **Tbsp** malt vinegar
- 1/2 **tsp** ginger, ground
- 1/4 **tsp** pepper

Place spinach in a bowl. Add orange sections, mushrooms, and onion. Toss lightly to mix. In a separate bowl, mix oil, vinegar, orange juice, ginger, and pepper. Pour over spinach. Toss to mix and chill; serve.

Exchanges/Choices

1/2 Fruit
1 Vegetable
1 1/2 Fat

Basic Nutritional Values

Calories 115
  Calories from Fat 65
Total Fat. . . . . .7.0 g
  Saturated Fat . . . . .0.5 g
  Trans Fat. . . . . .0.0 g
Cholesterol. . . . . .0 mg
Sodium. . . . . .25 mg
Total Carbohydrate . . .13 g
  Dietary Fiber. . . . . .3 g
  Sugars . . . . .8 g
Protein. . . . . .2 g

Potato Salad

Serves 4   Serving size: 1/4 recipe

- 2 **cups** potatoes, peeled, boiled, and cubed
- 1/4 **cup** onion, chopped and diced
- 1/4 **cup** light Italian salad dressing
- 1/2 **cup** canola mayonnaise
- 2 eggs, hard boiled and chopped

Wash and peel potatoes. Cook potatoes in boiling water for about 30 minutes. Drain and slice into small cubes. In a large bowl, combine the potatoes with all other ingredients and mix well. Serve chilled.

Exchanges/Choices

1 1/2 Starch
2 Fat

Basic Nutritional Values

Calories 215
  Calories from Fat 115
Total Fat. . . . . .13.0 g
  Saturated Fat . . . . .0.9 g
  Trans Fat. . . . . .0.0 g
Cholesterol. . . . . .105 mg
Sodium. . . . . .395 mg
Total Carbohydrate . . .20 g
  Dietary Fiber. . . . . .2 g
  Sugars . . . . .5 g
Protein. . . . . .5 g

Zesty Orange Oats Peach Crisp

Serves 9   Serving size: 1/9 recipe

Nonstick cooking spray

4 Tbsp Splenda

1 1/2 Tbsp whole-wheat flour

1 tsp ground ginger

1 tsp pure vanilla extract

6 cups fresh peach chunks

1 cup old-fashioned oats, uncooked

1/2 cup chopped walnuts

Dash allspice

Dash cinnamon

2 Tbsp Smart Balance margarine

1 small orange, peeled and chopped

1. Spray a 9-inch glass baking dish with nonstick cooking spray. Combine 2 Tbsp Splenda, flour, ginger, and vanilla until mixed well. Fold in peaches until evenly coated. Spoon peaches into prepared glass baking dish.

2. Combine oats, walnuts, allspice, cinnamon, 2 Tbsp Splenda, margarine, and orange; blend well. Sprinkle evenly over peach filling. Bake at 350°F for 35–40 minutes (or until golden brown and the filling is bubbly).

Exchanges/Choices

1 1/2 Carbohydrate
1 Fat

Basic Nutritional Values

Calories 150
  Calories from Fat 65
Total Fat . . . . .7.0 g
  Saturated Fat . . . . .1.1 g
  Trans Fat . . . . .0.0 g
Cholesterol . . . . .0 mg
Sodium . . . . .20 mg
Total Carbohydrate . . .20 g
  Dietary Fiber . . . . .3 g
  Sugars . . . . .10 g
Protein . . . . .4 g

Fried Bananas

Serves 4   Serving size: 1 banana

4 small bananas (or plantains)	1/4 **cup** whole-wheat flour
1/4 **cup** nonfat milk	1/4 **cup** Smart Balance Omega oil (for frying)
1/4 **cup** egg substitute	
1 **Tbsp** Splenda	

Peel the bananas and cut diagonally into half-inch-thick slices. Mix milk, egg substitute, Splenda, and flour until smooth. Heat oil in large skillet over medium heat. Dip each banana slice into batter and then drop into oil. Fry until browned, about 2 minutes on each side. Drain on paper towels. Serve warm or at room temperature.

Exchanges/Choices

1/2 Starch
1 1/2 Fruit
1 1/2 Fat

Basic Nutritional Values

Calories 190
  Calories from Fat 65
Total Fat . . . . 7.0 g
  Saturated Fat . . . . 0.6 g
  Trans Fat . . . . 0.0 g
Cholesterol . . . . 0 mg
Sodium . . . . 40 mg
Total Carbohydrate . . . 30 g
  Dietary Fiber . . . . 4 g
  Sugars . . . . 14 g
Protein . . . . 4 g

Barbecued Pork Sandwich

Serves 4   Serving size: 1 sandwich

3/4 **lb** pork tenderloin, trimmed of all visible fat	2 **Tbsp** water
1 **tsp** Smart Balance Omega oil	2 **Tbsp** apple cider vinegar
1/2 **cup** no-salt-added tomato sauce	2 **Tbsp** Worcestershire sauce
1 1/2 **Tbsp** Splenda	1/4 **tsp** dry mustard
	4 whole-wheat hamburger buns

Cut pork into thin slices and flatten, using a meat mallet or rolling pin. Heat oil in a large nonstick skillet over medium-high heat. Add pork; cook 3 minutes on each side until browned. Drain and coarsely chop. Wipe drippings from pan; add all other ingredients. Bring to a boil; add pork. Cover, reduce heat, and simmer 20 minutes, stirring often. Spoon 3/4 of the pork mixture onto each bun.

Exchanges/Choices

2 Starch
2 Lean Meat

Basic Nutritional Values

Calories 235
  Calories from Fat 45
Total Fat . . . . 5.0 g
  Saturated Fat . . . . 1.2 g
  Trans Fat . . . . 0.0 g
Cholesterol . . . . 45 mg
Sodium . . . . 345 mg
Total Carbohydrate . . . 26 g
  Dietary Fiber . . . . 4 g
  Sugars . . . . 7 g
Protein . . . . 20 g

Oven-Roasted Tomatoes

Serves 6   Serving size: 1 tomato

1 Tbsp Smart Balance Omega oil

6 medium tomatoes, sliced crosswise, 1/2- to 3/4-inch thick

2 Tbsp Splenda

Dash pepper

Preheat oven to 300°F. Line a baking sheet with aluminum foil; rub with oil. Arrange tomato slices in a single layer on the baking sheet. Sprinkle with Splenda and pepper. Roast until the tomatoes shrivel, the edges start to turn brown, and most of the liquid around the tomatoes has caramelized, about 1 hour. Roasted tomatoes will keep for 4–5 days in the refrigerator.

Exchanges/Choices

1 Vegetable
1/2 Fat

Basic Nutritional Values

Calories 45
  Calories from Fat 20
Total Fat . . . . 2.5 g
  Saturated Fat . . . . 0.2 g
  Trans Fat . . . . 0.0 g
Cholesterol . . . . 0 mg
Sodium . . . . 5 mg
Total Carbohydrate . . . 5 g
  Dietary Fiber . . . . 1 g
  Sugars . . . . 4 g
Protein . . . . 1 g

Skewered Chicken and Shrimp

Serves 4   Serving size: 1 skewer

6 Tbsp lime juice	**1** medium onion
3 Tbsp honey	**1/2 lb** boneless, skinless chicken breast (trimmed of all visible fat)
2 Tbsp rice wine vinegar	
2 tsp chopped cilantro	**4** medium kiwi fruit
1/4 oz gingerroot	**1/2 lb** shrimp
1/4 tsp red pepper flakes	
1 medium red pepper	

1. Combine lime juice, honey, vinegar, cilantro, gingerroot, and pepper flakes to make a marinade.

2. Cut chicken into 1-inch slices. Core and quarter pepper. Cut each quarter into four pieces. Peel and quarter onion. Cut each quarter into four pieces. Toss chicken, pepper, and onion with the lime-ginger marinade. Marinate 2 hours in refrigerator.

3. When ready to cook, peel kiwi fruit and cut into quarters. Peel and devein shrimp. Toss kiwis and shrimp with marinade until coated. Divide ingredients among four skewers. Grill or boil, 3–4 minutes per side, turning skewers once, until chicken and shrimp are cooked through.

Exchanges/Choices

1 Fruit
1 Carbohydrate
1 Vegetable
3 Lean Meat

Basic Nutritional Values

Calories	295
Calories from Fat	80
Total Fat	9.0 g
Saturated Fat	1.0 g
Trans Fat	0.0 g
Cholesterol	100 mg
Sodium	115 mg
Total Carbohydrate	34 g
Dietary Fiber	4 g
Sugars	25 g
Protein	21 g

Cold Pasta Salad

Serves 4   Serving size: 1/4 recipe

4 oz whole-wheat pasta, elbows or shells

1/2 cup diced tomatoes

1/2 cup diced cucumber

1/2 cup shredded carrot

1/4 cup canola mayonnaise

1/2 cup plain fat-free yogurt

Cook pasta according to package instructions. Drain and rinse with cold water. Toss all other ingredients together in a bowl with pasta. Refrigerate 3 hours and serve.

Exchanges/Choices

2 Starch
1/2 Fat

Basic Nutritional Values

Calories 170
  Calories from Fat 45
Total Fat . . . . 5.0 g
  Saturated Fat . . . . 0.1 g
  Trans Fat . . . . 0.0 g
Cholesterol . . . . 0 mg
Sodium . . . . 125 mg
Total Carbohydrate . . . 26 g
  Dietary Fiber . . . . 3 g
  Sugars . . . . 5 g
Protein . . . . 6 g

Carrots in Sherry Wine

Serves 4   Serving size: 1/4 recipe

2 cups baby carrots

2 Tbsp Smart Balance Light margarine

1/2 cup sherry cooking wine

Combine all ingredients and cook carrots over medium heat until tender.

Exchanges/Choices

2 Vegetable
1/2 Fat

Basic Nutritional Values

Calories 70
  Calories from Fat 20
Total Fat . . . . 2.5 g
  Saturated Fat . . . . 0.8 g
  Trans Fat . . . . 0.0 g
Cholesterol . . . . 0 mg
Sodium . . . . 85 mg
Total Carbohydrate . . . 8 g
  Dietary Fiber . . . . 2 g
  Sugars . . . . 4 g
Protein . . . . 1 g

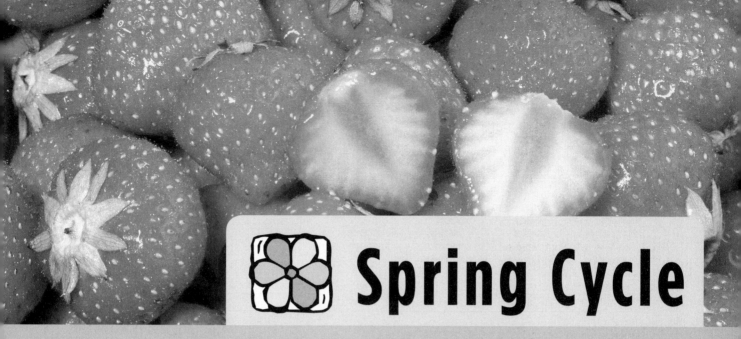

Spring Cycle

WEEK 1

FEATURED RECIPES

Whole-Wheat Pancakes or Waffles*

Pork with Orange Glaze

Apple Salad Dijon

Carrot Cake

Baked Sweet Potato Chips†

Lasagna

Spinach-Orange Salad*

Turkey and Swiss Roll-Up

Grilled Swordfish Steak

Cherry Crisp Dessert*

Marinated Vegetables

Cabbage Soup

Italian-Style Zucchini with Whole-Wheat Pasta

Roast Pork Stuffed with Fruit

German Potato Salad*

Carrots in Sherry Wine*

New Orleans Chilled Rice*

Beef Chow Mein

Whole-Wheat Blueberry Muffins*

Banana Walnut Bread

Fiesta Pasta Salad

Baked Fish and Zucchini

Perfection Salad

Potatoes au Gratin*

Strawberry Whip Parfaits*

Pumpkin Spice Muffins*

Ham and Swiss Roll-Up

Dilled Summer Squash

Quick and Easy Chili

Zesty Orange Oats Peach Crisp*

Sweet and Sour Chicken Salad

Zucchini Bread

Cinnamon Red Cabbage*

Asian Pork Chops

Raspberry Smoothie*

*Indicates that the recipe has been used previously.

†This recipe is used as a snack, but its ingredients are in the shopping list.

1500 calorie MEAL PLAN SPRING WEEK 1

	Sunday	Monday	Tuesday	Wednesday	Thursday	Friday	Saturday
Breakfast	**Whole-Wheat Pancakes or Waffles*** 1/4 cup sugar-free syrup 1 small orange 1 cup nonfat milk 1 oz lean turkey ham 1/2 tsp margarine	1/2 whole-wheat bagel 1 Tbsp jam 1 cup nonfat milk 1/4 cup egg substitute, scrambled 1 tsp margarine 3 almonds	Whole-wheat corn muffin 1/2 cup bran cereal 1 cup cantaloupe 1 cup nonfat milk 1/4 cup egg substitute, scrambled 1 tsp margarine	3/4 cup Chex cereal 1 slice multigrain bread 1 medium peach 1 cup nonfat milk 1 tsp margarine 3 macadamia nuts	**Whole-Wheat Blueberry Muffins*** 1/2 cup shredded wheat 1 cup cantaloupe 1 cup nonfat milk 2 pecans	**Pumpkin Spice Muffins*** 1/2 Tbsp 100% fruit spread 1 small banana 1 cup nonfat milk 1 oz lean turkey ham 1 tsp margarine 3 macadamia nuts	2 whole-grain waffles 3/4 cup pineapple 1 cup nonfat milk 1 oz Canadian bacon 1 Tbsp cashew butter
Lunch	**Pork with Orange Glaze Apple Salad Dijon Carrot Cake** 1 slice whole-wheat bread 1/2 cup cooked green beans	**Turkey and Swiss Roll-Up** 10 fat-free potato chips 3/4 cup pineapple	**Cabbage Soup Italian-Style Zucchini with Whole-Wheat Pasta** 2 oz canned salmon	**New Orleans Chilled Rice*** 1/2 cup peas 1 1/4 cup strawberries 2 oz grilled chicken	**Banana Walnut Bread Fiesta Pasta Salad** 1/2 cup green peas 1 small plum 1 oz reduced-fat cheese	**Ham and Swiss Roll-Up Dilled Summer Squash** 1 Tbsp raisins 2 small tangerines 1/2 cup cooked asparagus	**Sweet and Sour Chicken Salad** (1/2 serving) **Zucchini Bread Cinnamon Red Cabbage*** 2 graham cracker squares 6 almonds
Snack A							
Snack B							
Dinner	**Lasagna** (1/2 serving) **Spinach-Orange Salad*** 1 slice oatmeal bread 1 plum 1 cup nonfat milk 1/2 cup steamed green beans 1/2 tsp margarine	**Grilled Swordfish Steak Cherry Crisp Dessert* Marinated Vegetables** 1/4 large roasted potato 1 cup nonfat milk	**Roast Pork Stuffed with Fruit German Potato Salad* Carrots in Sherry Wine*** 1/2 cup nonfat milk 12 black olives	**Beef Chow Mein** 1 fortune cookie 3 dates 1 cup nonfat milk 15 peanuts	**Baked Fish and Zucchini Perfection Salad Potatoes au Gratin* Strawberry Whip Parfaits*** 17 grapes 20 peanuts	**Quick and Easy Chili Zesty Orange Oats Peach Crisp*** 1 slice wheat bread 1 cup nonfat milk 1/2 tsp margarine	**Asian Pork Chops Raspberry Smoothie*** 1 slice multigrain bread 1/2 cup nonfat milk 1/2 cup cooked broccoli 1 tsp margarine

*Indicates that the recipe has been used previously.

	Sunday	Monday	Tuesday	Wednesday	Thursday	Friday	Saturday
Breakfast	**Whole-Wheat Pancakes or Waffles*** 2 Tbsp sugar-free syrup 1 small orange 1 cup nonfat milk 1/2 tsp margarine	1/2 whole-wheat bagel 1 Tbsp jam 1 cup nonfat milk 1/4 cup egg substitute, scrambled 2 tsp margarine	Whole-wheat corn muffin 1/2 cup bran cereal 1 cup cantaloupe 1 cup nonfat milk 1/4 cup egg substitute, scrambled 1 tsp margarine	3/4 cup Chex cereal 1 slice multigrain bread 1 medium peach 1 cup nonfat milk 1/4 cup egg substitute, scrambled 1 tsp margarine 3 macadamia nuts	**Whole-Wheat Blueberry Muffins*** 1/2 cup shredded wheat 1 cup cantaloupe 1 cup nonfat milk 4 pecans	**Pumpkin Spice Muffins*** 1/2 Tbsp 100% fruit spread 1 small banana 1 cup nonfat milk 1 oz lean turkey ham 1 tsp margarine 3 macadamia nuts	2 whole-grain waffles 3/4 cup pineapple 1 cup nonfat milk 1 oz Canadian bacon 1 Tbsp cashew butter
Lunch	**Pork with Orange Glaze Apple Salad Dijon Carrot Cake** 1 slice whole-wheat bread 1/2 cup cooked green beans 1 tsp margarine	**Turkey and Swiss Roll-Up** 10 fat-free potato chips 3/4 cup pineapple 2 Tbsp avocado	**Cabbage Soup Italian-Style Zucchini with Whole-Wheat Pasta** 2 oz canned salmon 1 Tbsp pine nuts	**New Orleans Chilled Rice*** 1/2 cup peas 1 1/4 cup strawberries 2 oz grilled chicken 4 walnut halves	**Banana Walnut Bread Fiesta Pasta Salad** 1/2 cup green peas 1 small plum 2 oz reduced-fat cheese 1/2 tsp margarine	**Ham and Swiss Roll-Up Dilled Summer Squash** 1 Tbsp raisins 2 small tangerines 1/2 cup cooked asparagus	**Sweet and Sour Chicken Salad** (1/2 serving) **Zucchini Bread Cinnamon Red Cabbage*** 2 graham cracker squares 12 almonds
Snack A	6 cashews 1 cup cantaloupe	5 hazelnuts 12 cherries	1 1/2 tsp peanut butter 1 small piece of celery 2 Tbsp raisins	1 Tbsp pine nuts 1/2 cup mango	3 macadamia nuts 3/4 cup blueberries	4 pecans 1/2 large pear	1 oz dried fruit trail mix
Snack B	1 cup nonfat milk	1 cup nonfat milk	1 cup nonfat milk	1 cup nonfat milk	1 cup nonfat milk	1 cup nonfat milk	1 cup nonfat milk
Dinner	**Lasagna Spinach-Orange Salad*** 1 plum 1 cup nonfat milk 1 cup steamed green beans 1/2 tsp margarine	**Grilled Swordfish Steak Cherry Crisp Dessert* Marinated Vegetables** 1/4 large roasted potato 1 cup nonfat milk	**Roast Pork Stuffed with Fruit German Potato Salad* Carrots in Sherry Wine*** 1/2 cup nonfat milk 1 oz smoked fish, served on 3 cucumber slices 12 black olives	**Beef Chow Mein** 1 fortune cookie 3 dates 1 cup nonfat milk 15 peanuts	**Baked Fish and Zucchini Perfection Salad Potatoes au Gratin* Strawberry Whip Parfaits*** 17 grapes 20 peanuts	**Quick and Easy Chili Zesty Orange Oats Peach Crisp*** 1 slice wheat bread 1 cup nonfat milk 1 oz reduced-fat cheese 1/2 tsp margarine	**Asian Pork Chops Raspberry Smoothie*** 1/3 cup baked beans 1/2 cup nonfat milk 1/2 cup cooked broccoli 1 tsp margarine

*Indicates that the recipe has been used previously.

2000 calorie MEAL PLAN SPRING WEEK 1

	Sunday	Monday	Tuesday	Wednesday	Thursday	Friday	Saturday
Breakfast	Whole-Wheat Pancakes or Waffles* 2 Tbsp sugar-free syrup 1 small orange 1 cup nonfat milk 1/2 tsp margarine	1/2 whole-wheat bagel 1 Tbsp jam 1 cup nonfat milk 1/4 cup egg substitute, scrambled 2 tsp margarine	Whole-wheat corn muffin 1/2 cup bran cereal 1 cup cantaloupe 1 cup nonfat milk 1/4 cup egg substitute, scrambled 1 tsp margarine	3/4 cup Chex cereal 1 slice multigrain bread 1 medium peach 1 cup nonfat milk 1/4 cup egg substitute, scrambled 1 tsp margarine 3 macadamia nuts	Whole-Wheat Blueberry Muffins* 1/2 cup shredded wheat 1 cup cantaloupe 1 cup nonfat milk 4 pecans	Pumpkin Spice Muffins* 1/2 Tbsp 100% fruit spread 1 small banana 1 cup nonfat milk 1 oz lean turkey ham 1 tsp margarine 3 macadamia nuts	2 whole-grain waffles 3/4 cup pineapple 1 cup nonfat milk 1 oz Canadian bacon 1 Tbsp cashew butter
Lunch	Pork with Orange Glaze Apple Salad Dijon Carrot Cake 1 slice whole-wheat bread 17 grapes 1 cup cooked green beans 1 tsp margarine	Turkey and Swiss Roll-Up 10 fat-free potato chips 3/4 cup pineapple 1 cup raspberries 1 cup celery sticks 2 Tbsp avocado	Cabbage Soup Italian-Style Zucchini with Whole-Wheat Pasta 1/2 cup fruit cup 2 oz canned salmon 1 Tbsp pine nuts	New Orleans Chilled Rice* 1/2 cup peas 1 1/4 cup strawberries 1/2 cup cooked spinach 2 oz grilled chicken 4 walnut halves	Banana Walnut Bread Fiesta Pasta Salad 1/2 cup green peas 3 small plums 2 oz reduced-fat cheese 1/2 tsp margarine	Ham and Swiss Roll-Up Dilled Summer Squash 1 Tbsp raisins 2 small tangerines 3/4 cup blueberries 1 cup cooked asparagus	Sweet and Sour Chicken Salad (1/2 serving) Zucchini Bread Cinnamon Red Cabbage* 2 graham cracker squares 1 cup cantaloupe 1/2 cup cooked summer squash 12 almonds
Snack A	1 cup broccoli florets 1 Tbsp light salad dressing 1 cup cantaloupe	1 cup raw vegetable sticks 5 hazelnuts 12 cherries	1 cup celery 1 1/2 tsp peanut butter 2 Tbsp raisins	1 cup mixed raw vegetables 1 Tbsp pine nuts 1/2 cup mango	1 cup raw broccoli 3 macadamia nuts 3/4 cup blueberries	1 cup cucumber slices 4 pecans 1/2 large pear	1 cup raw vegetable sticks 1 oz dried fruit trail mix
Snack B	Baked Sweet Potato Chips 6 cashews 1 cup nonfat milk	2 sandwich cookies 1 cup nonfat milk	3/4 oz baked potato chips 1 oz avocado 1 cup nonfat milk	1/2 cup oatmeal 1 tsp margarine 1 cup nonfat milk	3 cup popcorn 1 tsp margarine 1 cup nonfat milk	3 ginger snaps 2 Brazil nuts 1 cup nonfat milk	5 vanilla wafers 1 cup nonfat milk
Dinner	Lasagna Spinach-Orange Salad* 1 plum 1 cup nonfat milk 1 cup steamed green beans 1/2 tsp margarine	Grilled Swordfish Steak Cherry Crisp Dessert* Marinated Vegetables 1/4 large roasted potato 1 cup nonfat milk	Roast Pork Stuffed with Fruit German Potato Salad* Carrots in Sherry Wine* 1/2 cup nonfat milk 1 oz smoked fish, served on 3 cucumber slices 12 black olives	Beef Chow Mein 1 fortune cookie 3 dates 1 cup nonfat milk 15 peanuts	Baked Fish and Zucchini Perfection Salad Potatoes au Gratin* Strawberry Whip Parfaits* 17 grapes 20 peanuts	Quick and Easy Chili Zesty Orange Oats Peach Crisp* 1 slice wheat bread 1 cup nonfat milk 1 oz reduced-fat cheese 1/2 tsp margarine	Asian Pork Chops Raspberry Smoothie* 1/3 cup baked beans 1/2 cup nonfat milk 1/2 cup cooked broccoli 1 tsp margarine

*Indicates that the recipe has been used previously.

	Sunday	Monday	Tuesday	Wednesday	Thursday	Friday	Saturday
Breakfast	**Whole-Wheat Pancakes or Waffles*** 2 Tbsp sugar-free syrup 1 small orange 1 cup nonfat milk 1 oz lean turkey ham 1/2 tsp margarine	1/2 whole-wheat bagel 1 Tbsp jam 1 cup nonfat milk 1/2 cup egg substitute, scrambled 2 tsp margarine	Whole-wheat corn muffin 1/2 cup bran cereal 1 cup cantaloupe 1 cup nonfat milk 1/2 cup egg substitute, scrambled 1 tsp margarine	3/4 cup Chex cereal 1 slice multigrain bread 1 medium peach 1 cup nonfat milk 1/2 cup egg substitute, scrambled 3 macadamia nuts	**Whole-Wheat Blueberry Muffins*** 1/2 cup shredded wheat 1 cup cantaloupe 1 cup nonfat milk 1 oz smoked salmon (lox) 4 pecans	**Pumpkin Spice Muffins*** 1/2 Tbsp 100% fruit spread 1 small banana 1 cup nonfat milk 2 oz lean turkey ham 1 tsp margarine 3 macadamia nuts	2 whole-grain waffles 3/4 cup pineapple 1 cup nonfat milk 1 oz Canadian bacon 1 Tbsp cashew butter
Lunch	**Pork with Orange Glaze Apple Salad Dijon Carrot Cake** 1 slice whole-wheat bread 17 grapes 1 cup cooked green beans 1 tsp margarine	**Turkey and Swiss Roll-Up** 10 fat-free potato chips 3/4 cup pineapple 1 cup raspberries 1 cup celery sticks 2 Tbsp avocado	**Cabbage Soup Italian-Style Zucchini with Whole-Wheat Pasta** 1/2 cup fruit cup 2 oz canned salmon 1 Tbsp pine nuts	**New Orleans Chilled Rice*** 1/2 cup peas 1 1/4 cup strawberries 1 kiwi fruit 2 oz grilled chicken 4 walnut halves	**Banana Walnut Bread Fiesta Pasta Salad** 1/2 cup green peas 3 small plums 2 oz reduced-fat cheese 1/2 tsp margarine	**Ham and Swiss Roll-Up Dilled Summer Squash** 1 Tbsp raisins 2 small tangerines 3/4 cup blueberries 1 cup cooked asparagus	**Sweet and Sour Chicken Salad** (1/2 serving) **Zucchini Bread Cinnamon Red Cabbage*** 2 graham cracker squares 1 cup cantaloupe 1/2 cup cooked summer squash 12 almonds
Snack A	1 cup broccoli florets 1 Tbsp light salad dressing 1 cup cantaloupe	1 cup raw vegetable sticks 5 hazelnuts 12 cherries	1 cup celery 1 1/2 tsp peanut butter 2 Tbsp raisins	1 cup mixed raw vegetables 1 Tbsp pine nuts 1/2 cup mango	1 cup raw broccoli 3 macadamia nuts 3/4 cup blueberries	1 cup cucumber slices 4 pecans 1/2 large pear	1 cup raw vegetable sticks 1 oz dried fruit trail mix
Snack B	**Baked Sweet Potato Chips** 6 cashews 1 cup nonfat milk	2 sandwich cookies 1 cup nonfat milk	3/4 oz baked potato chips 1 oz avocado 1 cup nonfat milk	1/2 cup oatmeal 1 tsp margarine 1 cup nonfat milk	3 cup popcorn 1 tsp margarine 1 cup nonfat milk	3 ginger snaps 2 Brazil nuts 1 cup nonfat milk	5 vanilla wafers 1 cup nonfat milk
Dinner	**Lasagna Spinach-Orange Salad*** 1 plum 1 cup nonfat milk 1 cup steamed green beans 1/2 tsp margarine	**Grilled Swordfish Steak Cherry Crisp Dessert* Marinated Vegetables** 1 slice whole-grain bread 1/4 large roasted potato 1 cup nonfat milk	**Roast Pork Stuffed with Fruit German Potato Salad* Carrots in Sherry Wine*** 1 1/2 oz corn bread 1/2 cup nonfat milk 1 oz smoked fish, served on 3 cucumber slices 12 black olives	**Beef Chow Mein** 1 fortune cookie 3/4 oz pretzels 3 dates 1 cup nonfat milk 15 peanuts	**Baked Fish and Zucchini Perfection Salad Potatoes au Gratin* Strawberry Whip Parfaits*** 17 grapes 20 peanuts	**Quick and Easy Chili Zesty Orange Oats Peach Crisp*** 2 oz low-fat corn bread 1 cup nonfat milk 1 oz reduced-fat cheese 1/2 tsp margarine	**Asian Pork Chops Raspberry Smoothie*** 2/3 cup baked beans 1/2 cup nonfat milk 1/2 cup cooked broccoli 1 tsp margarine

*Indicates that the recipe has been used previously.

SHOPPING LIST SPRING WEEK 1

VEGETABLES
_____ asparagus
_____ avocado
_____ bell peppers, green
_____ bell peppers, red
_____ bell peppers, yellow
_____ broccoli
_____ cabbage, green
_____ cabbage, red
_____ carrots
_____ celery
_____ cucumber
_____ garlic
_____ green beans
_____ lettuce, romaine
_____ mushrooms
_____ onions, green
_____ onions, red
_____ onions, yellow or white
_____ peas, green
_____ potatoes, red or russet
_____ potatoes, sweet
_____ shallots
_____ snow peas
_____ spinach
_____ summer squash
_____ tomatoes
_____ tomatoes, cherry
_____ zucchini

MEATS
_____ bacon, Canadian
_____ bacon, turkey
_____ beef, sirloin, lean
_____ canned salmon
_____ chicken breasts, boneless, skinless
_____ fish fillets, any white-meat fish
_____ ground beef, 96% lean
_____ ham, light
_____ pork chops, boneless sirloin
_____ smoked fish
_____ swordfish steaks
_____ turkey breast, lean
_____ turkey ham, lean

FRUITS
_____ apples
_____ bananas
_____ blueberries
_____ cantaloupe
_____ grapes
_____ lemon (for peel and juicing)
_____ oranges
_____ peaches
_____ pears
_____ pineapple
_____ plums
_____ raisins
_____ raspberries
_____ strawberries
_____ tangerines

DAIRY
_____ egg substitute
_____ milk, nonfat
_____ Smart Balance Light margarine
_____ Smart Balance Light spread
_____ whipped topping, fat-free
_____ yogurt, lemon, fat-free
_____ yogurt, plain, fat-free

CHEESE
_____ cheddar, reduced-fat
_____ cottage cheese, fat-free
_____ Parmesan, reduced-fat
_____ Swiss, reduced-fat

BREAD, GRAINS, & PASTA
_____ bagel, whole-wheat
_____ bread, whole-wheat, whole-grain
_____ muffin, corn, whole-wheat
_____ noodles, lasagna
_____ pasta, whole-wheat, macaroni or elbows
_____ rice, brown and/or whole-grain
_____ waffles, whole-grain, frozen

BEANS
_____ baked beans
_____ kidney beans, no-added-salt, 15-oz can

NUTS
_____ almonds
_____ dates
_____ macadamia nuts
_____ peanuts, dry roasted
_____ pecans
_____ pine nuts
_____ sesame seeds
_____ walnuts

CONDIMENTS

_____ canola mayonnaise
_____ hot sauce
_____ mustard, Dijon
_____ mustard, yellow
_____ salad dressing, Italian, light
_____ soy sauce, light
_____ stir-fry sauce

SPICES & HERBS

_____ allspice
_____ basil
_____ bay leaf
_____ black pepper
_____ cayenne pepper
_____ celery seed
_____ chili powder, no-added-salt
_____ cilantro
_____ cinnamon, ground
_____ cloves, ground
_____ coriander, ground
_____ cream of tartar
_____ cumin seed, ground
_____ dill weed
_____ dry mustard
_____ fennel seeds
_____ ginger, ground
_____ marjoram
_____ nutmeg, ground
_____ oregano
_____ paprika
_____ parsley
_____ red pepper flakes
_____ rosemary
_____ tarragon
_____ thyme

OTHER

_____ angel food cake
_____ applesauce, unsweetened
_____ black olives
_____ brown gravy mix
_____ canned pumpkin
_____ cashew butter
_____ cereal, bran
_____ cereal, Chex
_____ cereal, shredded wheat
_____ crackers, graham
_____ dill pickle
_____ fortune cookies
_____ frozen corn
_____ frozen oriental vegetables
_____ frozen vegetables mix (broccoli, carrots, water chestnuts, and red pepper)
_____ fruit cup or fruit cocktail in light syrup
_____ fruit spread, 100% fruit
_____ gelatin, raspberry, sugar-free, 0.3-oz box
_____ jam, any kind, no-added-sugar
_____ juice, pineapple
_____ juice, vegetable, low-sodium, 48-oz can
_____ maple syrup, sugar-free
_____ marmalade, orange, sugar-free
_____ noodles, chow mein, dry
_____ onion soup mix
_____ pie filling, cherry, light
_____ pineapple chunks, canned light
_____ pineapple, crushed, canned light
_____ potato chips, fat-free
_____ salsa, mild or hot
_____ spaghetti sauce, light
_____ tomato sauce, no-added-salt
_____ tomatoes, diced, no-added-salt, 28-oz can
_____ tomatoes, stewed, Italian-style
_____ tomatoes, stewed, no-added-salt, 14-oz can
_____ tortillas, corn, 6-inch

STAPLES

_____ almond extract
_____ baking powder
_____ baking soda
_____ bouillon, beef, sodium-free
_____ bouillon, chicken, sodium-free
_____ cornstarch
_____ flour, whole-wheat
_____ lemon juice
_____ nonstick cooking spray
_____ old-fashioned oats
_____ sherry, cooking
_____ Smart Balance Omega oil
_____ Splenda
_____ Splenda Brown Sugar Blend
_____ vanilla extract
_____ vinegar, cider
_____ vinegar, malt
_____ vinegar, red wine
_____ vinegar, white
_____ wine, red

Whole-Wheat Pancakes or Waffles

Serves 4   Serving size: 2 pancakes or waffles

1/2 **cup** rolled oats

1/2 **cup** whole-wheat flour, sifted

2 **tsp** baking powder

2 **Tbsp** Splenda

1/2 **cup** egg substitute, beaten well

3/4 **cup** nonfat milk

2 **Tbsp** Smart Balance Omega oil

Nonstick cooking spray

Exchanges/Choices

1 1/2 Starch
1 1/2 Fat

Basic Nutritional Values

Calories 185
  Calories from Fat 70
Total Fat . . . . 8.0 g
  Saturated Fat . . . . 0.7 g
  Trans Fat . . . . 0.0 g
Cholesterol . . . . 0 mg
Sodium . . . . 265 mg
Total Carbohydrate . . 22 g
  Dietary Fiber . . . . 3 g
  Sugars . . . . 3 g
Protein . . . . 8 g

Stir together dry ingredients. Combine egg substitute, milk, and oil; stir into flour mixture. Cook on a griddle lightly coated with nonstick spray until golden brown, then turn. Can also be made in a waffle iron.

Pork with Orange Glaze

Serves 4   Serving size: 1/4 recipe

1 **Tbsp** sodium-free chicken bouillon

1/2 **cup** water

1/4 **cup** sugar-free orange marmalade

3 **Tbsp** cooking sherry

3 **tsp** light soy sauce

1/2 **tsp** dried marjoram leaves

1/2 **tsp** lemon juice

3/4 **lb** boneless sirloin pork chops (trimmed of visible fat)

Nonstick cooking spray

Exchanges/Choices

1/2 Carbohydrate
2 Lean Meat

Basic Nutritional Values

Calories 110
  Calories from Fat 20
Total Fat . . . . 2.0 g
  Saturated Fat . . . . 0.3 g
  Trans Fat . . . . 0.0 g
Cholesterol . . . . 40 mg
Sodium . . . . 315 mg
Total Carbohydrate . . 6 g
  Dietary Fiber . . . . 0 g
  Sugars . . . . 3 g
Protein . . . . 15 g

1. In a 1 1/2-quart saucepan, combine the bouillon, water, marmalade, sherry, soy sauce, marjoram, and lemon juice. Heat over low heat until marmalade is just melted. Reserve 1/2 cup of the glaze.

2. Place pork in zip-top plastic bag. Add remaining glaze; seal and chill 2 hours, turning bag over once.

3. Prepare grill for medium-direct heat. Spray cooking grill with nonstick cooking spray. Place meat on grill and cook about 6 minutes per side. Brush with reserved glaze; grill 3 more minutes per side until pork reaches an internal temperature of 160°F.

Apple Salad Dijon

Serves 4   Serving size: 1/4 recipe

8	medium celery sticks	2 **tsp** cider vinegar
2	medium Granny Smith apples	1/2 **tsp** Splenda
4	**Tbsp** canola mayonnaise	2 **tsp** tarragon
2	**Tbsp** Dijon mustard	Black pepper, to taste

1. Cut the celery into 1 1/4-inch matchsticks and reserve celery leaves for garnish. Cut the apples into 1 1/2-inch slices.

2. In a bowl, whisk together the mayonnaise, mustard, vinegar, Splenda, tarragon, and pepper until the dressing is smooth. Add the celery and the apples. Toss the salad and serve garnished with celery leaves.

Exchanges/Choices

1 Fruit
1 Fat

Basic Nutritional Values

Calories	110
Calories from Fat	45
Total Fat	5.0 g
Saturated Fat	0.1 g
Trans Fat	0.0 g
Cholesterol	0 mg
Sodium	360 mg
Total Carbohydrate	16 g
Dietary Fiber	4 g
Sugars	11 g
Protein	1 g

Carrot Cake

Serves 6   Serving size: 1/6 recipe

	Nonstick cooking spray	1/4 **cup** fat-free plain yogurt
1 **cup**	whole-wheat flour	1 **cup** carrot, pureed in a blender
1 **cup**	Splenda	1 **cup** crushed pineapple (or canned light)
1 **tsp**	ground cinnamon	Splenda, powdered (pulse in a food processor or coffee grinder until very fine)
3/4 **tsp**	baking soda	
1/2 **cup**	egg substitute	
1 **tsp**	pure vanilla extract	
1/4 **cup**	unsweetened applesauce	

Preheat oven to 350°F. Spray a 12-cup fluted tube pan with nonstick cooking spray. In a large bowl, mix flour, Splenda, cinnamon, and baking soda. Stir in egg substitute, vanilla, applesauce, and yogurt until well blended. Stir in carrot and pineapple. Pour into pan. Bake for 55 minutes or until a toothpick inserted 2 inches from edge comes out clean. Cool in pan on a wire rack for 20 minutes. Remove cake from pan. Allow cake to cool completely. To serve, lightly sprinkle with powdered Splenda.

Exchanges/Choices

2 Carbohydrate

Basic Nutritional Values

Calories	135
Calories from Fat	0
Total Fat	0.0 g
Saturated Fat	0.1 g
Trans Fat	0.0 g
Cholesterol	0 mg
Sodium	220 mg
Total Carbohydrate	28 g
Dietary Fiber	4 g
Sugars	11 g
Protein	6 g

Baked Sweet Potato Chips

Serves 4   Serving size: 1/4 recipe

Nonstick cooking spray

1 **tsp** dried rosemary

1 bunch parsley

1 **tsp** dry mustard

1 **tsp** paprika

1 **tsp** cinnamon

Pepper, to taste

2 medium sweet potatoes, washed and unpeeled

Exchanges/Choices

1 Starch

Basic Nutritional Values

Calories 75
  Calories from Fat 5
Total Fat . . . . 0.5 g
  Saturated Fat . . . . 0.1 g
  Trans Fat . . . . 0.0 g
Cholesterol . . . . 0 mg
Sodium . . . . 35 mg
Total Carbohydrate . . . 17 g
  Dietary Fiber . . . . 4 g
  Sugars . . . . 5 g
Protein . . . . 2 g

Preheat the oven to 450°F. Lightly spray a baking sheet with the cooking spray. In a small bowl, combine the rosemary, parsley, mustard, paprika, cinnamon, and pepper. Cut the potatoes crosswise into 1/8-inch slices. Lightly spray the tops with cooking spray and sprinkle with the seasonings. Bake for about 25 minutes or until crisp-tender.

Lasagna

Serves 4   Serving size: 1/4 recipe

8 **oz** lasagna noodles

1 **lb** 96% lean ground beef

1/2 **cup** chopped onions

2/3 head garlic, large, minced

2 **cups** light spaghetti sauce, reserve 1/4 cup

2 **tsp** dried parsley

1 **tsp** dried basil leaves, crushed

1/2 **tsp** oregano

1/4 **tsp** black pepper

1 **cup** fat-free cottage cheese

1 **tsp** reduced-fat Parmesan cheese, grated

Exchanges

2 Starch
4 Lean Meat

Basic Nutritional Values

Calories 330
  Calories from Fat 45
Total Fat . . . . 5.0 g
  Saturated Fat . . . . 2.1 g
  Trans Fat . . . . 0.3 g
Cholesterol . . . . 65 mg
Sodium . . . . 660 mg
Total Carbohydrate . . . 33 g
  Dietary Fiber . . . . 3 g
  Sugars . . . . 13 g
Protein . . . . 36 g

1. Cook lasagna noodles according to package directions; set aside. Brown the ground beef. Drain the fat; add all remaining ingredients to the meat, except the cheeses and 1/4 cup reserved spaghetti sauce. Cook until garlic is just browned.

2. Layer the bottom of a baking dish with a layer of the noodles and then spoon the meat mixture over the noodles, followed by a layer of cottage cheese. Repeat layering and cover with a final layer of noodles. Spread reserved spaghetti sauce on top. Bake at 350°F for 30 minutes. Uncover, sprinkle with Parmesan. Bake 10 minutes more, until hot and bubbly. Let stand 10 minutes before serving.

This recipe is high in sodium.

Spinach-Orange Salad

Serves 4   Serving size: 1/4 recipe

- **4 cups** spinach, torn into pieces
- **2** medium oranges, peeled and sectioned, juice reserved (about 1/4 cup)
- **2/3 cup** mushrooms, sliced
- **1/2 cup** red onion, sliced
- **2 Tbsp** Smart Balance Omega oil
- **2 Tbsp** malt vinegar
- **1/2 tsp** ginger, ground
- **1/4 tsp** pepper

Place spinach in a bowl. Add orange sections, mushrooms, and onion. Toss lightly to mix. In a separate bowl, mix oil, vinegar, orange juice, ginger, and pepper. Pour over spinach. Toss to mix and chill; serve.

Exchanges/Choices

1/2 Fruit
1 Vegetable
1 1/2 Fat

Basic Nutritional Values

Calories 115
 Calories from Fat 65
Total Fat . . . . 7.0 g
 Saturated Fat . . . . 0.5 g
 Trans Fat . . . . 0.0 g
Cholesterol . . . . 0 mg
Sodium . . . . 25 mg
Total Carbohydrate . . . . 13 g
 Dietary Fiber . . . . 3 g
 Sugars . . . . 8 g
Protein . . . . 2 g

Turkey and Swiss Roll-Up

Serves 4   Serving size: 3 roll-ups

8 oz light turkey breast	**12** leaves romaine lettuce
4 slices reduced-fat Swiss cheese	**16** tomato slices, diced
4 Tbsp canola mayonnaise	**12** (**6-inch**) corn tortillas

Divide the turkey breast between 3 tortillas per person. Slice each cheese slice into three pieces and place one on each tortilla. Place a lettuce leaf on top of each, followed by diced tomatoes. Place 1/3 tsp mayonnaise on top; roll up the tortilla and serve.

Exchanges/Choices

2 1/2 Starch
1 Vegetable
2 Lean Meat
1 1/2 Fat

Basic Nutritional Values

Calories 375
 Calories from Fat 100
Total Fat . . . . 11.0 g
 Saturated Fat . . . . 2.8 g
 Trans Fat . . . . 0.0 g
Cholesterol . . . . 40 mg
Sodium . . . . 375 mg
Total Carbohydrate . . . 42 g
 Dietary Fiber . . . . 5 g
 Sugars . . . . 7 g
Protein . . . . 24 g

Grilled Swordfish Steak

Serves 4   Serving size: 1/4 recipe

2 Tbsp Smart Balance Omega oil	**1/4 tsp** ginger, ground
2 Tbsp lemon juice	**1 Tbsp** grated lemon peel
1 Tbsp cooking sherry	**1/4 tsp** pepper
2 medium garlic cloves, minced	**1 lb** swordfish steaks

Combine the oil, lemon juice, sherry, garlic, ginger, lemon peel, and pepper; set aside. Lay the swordfish steaks in a shallow baking pan just large enough to hold them; pour on the marinade and turn steaks to coat well. Cover and refrigerate for 2 hours. Place a skillet over medium-high heat for 30 seconds. Add swordfish steaks and cook uncovered for 3 minutes on each side until firm.

Exchanges/Choices

3 Lean Meat
1 Fat

Basic Nutritional Values

Calories 205
 Calories from Fat 110
Total Fat . . . . 12.0 g
 Saturated Fat . . . . 1.7 g
 Trans Fat . . . . 0.0 g
Cholesterol . . . . 45 mg
Sodium . . . . 105 mg
Total Carbohydrate . . . 2 g
 Dietary Fiber . . . . 0 g
 Sugars . . . . 0 g
Protein . . . . 22 g

Cherry Crisp Dessert
Serves 8   Serving size: 1/8 recipe

1 (20-oz) can light cherry pie filling

3/8 tsp almond extract

3 1/2 Tbsp Smart Balance margarine, melted

2 cups rolled oats, dry

1/4 cup Splenda

Place pie filling and almond extract in a baking dish that has sides about 2 inches high. Stir until blended; set aside. Place melted margarine in a small bowl; add oats and Splenda. Stir until well mixed. Spoon mixture evenly over pie filling. Bake at 350°F for about 30 minutes. Serve warm.

Exchanges/Choices

2 Carbohydrate
1 Fat

Basic Nutritional Values

Calories 165
  Calories from Fat 45
Total Fat . . . . 5 g
  Saturated Fat . . . . 1.3 g
  Trans Fat . . . . 0 g
Cholesterol . . . . 0 mg
Sodium . . . . 55 mg
Total Carbohydrate . . . 27 g
  Dietary Fiber . . . . 3 g
  Sugars . . . . 13 g
Protein . . . . 4 g

Marinated Vegetables
Serves 4   Serving size: 1/4 recipe

1/2 cup carrots, sliced

1/2 medium yellow bell pepper

1/2 cup light Italian dressing

1 Tbsp Dijon mustard

1/2 cup broccoli

1/2 cucumber, sliced

10 small cherry tomatoes

1 Tbsp parsley

Diagonally slice the carrots. Cut yellow pepper into strips. Combine dressing and mustard. Combine all other ingredients in a bowl, and pour the dressing and mustard mixture over all remaining ingredients; cover. Refrigerate 2 hours to marinate. Serve immediately.

Exchanges/Choices

2 Vegetable

Basic Nutritional Values

Calories 65
  Calories from Fat 20
Total Fat . . . . 2.5 g
  Saturated Fat . . . . 0.3 g
  Trans Fat . . . . 0.0 g
Cholesterol . . . . 0 mg
Sodium . . . . 460 mg
Total Carbohydrate . . . 11 g
  Dietary Fiber . . . . 2 g
  Sugars . . . . 7 g
Protein . . . . 2 g

Cabbage Soup

Serves 8   Serving size: 1/8 recipe

- 1 **Tbsp** Smart Balance Omega oil
- 3 medium onions, sliced
- 1 **Tbsp** minced garlic
- 1 celery stalk, diced
- 1 medium carrot, diced
- 3 **Tbsp** sodium-free chicken bouillon
- 3 **cups** water
- 1 bay leaf
- 1/4 **cup** finely chopped parsley

- 1 (**28-oz**) can no-added-salt diced tomatoes with juice
- 1 **tsp** thyme
- 2 **cups** shredded cabbage
- 2 small green peppers, seeded and chopped
- 1/2 **cup** mushrooms
- 1 (**48-oz**) can low-sodium vegetable juice
- 1 1/2 **cup** cooked brown rice

Exchanges/Choices

1/2 Starch
4 Vegetable
1/2 Fat

Basic Nutritional Values

Calories 165
  Calories from Fat 20
Total Fat . . . . 2.5 g
  Saturated Fat . . . . 0.3 g
  Trans Fat . . . . 0.0 g
Cholesterol . . . . 0 mg
Sodium . . . . 170 mg
Total Carbohydrate . . . 35 g
  Dietary Fiber . . . . 6 g
  Sugars . . . . 15 g
Protein . . . . 3 g

Heat oil in a medium skillet. Cook the onion, garlic, celery, and carrot until the onion is softened. In a large stockpot, combine the water and bouillon to make a stock. Add bay leaf, parsley, tomatoes, thyme, cabbage, peppers, mushrooms, and vegetable juice. Add cooked ingredients; bring soup to a simmer. Simmer about 2 hours, until all ingredients are softened; add cooked rice and serve.

Italian-Style Zucchini with Whole-Wheat Pasta
Serves 6   Serving size: 1/6 recipe

6 **oz** whole-wheat pasta, macaroni or elbows

1 large onion, chopped

1 clove garlic, minced

1 medium carrot, thinly chopped

2 **Tbsp** Smart Balance Omega oil

1 **(16-oz)** can Italian-style stewed tomatoes

1 zucchini, halved lengthwise and sliced in 1/4-inch pieces

1/2 **tsp** fennel seeds, crushed

1/4 **tsp** red pepper flakes

Exchanges/Choices
1 1/2 Starch
2 Vegetable
1/2 Fat

Basic Nutritional Values
Calories 185
  Calories from Fat 45
Total Fat. . . . . .5.0 g
  Saturated Fat . . . . .0.5 g
  Trans Fat. . . . . .0.0 g
Cholesterol. . . . . .0 mg
Sodium. . . . . .255 mg
Total Carbohydrate . . .33 g
  Dietary Fiber. . . . . .5 g
  Sugars . . . . .8 g
Protein . . . . .6 g

Cook the pasta according to package directions; drain and set aside. In a large skillet, cook the onion, garlic, and carrot in hot oil for 5 minutes or until tender. Add tomatoes, zucchini, fennel seeds, and red pepper flakes. Bring to a boil and reduce heat. Simmer uncovered for about 3 minutes. Stir in pasta and heat through.

Roast Pork Stuffed with Fruit
Serves 4   Serving size: 1/4 recipe

2 **cups** crushed pineapple (fresh, frozen, or canned light, well drained)

1/2 **cup** chopped apple

1/4 **cup** sugar-free orange marmalade, divided

1 **Tbsp** raisins

1 **Tbsp** green onion, sliced

2 **tsp** light soy sauce

1/2 **tsp** ground coriander

3/4 **lb** boneless sirloin pork chops (trimmed of visible fat)

1/4 **tsp** freshly ground black pepper
     Nonstick cooking spray

3/4 **tsp** sesame seeds, toasted

Exchanges/Choices
1 1/2 Fruit
2 Lean Meat

Basic Nutritional Values
Calories 175
  Calories from Fat 20
Total Fat. . . . . .2.5 g
  Saturated Fat . . . . .0.4 g
  Trans Fat. . . . . .0.0 g
Cholesterol. . . . . .40 mg
Sodium. . . . . .300 mg
Total Carbohydrate . . .25 g
  Dietary Fiber. . . . . .2 g
  Sugars . . . . .20 g
Protein . . . . .16 g

In a small bowl, combine the pineapple, apple, 1 Tbsp marmalade, raisins, green onion, soy sauce, and coriander. Slit each pork chop lengthwise to form a pocket. Rub inside of pockets evenly with pepper. Fill pockets evenly with stuffing. Secure openings with toothpicks. Prepare grill for medium direct heat. Spray cooking grill with nonstick cooking spray. Place pork on grill; cook covered for 6 minutes per side; brush fillets with remaining 3 Tbsp marmalade and sprinkle with sesame seeds. Grill 3 more minutes per side or until pork reaches an internal temperature of 160°F.

German Potato Salad

Serves 4   Serving size: 1/4 recipe

4 cups potatoes	**1 cup** water
4 slices turkey bacon	**1/2 cup** cider vinegar
1/2 cup chopped onions	**2 1/2 Tbsp** Splenda
2 Tbsp whole-wheat flour	**1/16 tsp** black pepper

Peel and dice the potatoes; place in boiling water. Cook until just soft. Fry bacon in a large skillet until crisp; remove and drain. Place the onions in the skillet and cook until tender. Slowly stir in flour; blend well. Add water and vinegar; cook, stirring, until bubbly and slightly thick. Stir in Splenda and pepper; simmer for 10 minutes. Crumble bacon. Carefully stir bacon and potatoes into hot mixture. Heat through, stirring gently to coat potato slices. Serve warm.

Exchanges/Choices
2 Starch

Basic Nutritional Values
Calories 160
 Calories from Fat 25
Total Fat . . . . 3.0 g
 Saturated Fat . . . . 0.8 g
 Trans Fat . . . . 0.0 g
Cholesterol . . . . 15 mg
Sodium . . . . 180 mg
Total Carbohydrate . . . 28 g
 Dietary Fiber . . . . 3 g
 Sugars . . . . 4 g
Protein . . . . 5 g

Carrots in Sherry Wine

Serves 4   Serving size: 1/4 recipe

2 cups baby carrots	**1/2 cup** sherry cooking wine
2 Tbsp Smart Balance Light margarine	

Combine all ingredients and cook carrots over medium heat until tender.

Exchanges/Choices
2 Vegetable
1/2 Fat

Basic Nutritional Values
Calories 70
 Calories from Fat 20
Total Fat . . . . 2.5 g
 Saturated Fat . . . . 0.8 g
 Trans Fat . . . . 0.0 g
Cholesterol . . . . 0 mg
Sodium . . . . 85 mg
Total Carbohydrate . . . 8 g
 Dietary Fiber . . . . 2 g
 Sugars . . . . 4 g
Protein . . . . 1 g

New Orleans Chilled Rice

Serves 4   Serving size: 1/4 recipe

3/4 **cups** whole-grain rice

1 **Tbsp** Smart Balance Omega oil

1/2 **cup** chopped dill pickle

1/2 **cup** celery, diced

1/2 **cup** onion

1/2 **cup** shallots, chopped

1/2 medium red pepper, chopped

1/4 **cup** canola mayonnaise

1/4 **cup** fat-free plain yogurt

1/2 **Tbsp** vinegar

Cook rice according to package directions. In a large bowl, combine all other ingredients with the cooked rice; chill before serving.

Exchanges/Choices

2 Starch
2 Vegetable
1 Fat

Basic Nutritional Values

Calories 255
 Calories from Fat 70
Total Fat. . . . . 8.0 g
 Saturated Fat . . . . 0.4 g
 Trans Fat . . . . 0.0 g
Cholesterol . . . . 0 mg
Sodium. . . . . 345 mg
Total Carbohydrate . . . 39 g
 Dietary Fiber . . . . 2 g
 Sugars . . . . 5 g
Protein . . . . 5 g

Beef Chow Mein

Serves 4   Serving size: 1/4 recipe

1 **lb** lean sirloin beef (trimmed of visible fat), cut into thin strips

1 **Tbsp** Smart Balance Omega oil

1 **Tbsp** sodium-free beef bouillon

1 **cup** water

2 **Tbsp** cornstarch

1 **Tbsp** brown gravy mix, dry

1 **Tbsp** light soy sauce

1/2 **cup** celery, diced

1/2 **cup** onion, diced

1/2 **cup** mushrooms, sliced

1 **lb** frozen oriental vegetables

2 **cups** dry chow mein noodles

Heat oil in a large skillet over medium heat. Add beef strips, cooking and stirring constantly. In a separate bowl, combine beef bouillon, water, cornstarch, gravy mix, and soy sauce; pour over meat. Heat to boiling and then simmer for 30 minutes. Add celery, onions, mushrooms, and vegetables; heat to boiling, stirring frequently. Boil for 1 minute. Pour mixture over dry chow mein noodles. Serve hot.

Exchanges/Choices

1 1/2 Starch
2 Vegetable
3 Lean Meat
1/2 Fat

Basic Nutritional Values

Calories 325
 Calories from Fat 70
Total Fat. . . . . 8.0 g
 Saturated Fat . . . . 2.0 g
 Trans Fat . . . . 0.1 g
Cholesterol . . . . 45 mg
Sodium. . . . . 545 mg
Total Carbohydrate . . . 31 g
 Dietary Fiber . . . . 5 g
 Sugars . . . . 7 g
Protein . . . . 28 g

Whole-Wheat Blueberry Muffins
Serves 12   Serving size: 1 muffin

1 cup whole-wheat flour	**3 Tbsp** Smart Balance margarine
5 1/2 Tbsp Splenda	**1/2 cup** egg substitute
1 tsp baking powder	**1/2 cup** blueberries
6 Tbsp nonfat milk	

Preheat oven to 400°F. In a medium bowl, combine flour, Splenda, and baking powder. In a small bowl, beat milk, margarine, and egg substitute; stir into dry ingredients until just moist. Fold in blueberries and spoon batter into 12 paper-lined muffin cups. Bake for 20–25 minutes or until golden brown. Serve immediately.

Exchanges/Choices
1/2 Starch
1/2 Fat

Basic Nutritional Values
Calories 70
 Calories from Fat 20
Total Fat. . . . . .2.5 g
 Saturated Fat . . . . .0.7 g
 Trans Fat. . . . . .0.0 g
Cholesterol. . . . . .0 mg
Sodium. . . . . .75 mg
Total Carbohydrate . . .9 g
 Dietary Fiber. . . . . .1 g
 Sugars . . . . .2 g
Protein . . . . .3 g

Banana Walnut Bread
Serves 18   Serving size: 1 slice

Nonstick cooking spray	**1 1/2 cups** whole-wheat flour
3 ripe bananas	**1 tsp** baking soda
1/2 cup egg substitute	**1 tsp** cream of tartar
3/4 cup Splenda	**1/4 cup** shelled walnuts, crushed
1/2 cup Smart Balance margarine	

Preheat oven to 350°F. Spray a 9 × 5 × 3-inch loaf pan with nonstick cooking spray. Mash the bananas and egg substitute together by hand or with an electric mixer. Add the Splenda and margarine, mixing by hand or electric mixer. Add remaining ingredients and blend well. Pour into the loaf pan and bake for 50 minutes. When done, a toothpick inserted in the center will come out clean. Let cool for 10 minutes before turning it out. Let cool completely. Makes one 9-inch loaf.

Exchanges/Choices
1/2 Starch
1/2 Fruit
1 Fat

Basic Nutritional Values
Calories 105
 Calories from Fat 45
Total Fat. . . . . .5.0 g
 Saturated Fat . . . . .1.3 g
 Trans Fat. . . . . .0.0 g
Cholesterol. . . . . .0 mg
Sodium. . . . . .125 mg
Total Carbohydrate . . .13 g
 Dietary Fiber. . . . . .2 g
 Sugars . . . . .4 g
Protein . . . . .3 g

Fiesta Pasta Salad

Serves 4   Serving size: 1/4 recipe

4 **oz** whole-wheat pasta

1/2 **cup** tomato, peeled and diced

1/2 medium red pepper

1/2 medium green pepper

1/2 medium yellow pepper

1/2 medium red onion

1/2 **cup** corn, frozen

1/4 **cup** salsa, mild or hot

1 medium garlic clove, minced

1/2 **cup** carrot, shredded

1 **Tbsp** cilantro, chopped

1 **Tbsp** Smart Balance Omega oil

1 **tsp** ground cumin seed

1/4 **tsp** cayenne pepper

1/4 **tsp** chili powder

Exchanges/Choices

1 1/2 Starch
2 Vegetable
1/2 Fat

Basic Nutritional Values

Calories	185
Calories from Fat	40
Total Fat	4.5 g
Saturated Fat	0.4 g
Trans Fat	0.0 g
Cholesterol	0 mg
Sodium	115 mg
Total Carbohydrate	34 g
Dietary Fiber	6 g
Sugars	5 g
Protein	5 g

Cook pasta according to package directions; rinse and drain. Dice tomatoes, chop peppers and red onion. Thaw corn; cook in microwave for about 2 minutes. Place pasta in a large bowl; add all other ingredients and mix to blend. Chill for 1 hour before serving.

Baked Fish and Zucchini

Serves 4   Serving size: 1/4 recipe

1/4 **cup** no-added-salt tomato sauce

1 **tsp** lemon juice

1/2 **tsp** basil

Pepper, to taste

1 small zucchini, cut into 1/2-inch slices

1 **lb** fish fillets, any white-meat fish

1 **tsp** Smart Balance Omega oil

Exchanges/Choices

3 Lean Meat

Basic Nutritional Values

Calories	110
Calories from Fat	20
Total Fat	2.0 g
Saturated Fat	0.2 g
Trans Fat	0.0 g
Cholesterol	50 mg
Sodium	75 mg
Total Carbohydrate	2 g
Dietary Fiber	1 g
Sugars	1 g
Protein	21 g

Combine tomato sauce, lemon juice, basil, pepper, and zucchini. Place fish in an oven-safe pan and add oil. Cover each fillet with a portion of the mixture; bake at 375°F for 12 minutes or until fish flakes easily when pierced with a fork.

Perfection Salad

Serves 4   Serving size: 1/4 recipe

1 (0.3-oz) box sugar-free raspberry gelatin

2 **tsp** vinegar

1/2 head cabbage, shredded

2 carrots, shredded

Make gelatin according to package directions. Add vinegar, cabbage, and carrots. Refrigerate 2 hours before serving.

Exchanges/Choices

2 Vegetable

Basic Nutritional Values

Calories	50
Calories from Fat	0
Total Fat	0.0 g
Saturated Fat	0.0 g
Trans Fat	0.0 g
Cholesterol	0 mg
Sodium	105 mg
Total Carbohydrate	10 g
Dietary Fiber	4 g
Sugars	6 g
Protein	3 g

Potatoes Au Gratin

Serves 4   Serving size: 1/4 recipe

Nonstick cooking spray

2 **cups** red or russet potatoes, peeled and cubed

1/2 **cup** nonfat milk

1/2 **Tbsp** whole-wheat flour

3/16 **tsp** pepper

2 **oz** fat-free shredded cheddar cheese

1 1/2 **oz** reduced-fat shredded cheddar cheese

1. Preheat oven to 375°F. Lightly spray a 9-inch baking dish with nonstick cooking spray.

2. In a mixing bowl, add potato cubes, cover with cold water, and set aside.

3. In a saucepan, whisk together the milk, flour, and pepper until well blended. Stirring constantly over medium-high heat, bring to a full boil. Reduce heat to low and stir in the cheeses; simmer until cheese is melted.

4. Drain potatoes and place in baking dish. Pour cheese mixture on top of potatoes. Bake for 1 hour or until potatoes are tender.

Exchanges/Choices

1 Starch
1 Lean Meat

Basic Nutritional Values

Calories	135
Calories from Fat	20
Total Fat	2.5 g
Saturated Fat	1.4 g
Trans Fat	0.0 g
Cholesterol	10 mg
Sodium	245 mg
Total Carbohydrate	19 g
Dietary Fiber	2 g
Sugars	3 g
Protein	10 g

Strawberry Whip Parfaits

Serves 4   Serving size: 1/4 recipe

2 **cups** sliced strawberries

2 **cups** fat-free whipped topping

4 (**1-oz**) slices angel food cake

Place sliced strawberries in an electric blender. Cover and blend until smooth, stopping once to scrape the sides. Fold strawberry puree into whipped topping. Tear angel food cake into pieces and fold into strawberry mixture. Spoon into parfait glasses, cover, and serve chilled.

Exchanges/Choices

2 Carbohydrate

Basic Nutritional Values

Calories 125
  Calories from Fat 15
Total Fat . . . . .1.5 g
  Saturated Fat . . . . .0.6 g
  Trans Fat . . . . .0.0 g
Cholesterol . . . . .5 mg
Sodium . . . . .160 mg
Total Carbohydrate . . .27 g
  Dietary Fiber . . . . .2 g
  Sugars . . . . .16 g
Protein . . . . .3 g

Pumpkin Spice Muffins

Serves 8   Serving size: 2 muffins

1 **cup** whole-wheat flour	1 **cup** canned pumpkin
3 **tsp** baking powder	1/2 **cup** nonfat milk
2 **tsp** ground cinnamon	1/4 **cup** unsweetened
2 **tsp** ground nutmeg	applesauce
1/4 **cup** egg substitute	1/4 **cup** raisins or chopped nuts
2 **Tbsp** Splenda	

Preheat oven to 400°F. Line sixteen muffin-pan cups with paper liners or spray with nonstick cooking spray. In a large bowl, stir together the flour, baking powder, cinnamon, and nutmeg. In a medium bowl, beat egg substitute with a whisk. Add Splenda, pumpkin, milk, and applesauce; stir until well blended. Stir in raisins. Stir into flour mixture until just blended. Fill muffin-pan cups 2/3 full. Bake 20–25 minutes until a wooden toothpick inserted in the center comes out clean. Remove muffins from muffin pans. Serve warm or at room temperature.

Exchanges/Choices

1 1/2 Carbohydrate

Basic Nutritional Values

Calories 95
 Calories from Fat 5
Total Fat . . . . 0.5 g
 Saturated Fat . . . . 0.2 g
 Trans Fat . . . . 0.0 g
Cholesterol . . . . 0 mg
Sodium . . . . 160 mg
Total Carbohydrate . . . 20 g
 Dietary Fiber . . . . 3 g
 Sugars . . . . 6 g
Protein . . . . 4 g

Ham and Swiss Roll-Up

Serves 4   Serving size: 3 roll-ups

12 (**6-inch**) corn tortillas	1 **cup** shredded lettuce
8 **oz** light ham	4 slices tomato, diced
4 slices reduced-fat Swiss cheese	4 **Tbsp** yellow mustard

Lay each tortilla on a flat surface and the place equal portions of the ham on each one. Slice the cheese into 3 equal slices and place on the ham. Place the lettuce and mustard on top. Roll up the tortillas.

This recipe is high in sodium.

Exchanges/Choices

2 1/2 Starch
2 Lean Meat

Basic Nutritional Values

Calories 300
 Calories from Fat 65
Total Fat . . . . 7.0 g
 Saturated Fat . . . . 2.5 g
 Trans Fat . . . . 0.0 g
Cholesterol . . . . 40 mg
Sodium . . . . 640 mg
Total Carbohydrate . . . 38 g
 Dietary Fiber . . . . 4 g
 Sugars . . . . 4 g
Protein . . . . 23 g

Dilled Summer Squash

Serves 4   Serving size: 1/4 recipe

1 **cup** yellow summer squash, sliced thin

1 **cup** zucchini, sliced thin

2 **Tbsp** Smart Balance Light Spread

1 **Tbsp** dill weed

1 **Tbsp** lemon juice

Cook squash and zucchini together in water for a few minutes; drain. Add margarine, dill weed, and lemon juice. Serve hot.

Exchanges/Choices
1/2 Fat

Basic Nutritional Values

Calories	30
Calories from Fat	20
Total Fat	2.5 g
Saturated Fat	0.8 g
Trans Fat	0.0 g
Cholesterol	0 mg
Sodium	45 mg
Total Carbohydrate	2 g
Dietary Fiber	1 g
Sugars	1 g
Protein	1 g

Quick and Easy Chili

Serves 6   Serving size: 1/6 recipe

Nonstick cooking spray

1 **lb** 96% lean ground beef

1/2 **cup** chopped onion (about 1 large)

1/2 **cup** chopped green bell pepper (about 2 small)

6 garlic cloves, minced

1 **(14-oz)** can no-added-salt stewed tomatoes, chopped and juice reserved

1 **(15-oz)** can no-added-salt kidney beans, rinsed and drained

1 **(8-oz)** can no-added-salt tomato sauce

1 **(1-oz)** envelope onion soup mix

1 **cup** water

1 **Tbsp** no-added-salt chili powder

1 **Tbsp** paprika

1 **tsp** hot sauce

Exchanges/Choices
1 Starch
2 Vegetable
2 Lean Meat
1/2 Fat

Basic Nutritional Values

Calories	240
Calories from Fat	65
Total Fat	7.0 g
Saturated Fat	2.5 g
Trans Fat	0.4 g
Cholesterol	45 mg
Sodium	545 mg
Total Carbohydrate	24 g
Dietary Fiber	6 g
Sugars	9 g
Protein	21 g

Lightly spray a Dutch oven with nonstick cooking spray; heat over medium-high heat. Add beef, onion, pepper, and garlic. Cook until meat is browned, stirring until it crumbles. Drain away fat. Return mixture to pan; add all remaining ingredients. Bring to a boil; cover, reduce heat, and simmer 20 minutes, stirring occasionally. To serve, ladle chili into bowls.

Zesty Orange Oats Peach Crisp

Serves 9   Serving size: 1/9 recipe

Nonstick cooking spray

4 Tbsp Splenda

1 1/2 Tbsp whole-wheat flour

1 tsp ground ginger

1 tsp pure vanilla extract

6 cups fresh peach chunks

1 cup old-fashioned oats, uncooked

1/2 cup chopped walnuts

Dash allspice

Dash cinnamon

2 Tbsp Smart Balance margarine

1 small orange, peeled and chopped

Exchanges/Choices

1 1/2 Carbohydrate
1 Fat

Basic Nutritional Values

Calories 150
  Calories from Fat 65
Total Fat . . . . 7.0 g
  Saturated Fat . . . . 1.1 g
  Trans Fat . . . . 0.0 g
Cholesterol . . . . 0 mg
Sodium . . . . 20 mg
Total Carbohydrate . . . 20 g
  Dietary Fiber . . . . 3 g
  Sugars . . . . 10 g
Protein . . . . 4 g

1. Spray a 9-inch glass baking dish with nonstick cooking spray. Combine 2 Tbsp Splenda, flour, ginger, and vanilla until mixed well. Fold in peaches until evenly coated. Spoon peaches into prepared glass baking dish.

2. Combine oats, walnuts, allspice, cinnamon, 2 Tbsp Splenda, margarine, and orange; blend well. Sprinkle evenly over peach filling. Bake at 350°F for 35–40 minutes (or until golden brown and the filling is bubbly).

Sweet and Sour Chicken Salad

Serves 4   Serving size: 1/4 recipe

3/4 **lb** boneless, skinless chicken breast (trimmed of any visible fat), cooked and cut into 1/2-inch cubes

1 **cup** celery, sliced diagonally

3/4 **cup** snow peas

1/2 **cup** diced red pepper

3/4 **cup** apples, cored and diced

1/4 **cup** cider vinegar

1 **Tbsp** Smart Balance Omega oil

2 **Tbsp** Splenda

1 **tsp** celery seeds

1 **tsp** paprika

Pepper, to taste

Exchanges/Choices

1/2 Carbohydrate
4 Lean Meat

Basic Nutritional Values

Calories 205
  Calories from Fat 65
Total Fat . . . . 7.0 g
  Saturated Fat . . . . 1.2 g
  Trans Fat . . . . 0.0 g
Cholesterol . . . . 70 mg
Sodium . . . . 90 mg
Total Carbohydrate . . . 8 g
  Dietary Fiber . . . . 2 g
  Sugars . . . . 5 g
Protein . . . . 27 g

Combine all ingredients; let cool before serving.

Zucchini Bread

Serves 8   Serving size: 1 slice

Nonstick cooking spray

1 **cup** whole-wheat flour

1/2 **cup** Splenda Brown Sugar Blend

1 **tsp** baking powder

1 **tsp** ground cinnamon

1/4 **tsp** baking soda

1 **cup** shredded zucchini

1 **Tbsp** finely chopped walnuts

1/4 **cup** egg substitute

1 **Tbsp** Smart Balance Omega oil

1/2 **tsp** vanilla extract

1/2 **cup** pineapple juice

Exchanges/Choices

2 Carbohydrate

Basic Nutritional Values

Calories 140
  Calories from Fat 20
Total Fat . . . . 2.5 g
  Saturated Fat . . . . 0.2 g
  Trans Fat . . . . 0.0 g
Cholesterol . . . . 0 mg
Sodium . . . . 105 mg
Total Carbohydrate . . . 26 g
  Dietary Fiber . . . . 2 g
  Sugars . . . . 14 g
Protein . . . . 3 g

Preheat the oven to 350°F. Spray a 9 × 5 × 3-inch loaf pan with nonstick cooking spray. In a large bowl, combine the flour, Splenda, baking powder, cinnamon, and baking soda. Then stir in the zucchini and walnuts. In a small bowl, combine the egg substitute with the oil, vanilla extract, and the pineapple juice. Combine ingredients from both bowls and stir until moistened. Pour the batter into the baking dish. Bake about 1 hour or until a toothpick inserted into the center of the loaf comes out clean.

Cinnamon Red Cabbage

Serves 4   Serving size: 1/4 recipe

4 **cups** red cabbage

1 medium Granny Smith apple

1 medium pear

1/4 **cup** sugar-free orange marmalade

1 **tsp** cinnamon

1 **tsp** ground cloves

3 **Tbsp** red wine vinegar

3 **Tbsp** red table wine

Thinly slice the cabbage. Peel and slice the apple. Peel and chop the pear. In a large pot, combine the cabbage, apple, pear, marmalade, cinnamon, cloves, vinegar, wine, and 1 cup water. Bring to a boil and cook the mixture, covered, over moderately low heat, stirring occasionally, for 3 hours. Serve the cabbage chilled as an accompaniment to cold sliced meats.

Exchanges/Choices

1 Fruit
1 Vegetable

Basic Nutritional Values

Calories	80
Calories from Fat	0
Total Fat	0.0 g
Saturated Fat	0.1 g
Trans Fat	0.0 g
Cholesterol	0 mg
Sodium	15 mg
Total Carbohydrate	22 g
Dietary Fiber	4 g
Sugars	14 g
Protein	1 g

Asian Pork Chops

Servings 4   Serving size: 1/4 recipe

3/4 **lb** boneless sirloin pork chops (trimmed of visible fat)

1 **Tbsp** Smart Balance Omega oil

1 (**16-oz**) pkg frozen vegetables, including broccoli, carrots, water chestnuts, and red pepper

1/4 **cup** stir-fry sauce

2 **cups** canned light pineapple chunks, drained and syrup reserved

2 **Tbsp** Splenda

1/2 **tsp** cornstarch

Heat a nonstick skillet over medium-high heat. Brush chops lightly with oil. Cook for 6 minutes, turning once, until evenly browned. Add vegetables to skillet. In a small bowl, stir together stir-fry sauce, pineapple juice, Splenda, and cornstarch; add to skillet with vegetables. Reduce heat to low; cover and cook for 8–10 minutes or until vegetables are crisp-tender. Stir in pineapple chunks. Cook for 3–5 minutes or until sauce thickens slightly.

Exchanges/Choices

1 1/2 Fruit
1 Vegetable
2 Lean Meat
1 Fat

Basic Nutritional Values

Calories	260
Calories from Fat	65
Total Fat	7.0 g
Saturated Fat	0.8 g
Trans Fat	0.0 g
Cholesterol	40 mg
Sodium	495 mg
Total Carbohydrate	31 g
Dietary Fiber	4 g
Sugars	27 g
Protein	17 g

Raspberry Smoothie

Serves 4   Serving size: 1/4 recipe

8 **oz** fat-free lemon yogurt   2 **cups** raspberries

1 **cup** fat-free whipped topping   4 ice cubes

Combine ingredients in a blender; cover and process until smooth.

Exchanges/Choices

1 Carbohydrate

Basic Nutritional Values

Calories 85
 Calories from Fat 0
Total Fat . . . . 0.0 g
 Saturated Fat . . . . 0.0 g
 Trans Fat . . . . 0.0 g
Cholesterol . . . . 0 mg
Sodium . . . . 30 mg
Total Carbohydrate . . . 18 g
 Dietary Fiber . . . . 4 g
 Sugars . . . . 9 g
Protein . . . . 2 g

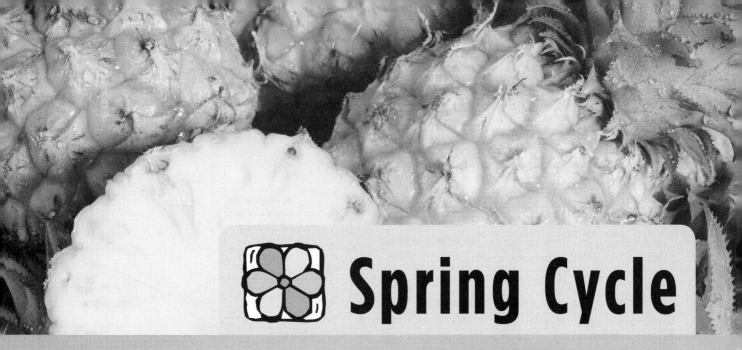

Spring Cycle

WEEK 2

FEATURED RECIPES

French Toast*
Sizzlin' Fruit Salad*
Sweet Potatoes and Walnuts
Low-Fat, Low-Sugar Carrot Cake
Grilled Marinated Fish
Multigrain Rice Pilaf
Green Beans, Celery, and Onions
Shredded Wheat Custard
Beef Pita Tacos
Tex-Mex Salad
Green Bean Sesame Salad
Chipotle Chicken Skewers with Dipping Sauce
Corn and Zucchini Combo
Waldorf Salad
Bran Muffins
Peach and Apple Crisp*
Southwestern Black-Eyed Pea Salad
Citrus Halibut Steak

Parmesan Potatoes*
Tuna Melt Muffin
Texas Marinated Flank Steak
Blackberry Cobbler
Fruit Salad Medley*
Low-Fat Corn Bread*
Grilled Portobello on Whole-Wheat Bread
Sweet and Sour Red Cabbage
Baked Chicken and Pineapple
Vegetable Salad
Apple Oatmeal Squares
Chicken Soft Tacos
Dijon Pork Cutlets
Three Bean Salad
Grilled Marinated Pineapple
Chicken Macaroni Salad
Sliced Tomato Salad
Spicy Chicken and Brown Rice
Oven-Roasted Tomatoes*

*Indicates that the recipe has been used previously.

1500 calorie MEAL PLAN SPRING WEEK 2

	Sunday	Monday	Tuesday	Wednesday	Thursday	Friday	Saturday
Breakfast	French Toast* Sizzlin' Fruit Salad* 1 cup nonfat milk 1 oz lean turkey sausage 1 tsp margarine	Shredded Wheat Custard (1/2 serving) 1/3 cup baked beans 1/2 Tbsp dried cranberries 1/2 cup nonfat milk 4 Brazil nuts	Bran Muffins Peach and Apple Crisp* 1 cup nonfat milk 1 1/2 tsp margarine	1/4 cup Grape Nuts cereal 1 slice oatmeal bread 1/2 cup mango 3/4 cup fat-free yogurt 1 tsp margarine 4 pecans	Fruit Salad Medley* Low-Fat Corn Bread* 1/2 tsp margarine	Apple Oatmeal Squares 1/2 cup shredded wheat 1 cup nonfat milk 9 almonds	Grilled Marinated Pineapple 1 cup cream of wheat cereal 1 cup nonfat milk 1/2 tsp margarine
Lunch	Sweet Potatoes and Walnuts Low-Fat, Low-Sugar Carrot Cake 1 slice whole-wheat bread 1/2 cup collard greens 2 oz roasted pork tenderloin 1 tsp margarine	Beef Pita Tacos Tex-Mex Salad Green Bean Sesame Salad 1/2 cup fat-free, no-added-sugar ice cream	Southwestern Black-Eyed Pea Salad (2 servings) 6 saltine crackers 1 small apple	Tuna Melt Muffin 1/2 cup peas 1 kiwi fruit 1 tsp margarine	Grilled Portobello on Whole-Wheat Bread Sweet and Sour Red Cabbage 1/2 large pear 1/2 cup fat-free cottage cheese	Chicken Soft Tacos 5 oz corn on the cob 3/4 oz baked tortilla chips 3/4 cup mandarin oranges packed in juice 1 tsp margarine	Chicken Macaroni Salad (1/2 serving) Sliced Tomato Salad (1/2 serving) 2 small dinner rolls 1 medium banana 1/2 cup celery sticks
Snack A							
Snack B							
Dinner	Grilled Marinated Fish Multigrain Rice Pilaf Green Beans, Celery, and Onions 1 cup nonfat milk 2 Tbsp pine nuts	Chipotle Chicken Skewers with Dipping Sauce Corn and Zucchini Combo Waldorf Salad 1/2 cup boiled red potatoes 1 cup nonfat milk 1/2 cup cooked spinach 1/2 tsp margarine	Citrus Halibut Steak Parmesan Potatoes* 1/2 cup nonfat milk 2 tsp margarine	Texas Marinated Flank Steak Blackberry Cobbler 1 medium peach 1 cup nonfat milk 1 cup cooked broccoli and cauliflower 1/2 tsp margarine	Baked Chicken and Pineapple Vegetable Salad 2 oz avocado	Dijon Pork Cutlets Three Bean Salad 1/2 slice oatmeal bread 3/4 cup blueberries 1 cup nonfat milk 1/2 cup cooked cabbage 1/2 tsp margarine	Spicy Chicken and Brown Rice Oven-Roasted Tomatoes* 9 cashews

*Indicates that the recipe has been used previously.

	Sunday	Monday	Tuesday	Wednesday	Thursday	Friday	Saturday
Breakfast	French Toast* Sizzlin' Fruit Salad* 1 cup nonfat milk 1 oz lean turkey sausage 1 tsp margarine	Shredded Wheat Custard (1/2 serving) 1/3 cup baked beans 1/2 Tbsp dried cranberries 1/2 cup nonfat milk 4 Brazil nuts	Bran Muffins Peach and Apple Crisp* 1 cup nonfat milk 1 oz smoked salmon (lox) 1 1/2 tsp margarine	1/4 cup Grape Nuts cereal 1 slice oatmeal bread 1/2 cup mango 3/4 cup fat-free yogurt 1 oz lean ham 1 tsp margarine 4 pecans	Fruit Salad Medley* Low-Fat Corn Bread* 1/4 cup egg substitute, scrambled 1 1/2 tsp margarine	Apple Oatmeal Squares 1/2 cup shredded wheat 1 cup nonfat milk 9 almonds	Grilled Marinated Pineapple 1 cup cream of wheat cereal 1 cup nonfat milk 1/4 cup cottage cheese 1 tsp margarine
Lunch	Sweet Potatoes and Walnuts Low-Fat, Low-Sugar Carrot Cake 1 slice whole-wheat bread 1/2 cup collard greens 2 oz roasted pork tenderloin 2 tsp margarine	Beef Pita Tacos Tex-Mex Salad Green Bean Sesame Salad 1/2 cup fat-free, no-added-sugar ice cream	Southwestern Black-Eyed Pea Salad (2 servings) 6 saltine crackers 1 small apple 1 cup salad greens 2 Tbsp light salad dressing	Tuna Melt Muffin 1/2 cup refried beans 1 kiwi fruit 1 tsp margarine 10 stuffed green olives	Grilled Portobello on Whole-Wheat Bread Sweet and Sour Red Cabbage 1/2 large pear 1/2 cup fat-free cottage cheese	Chicken Soft Tacos 5 oz corn on the cob 3/4 oz baked tortilla chips 3/4 cup mandarin oranges packed in juice 1 tsp margarine 8 large black olives	Chicken Macaroni Salad (1/2 serving) Sliced Tomato Salad (1/2 serving) 2 small dinner rolls 1 medium banana 1/2 cup celery sticks 1/2 tsp margarine
Snack A	1 cup raspberries	16 pistachios 3/4 oz chewy fruit snack	3 macadamia nuts 3 prunes	5 hazelnuts 1 medium peach	2 Tbsp sunflower seeds 1 1/4 cups strawberries	4 walnut halves 2 medium figs	1 Tbsp pine nuts 2 small plums
Snack B	1/2 cup frozen yogurt	3/4 cup fat-free yogurt	1 cup nonfat buttermilk	1 cup nonfat milk	1 cup nonfat milk	1 cup nonfat milk	1 cup nonfat milk
Dinner	Grilled Marinated Fish Multigrain Rice Pilaf Green Beans, Celery, and Onions 1 cup nonfat milk 2 Tbsp pine nuts	Chipotle Chicken Skewers with Dipping Sauce Corn and Zucchini Combo Waldorf Salad 1/4 cup boiled red potatoes 1 cup nonfat milk 1/2 cup cooked spinach 1/2 tsp margarine	Citrus Halibut Steak Parmesan Potatoes* 1/2 cup nonfat milk 1 cup steamed asparagus 2 tsp margarine	Texas Marinated Flank Steak Blackberry Cobbler 1 medium peach 1 cup nonfat milk 1 cup cooked broccoli and cauliflower 1/2 tsp margarine	Baked Chicken and Pineapple Vegetable Salad 2 oz avocado	Dijon Pork Cutlets Three Bean Salad 1/2 slice oatmeal bread 3/4 cup blueberries 1 cup nonfat milk 1/2 cup cooked cabbage 1/2 tsp margarine	Spicy Chicken and Brown Rice Oven-Roasted Tomatoes* 1 cup salad greens 1 1/2 Tbsp light salad dressing

*Indicates that the recipe has been used previously.

2000 calorie MEAL PLAN SPRING WEEK 2

	Sunday	Monday	Tuesday	Wednesday	Thursday	Friday	Saturday
Breakfast	French Toast* Sizzlin' Fruit Salad* 1 cup nonfat milk 1 oz lean turkey sausage 1 tsp margarine	Shredded Wheat Custard (1/2 serving) 1/3 cup baked beans 1/2 Tbsp dried cranberries 1/2 cup nonfat milk 4 Brazil nuts	Bran Muffins Peach and Apple Crisp* 1 cup nonfat milk 1 oz smoked salmon (lox) 1 1/2 tsp margarine	1/4 cup Grape Nuts cereal 1 slice oatmeal bread 1/2 cup mango 3/4 cup fat-free yogurt 1 oz lean ham 1 tsp margarine 4 pecans	Fruit Salad Medley* Low-Fat Corn Bread* 1/4 cup egg substitute, scrambled 1 1/2 tsp margarine	Apple Oatmeal Squares 1/2 cup shredded wheat 1 cup nonfat milk 9 almonds	Grilled Marinated Pineapple 1 cup cream of wheat cereal 1 cup nonfat milk 1/4 cup cottage cheese 1 tsp margarine
Lunch	Sweet Potatoes and Walnuts Low-Fat, Low-Sugar Carrot Cake 1 slice whole-wheat bread 1 small orange 1 cup collard greens 2 oz roasted pork tenderloin 2 tsp margarine	Beef Pita Tacos Tex-Mex Salad Green Bean Sesame Salad 1/2 cup fat-free, no-added-sugar ice cream 1 small apple	Southwestern Black-Eyed Pea Salad (2 servings) 6 saltine crackers 1 large apple 2 cups salad greens 2 Tbsp light salad dressing	Tuna Melt Muffin 1/2 cup refried beans 1 kiwi fruit 1/2 cup canned picked beets 1 tsp margarine 10 stuffed green olives	Grilled Portobello on Whole-Wheat Bread Sweet and Sour Red Cabbage 1 large pear 1/2 cup cooked Brussels sprouts 1/2 cup fat-free cottage cheese	Chicken Soft Tacos 5 oz corn on the cob 3/4 oz baked tortilla chips 1 1/2 cups mandarin oranges packed in juice 1 cup tomato slices 1 tsp margarine 8 large black olives	Chicken Macaroni Salad (1/2 serving) Sliced Tomato Salad (1/2 serving) 2 small dinner rolls 1 large banana 1/2 cup celery sticks 1/2 cup cooked spinach 1/2 tsp margarine
Snack A	1 cup cauliflower 1 cup raspberries	1/2 small bagel 16 pistachios 3/4 oz chewy fruit snack	1 cup tomato juice 3 macadamia nuts 3 prunes	1 cup mixed raw vegetables 5 hazelnuts 1 medium peach	1 cup mixed vegetable sticks 2 Tbsp sunflower seeds 1 1/4 cup strawberries	1 cup cucumber sticks 4 walnut halves 2 medium figs	1/2 cup steamed green beans 1 Tbsp pine nuts 2 small plums
Snack B	1 small muffin 1/2 tsp margarine 1/2 cup frozen yogurt	1 cup mixed raw vegetables 1 tsp margarine 3/4 cup fat-free yogurt	2 rice cakes 1 1/2 tsp almond butter 1 cup nonfat buttermilk	8 animal crackers 10 peanuts 1 cup nonfat milk	1 cup tomato soup 1 cup nonfat milk	3/4 oz whole-wheat crackers 1 Tbsp light salad dressing 1 cup nonfat milk	1/2 whole-wheat bagel 1 Tbsp margarine 1 cup nonfat milk
Dinner	Grilled Marinated Fish Multigrain Rice Pilaf Green Beans, Celery, and Onions 1 cup nonfat milk 2 Tbsp pine nuts	Chipotle Chicken Skewers with Dipping Sauce Corn and Zucchini Combo Waldorf Salad 1/4 cup boiled red potatoes 1 cup nonfat milk 1/2 cup cooked spinach 1/2 tsp margarine	Citrus Halibut Steak Parmesan Potatoes* 1/2 cup nonfat milk 1 cup steamed asparagus 2 tsp margarine	Texas Marinated Flank Steak Blackberry Cobbler 1 medium peach 1 cup nonfat milk 1 cup cooked broccoli and cauliflower 1/2 tsp margarine	Baked Chicken and Pineapple Vegetable Salad 2 oz avocado	Dijon Pork Cutlets Three Bean Salad 1/2 slice oatmeal bread 3/4 cup blueberries 1 cup nonfat milk 1/2 cup cooked cabbage 1/2 tsp margarine	Spicy Chicken and Brown Rice Oven-Roasted Tomatoes* 1 cup salad greens 1 1/2 Tbsp light salad dressing

*Indicates that the recipe has been used previously.

	Sunday	Monday	Tuesday	Wednesday	Thursday	Friday	Saturday
Breakfast	French Toast* Sizzlin' Fruit Salad* 1 cup nonfat milk 2 oz lean turkey sausage 1 tsp margarine	Shredded Wheat Custard (1/2 serving) 1/3 cup baked beans 1/2 Tbsp dried cranberries 1/2 cup nonfat milk 1 oz reduced-fat cheese 4 Brazil nuts	Bran Muffins Peach and Apple Crisp* 1 cup nonfat milk 2 oz smoked salmon (lox) 1 1/2 tsp margarine	1/4 cup Grape Nuts cereal 1 slice oatmeal bread 1/2 cup mango 3/4 cup fat-free yogurt 2 oz lean ham 1 tsp margarine 4 pecans	Fruit Salad Medley* Low-Fat Corn Bread* 1/2 cup egg substitute, scrambled 1 1/2 tsp margarine	Apple Oatmeal Squares 1/2 cup shredded wheat 1 cup nonfat milk 1 oz lean sausage 9 almonds	Grilled Marinated Pineapple 1 cup cream of wheat cereal 1 cup nonfat milk 1/2 cup cottage cheese 1 tsp margarine
Lunch	Sweet Potatoes and Walnuts Low-Fat, Low-Sugar Carrot Cake 1 slice whole-wheat bread 1 small orange 1 cup collard greens 2 oz roasted pork tenderloin 2 tsp margarine	Beef Pita Tacos Tex-Mex Salad Green Bean Sesame Salad 1/2 cup fat-free, no-added-sugar ice cream 1 small apple	Southwestern Black-Eyed Pea Salad (2 servings) 6 saltine crackers 1 large apple 2 cups salad greens 2 Tbsp light salad dressing	Tuna Melt Muffin 1/2 cup refried beans 1 kiwi fruit 1/2 cup canned picked beets 1 tsp margarine 10 stuffed green olives	Grilled Portobello on Whole-Wheat Bread Sweet and Sour Red Cabbage 1 large pear 1/2 cup cooked Brussels sprouts 1/2 cup fat-free cottage cheese	Chicken Soft Tacos 5 oz corn on the cob 3/4 oz baked tortilla chips 1 1/2 cups mandarin oranges packed in juice 1 cup tomato slices 1 tsp margarine 8 large black olives	Chicken Macaroni Salad (1/2 serving) Sliced Tomato Salad (1/2 serving) 2 small dinner rolls 1 large banana 1/2 cup celery sticks 1/2 cup cooked spinach 1/2 tsp margarine
Snack A	1 cup cauliflower 1 cup raspberries	1/2 small bagel 16 pistachios 3/4 oz chewy fruit snack	1 cup tomato juice 3 macadamia nuts 3 prunes	1 cup mixed raw vegetables 5 hazelnuts 1 medium peach	1 cup mixed vegetable sticks 2 Tbsp sunflower seeds 1 1/4 cup strawberries	1 cup cucumber sticks 4 walnut halves 2 medium figs	1/2 cup steamed green beans 1 Tbsp pine nuts 2 small plums
Snack B	1 small muffin 1/2 tsp margarine 1/2 cup frozen yogurt	1 cup mixed raw vegetables 1 tsp margarine 3/4 cup fat-free yogurt	2 rice cakes 1 1/2 tsp almond butter 1 cup nonfat buttermilk	8 animal crackers 10 peanuts 1 cup nonfat milk	1 cup tomato soup 1 cup nonfat milk	3/4 oz whole-wheat crackers 1 Tbsp light salad dressing 1 cup nonfat milk	1/2 whole-wheat bagel 1 Tbsp margarine 1 cup nonfat milk
Dinner	Grilled Marinated Fish Multigrain Rice Pilaf Green Beans, Celery, and Onions 17 grapes 1 cup nonfat milk 2 Tbsp pine nuts	Chipotle Chicken Skewers with Dipping Sauce Corn and Zucchini Combo Waldorf Salad 3/4 cup boiled red potatoes 1 cup nonfat milk 1/2 cup cooked spinach 1/2 tsp margarine	Citrus Halibut Steak Parmesan Potatoes* 1 small dinner roll 1/2 cup nonfat milk 1 cup steamed asparagus 2 tsp margarine	Texas Marinated Flank Steak Blackberry Cobbler 1 slice wheat bread 1 medium peach 1 cup nonfat milk 1 cup cooked broccoli and cauliflower 1/2 tsp margarine	Baked Chicken and Pineapple Vegetable Salad 1/2 cup parsnips 2 oz avocado	Dijon Pork Cutlets Three Bean Salad 1 1/2 slices oatmeal bread 3/4 cup blueberries 1 cup nonfat milk 1/2 cup cooked cabbage 1/2 tsp margarine	Spicy Chicken and Brown Rice Oven-Roasted Tomatoes* 1 cup salad greens 1 1/2 Tbsp light salad dressing

*Indicates that the recipe has been used previously.

SHOPPING LIST SPRING WEEK 2

VEGETABLES
____ asparagus
____ avocado
____ bell peppers, green
____ broccoli
____ Brussels sprouts
____ cabbage, red
____ carrots
____ cauliflower
____ celery
____ chili, chipotle
____ collard greens
____ corn on the cob
____ corn, whole-kernel, frozen
____ cucumber
____ garlic
____ green beans
____ jalapeño pepper
____ lettuce, romaine
____ mushrooms, Portobello
____ onions, green
____ onions, red
____ onions, yellow or white
____ potatoes, red
____ potatoes, sweet
____ salad greens
____ spinach
____ tomatoes
____ tomatoes, grape
____ zucchini squash

MEATS
____ beef flank steak
____ chicken breasts, boneless, skinless
____ fish fillets, your choice
____ ground beef, 96% lean
____ halibut steaks
____ ham, lean
____ pork chops, boneless sirloin
____ pork tenderloin, roasted
____ sausage, lean, turkey
____ smoked salmon (lox)
____ tuna, packed in water, 6-oz can

FRUITS
____ apples
____ apples, Red Delicious
____ bananas
____ blackberries
____ blueberries
____ cherries
____ cranberries, dried
____ grapefruit
____ kiwi fruit
____ lemon
____ lime (for zest)
____ mango
____ oranges
____ peaches
____ pears
____ pineapple
____ prunes, pitted
____ raisins
____ strawberries

DAIRY
____ egg substitute
____ egg whites
____ ice cream, fat-free, no-added-sugar
____ milk, nonfat
____ Smart Balance Light margarine
____ Smart Balance Light spread
____ sour cream, fat-free
____ whipped topping, fat-free
____ yogurt, fat-free, plain

CHEESE
____ cheddar, shredded, reduced-fat
____ cheddar, slices, reduced-fat
____ cottage cheese, fat-free
____ mozzarella, shredded, fat-free
____ Parmesan, grated, reduced-fat

BREAD, GRAINS, & PASTA
____ barley, pearl
____ bread, oatmeal
____ bread, whole-wheat, whole-grain
____ dinner rolls
____ English muffins, whole-wheat
____ macaroni, elbows or shells
____ pita bread, whole-wheat, 6-inch
____ rice, brown
____ rice, wild

BEANS

____ baked beans
____ black beans, no-added-salt, 15-oz can
____ black-eyed peas
____ garbanzo beans
____ kidney beans
____ refried beans

NUTS

____ almonds
____ Brazil nuts
____ pecans
____ pine nuts
____ walnuts

CONDIMENTS

____ canola mayonnaise
____ mustard, Dijon

SPICES & HERBS

____ basil
____ chili powder, no-added-salt
____ cilantro
____ cinnamon, ground
____ cloves, ground
____ cumin, ground
____ dill weed
____ dry mustard
____ garlic powder
____ ginger, ground
____ gingerroot
____ marjoram
____ mint
____ nutmeg, ground
____ onion powder
____ oregano
____ paprika
____ parsley
____ pepper
____ peppercorns, green
____ rosemary
____ thyme

OTHER

____ applesauce, unsweetened
____ beets, pickled, canned
____ biscuit mix
____ bread crumbs
____ cereal, all-bran
____ cereal, cream of wheat
____ cereal, Grape Nuts
____ cereal, shredded wheat
____ crackers, butter-flavored, reduced-fat
____ crackers, saltine
____ gelatin, unflavored
____ honey
____ oats, old-fashioned
____ olives, black
____ olives, green, stuffed
____ orange juice
____ orange juice, frozen, from concentrate
____ oranges, mandarin, packed in juice
____ pineapple chunks, canned, no-added-sugar
____ pineapple, crushed, canned light
____ roasted red peppers, 7-oz jar
____ salad dressing, Italian, light
____ salsa, no-added-salt
____ sesame seeds
____ tortilla chips, baked
____ tortillas, flour, 6-inch

STAPLES

____ baking powder
____ baking soda
____ bouillon, chicken, sodium-free
____ cornmeal
____ cornstarch
____ flour, whole-wheat
____ lemon juice
____ lime juice
____ nonstick cooking spray
____ sherry, dry cooking
____ Smart Balance Omega oil
____ Splenda
____ Splenda Brown Sugar Blend
____ vanilla extract
____ vinegar, balsamic
____ vinegar, cider
____ vinegar, red wine
____ vinegar, white

French Toast

Serves 4   Serving size: 2 slices

1 **Tbsp** Splenda

1/2 **tsp** pure vanilla extract

2 **cups** nonfat milk

1 **cup** egg substitute

8 **slices** whole-grain bread

2 **Tbsp** Smart Balance Light Spread

Beat Splenda, vanilla, milk, and egg substitute with a beater until well blended and smooth. Soak bread in batter. Heat margarine in skillet and carefully transfer bread to the skillet. Cook bread over medium heat until browned and then flip to cook the other side.

Exchanges/Choices

1 1/2 Starch
1/2 Fat-Free Milk
1 Lean Meat
1/2 Fat

Basic Nutritional Values

Calories 240
  Calories from Fat 40
Total Fat . . . . .4.5 g
  Saturated Fat . . . . .1.2 g
  Trans Fat . . . . .0.0 g
Cholesterol . . . . .0 mg
Sodium . . . . .485 mg
Total Carbohydrate . . .31 g
  Dietary Fiber . . . . .4 g
  Sugars . . . . .10 g
Protein . . . . .18 g

Sizzlin' Fruit Salad

Serves 4   Serving size: 1/4 recipe

1/2 **cup** sliced pears
(can use fresh, frozen,
or canned light, drained)

1/2 **cup** fresh cherries
(or canned light, drained)

1/2 **cup** fresh cubed pineapple
(or canned light, drained)

2 medium oranges, peeled
and cut into cubes

1 **cup** water

1/2 **cup** Splenda

2 **Tbsp** Smart Balance
margarine

1 **Tbsp** cornstarch

1 **Tbsp** lemon juice

1/4 **cup** dry cooking sherry

1/2 **cup** raisins

Exchanges/Choices

3 Fruit
1 Fat

Basic Nutritional Values

Calories	205
Calories from Fat	45
Total Fat	5.0 g
Saturated Fat	1.3 g
Trans Fat	0.0 g
Cholesterol	0 mg
Sodium	55 mg
Total Carbohydrate	42 g
Dietary Fiber	4 g
Sugars	34 g
Protein	2 g

1. Combine pears, cherries, and pineapple in an ovenproof glass bowl.

2. Combine orange cubes and water in a saucepan. Heat to boiling and simmer 5–10 minutes or until oranges are tender. Strain; add to pears, cherries, and pineapple. Sprinkle the Splenda on top.

3. Melt the margarine and combine with cornstarch in a saucepan. Add lemon juice, sherry, and raisins; cook, stirring consistently, until thickened. Pour over fruit and bake at 350°F for 30–45 minutes. Cool slightly before serving.

Sweet Potatoes and Walnuts

Serves 4   Serving size: 1/4 recipe

3/4 **lb** small sweet potatoes

1/4 **cup** orange juice

1 **Tbsp** chopped walnuts

1/4 **tsp** ground nutmeg

1/2 **tsp** ground cinnamon

Exchanges/Choices

1 1/2 Starch

Basic Nutritional Values

Calories	100
Calories from Fat	15
Total Fat	1.5 g
Saturated Fat	0.2 g
Trans Fat	0.0 g
Cholesterol	0 mg
Sodium	10 mg
Total Carbohydrate	21 g
Dietary Fiber	2 g
Sugars	6 g
Protein	2 g

Boil potatoes for about 30 minutes or until tender. Using a slotted spoon, transfer the potatoes to a large bowl of cold water and soak until cool enough to handle and peel. Heat the oven to 375°F. In a large bowl, mash the potatoes and stir in the remaining ingredients. Bake about 30 minutes or until heated through.

Low-Fat, Low-Sugar Carrot Cake

Serves 12   Serving size: 1 slice

- **1 cup** pitted prunes
- **3 Tbsp** water
- **4 cups** carrots, coarsely shredded
- **2 cups** Splenda
- **1 tsp** pure vanilla extract
- **1 cup** egg white substitute
- **1 cup** crushed pineapple (fresh, frozen, or canned light, drained)
- **2 cups** whole-wheat flour
- **2 tsp** baking powder
- **2 tsp** ground cinnamon
- **1/2 tsp** baking soda

Place prunes and water in a blender or food processor and process until smooth. Combine the prunes, carrots, Splenda, vanilla, egg white substitute, and pineapple; mix well. Sift together the whole-wheat flour, baking powder, cinnamon, and baking soda. Stir into carrot mixture. Spoon batter into a 9 × 13-inch baking dish. Bake at 375°F for 45 minutes.

Exchanges/Choices

2 Carbohydrate

Basic Nutritional Values

Calories	150
Calories from Fat	5
Total Fat	0.5 g
Saturated Fat	0.1 g
Trans Fat	0.0 g
Cholesterol	0 mg
Sodium	175 mg
Total Carbohydrate	33 g
Dietary Fiber	5 g
Sugars	14 g
Protein	6 g

Grilled Marinated Fish

Serves 4   Serving size: 1/4 recipe

- **1/2 cup** light Italian salad dressing
- **1/4 cup** green onions, chopped
- **2 Tbsp** lemon juice
  Pepper, to taste
- **1 lb** fish (fillet of sole, perch, halibut, turbot, or other)
- **1/4 cup** bread crumbs
- **1/4 cup** dried parsley
- **1 Tbsp** Smart Balance Light margarine, melted

Combine the salad dressing, green onions, lemon juice, and pepper. Pour over fish fillets and marinate in the refrigerator for at least 6 hours. Drain. Top with bread crumbs and parsley; drizzle melted margarine on top. Broil until the fish flakes easily with a fork, about 8–10 minutes.

Exchanges/Choices

1/2 Starch
3 Lean Meat

Basic Nutritional Values

Calories	165
Calories from Fat	35
Total Fat	4.0 g
Saturated Fat	0.9 g
Trans Fat	0.0 g
Cholesterol	60 mg
Sodium	345 mg
Total Carbohydrate	8 g
Dietary Fiber	1 g
Sugars	3 g
Protein	23 g

Multigrain Rice Pilaf

Serves 6   Serving size: 1/6 recipe

1/2 **cup** pearl barley	1/4 **cup** diced celery
1/2 **cup** parsley	1 **Tbsp** sodium-free chicken bouillon
1/2 **cup** wild rice, uncooked	1 **cup** water
1/2 **cup** brown rice, uncooked	1/2 **tsp** ground thyme
2 **Tbsp** Smart Balance Light margarine	1/2 **tsp** pepper
1/2 **cup** diced onion	

Rinse the pearl barley. Chop the parsley. Bring a large pot of water to a full boil and add the wild rice first. Let it cook for about 10 minutes and then add the barley and the brown rice (wild rice takes longer to cook). Reduce heat; simmer until tender. Drain and rinse under cold water. Melt margarine in a large skillet over medium heat. Add onions and celery; cook until tender, about 4 minutes. In a small bowl, combine the bouillon and water to create a broth. Add cooked rice mixture, broth, thyme, and pepper to the skillet; cook, stirring occasionally, until heated through, about 5 minutes. Add parsley just before serving.

Exchanges/Choices
2 1/2 Starch

Basic Nutritional Values
Calories 190
  Calories from Fat 20
Total Fat. . . . . 2.5 g
  Saturated Fat . . . . 0.7 g
  Trans Fat . . . . 0.0 g
Cholesterol . . . . 0 mg
Sodium. . . . . 40 mg
Total Carbohydrate . . . 38 g
  Dietary Fiber . . . . 4 g
  Sugars . . . . 2 g
Protein . . . . 4 g

Green Beans, Celery, and Onions

Serves 4   Serving size: 1/4 recipe

1 **lb** cut green beans, frozen or fresh	1/2 **cup** celery, sliced and diced
1 **Tbsp** Smart Balance Light margarine	1/2 **cup** onions, diced
	1 **Tbsp** dill weed

Steam the green beans until tender. Melt the margarine in a large skillet over medium heat; add celery and onions and cook until tender, about 2 minutes. Add steamed green beans and dill weed; toss to combine. Serve hot.

Exchanges/Choices
2 Vegetable

Basic Nutritional Values
Calories 50
  Calories from Fat 15
Total Fat. . . . . 1.5 g
  Saturated Fat . . . . 0.4 g
  Trans Fat . . . . 0.0 g
Cholesterol . . . . 0 mg
Sodium. . . . . 45 mg
Total Carbohydrate . . . 9 g
  Dietary Fiber . . . . 3 g
  Sugars . . . . 4 g
Protein . . . . 2 g

Shredded Wheat Custard

Serves 4 · Serving size: 1/4 recipe

1 quart nonfat milk, warm

6 shredded wheat biscuits, crushed

4 egg whites, beaten

1 tsp pure vanilla extract

1/2 cup Splenda

3/4 cup raisins

Combine the warm milk and crushed shredded wheat. Add egg whites, vanilla, Splenda, and raisins. Bake at 350°F for 60 minutes or until fully set (a knife inserted in the center comes out clean).

Exchanges/Choices

2 Starch
1 1/2 Fruit
1 Fat-Free Milk

Basic Nutritional Values

Calories 325
  Calories from Fat 5
Total Fat. . . . . 0.5 g
  Saturated Fat . . . . 0.2 g
  Trans Fat. . . . . 0.0 g
Cholesterol . . . . 5 mg
Sodium. . . . . 190 mg
Total Carbohydrate . . . 67 g
  Dietary Fiber . . . . 5 g
  Sugars . . . . 33 g
Protein . . . . 17 g

Beef Pita Tacos

Serves 4   Serving size: 1 taco

3/4 **lb** 96% lean ground beef

2 **Tbsp** whole-wheat flour

1/2 **cup** water

1 **tsp** no-added-salt chili powder

1/2 **tsp** ground cumin

1/4 **tsp** garlic powder

1/4 **tsp** onion powder

1/4 **tsp** pepper

2 **(6-inch)** whole-wheat pita breads, halved

1 1/2 **cups** shredded lettuce

2 chopped medium tomatoes (about 1 cup)

1/2 **cup** chopped green bell pepper

1/2 **cup** chopped onion

Exchanges/Choices

1 Starch
2 Vegetable
2 Lean Meat
1/2 Fat

Basic Nutritional Values

Calories 245
  Calories from Fat 55
Total Fat . . . . .6.0 g
  Saturated Fat . . . . .2.2 g
  Trans Fat . . . . .0.1 g
Cholesterol . . . . .50 mg
Sodium . . . . .235 mg
Total Carbohydrate . . .28 g
  Dietary Fiber . . . . .5 g
  Sugars . . . . .4 g
Protein . . . . .22 g

1. In a large nonstick skillet, cook beef over medium-high heat until brown, 8–10 minutes, stirring occasionally. Put beef in a colander and rinse with hot water to remove excess fat; drain well. Drain fat from the skillet and return beef. Sprinkle flour over meat, stirring to combine. Stir in water, chili powder, cumin, garlic powder, onion powder, and pepper. Bring to a simmer over medium-high heat, stirring occasionally. Cook for 3–4 minutes or until mixture is thickened, stirring occasionally.

2. Wrap pitas in aluminum foil and heat in the oven for 5 minutes to soften.

3. To serve, spoon about 2 Tbsp meat mixture into each pita half. Top each pita taco with lettuce, tomatoes, green pepper, and onion.

Tex-Mex Salad

Serves 4   Serving size: 1/4 recipe

1 (15-oz) can no-added-salt black beans, drained and rinsed

1/4 cup chopped green onions

1/4 cup frozen whole-kernel corn, thawed

1/2 cup no-added-salt salsa

4 large romaine lettuce leaves

Combine all ingredients, except lettuce, in a small bowl. Spoon bean mixture over torn romaine lettuce leaves.

Exchanges/Choices

1 Starch
1 Vegetable

Basic Nutritional Values

Calories 115
 Calories from Fat 0
Total Fat . . . . 0.0 g
 Saturated Fat . . . . 0.1 g
 Trans Fat . . . . 0.0 g
Cholesterol . . . . 0 mg
Sodium . . . . 75 mg
Total Carbohydrate . . . 22 g
 Dietary Fiber . . . . 5 g
 Sugars . . . . 4 g
Protein . . . . 7 g

Green Bean Sesame Salad

Serves 4   Serving size: 1/4 recipe

2 tsp Smart Balance Light margarine

2 Tbsp sesame seeds

2 cups cut green beans

2 Tbsp lemon juice
Pepper, to taste

Melt margarine in a skillet and add sesame seeds; cook for about 3 minutes. Bring a pot of water to a boil. Add the green beans and cook until tender, about 5 minutes; drain and rinse under cold water. Place in a bowl and toss with the sesame seeds, lemon juice, and margarine. Season to taste with pepper.

Exchanges/Choices

2 Vegetable
1/2 Fat

Basic Nutritional Values

Calories 70
 Calories from Fat 30
Total Fat . . . . 3.5 g
 Saturated Fat . . . . 0.6 g
 Trans Fat . . . . 0.0 g
Cholesterol . . . . 0 mg
Sodium . . . . 20 mg
Total Carbohydrate . . . 9 g
 Dietary Fiber . . . . 4 g
 Sugars . . . . 2 g
Protein . . . . 3 g

Chipotle Chicken Skewers with Dipping Sauce

Serves 4   Serving size: 1/4 recipe

3/4 **lb** boneless, skinless chicken breast (trimmed of fat)

1/4 **cup** Splenda Brown Sugar Blend

2 **Tbsp** minced cilantro leaves

1 chipotle chili, minced

1/2 **tsp** chili powder

1/4 **tsp** garlic powder

1/2 **tsp** ground black pepper

3/4 **cup** fat-free sour cream

1/4 **cup** canola mayonnaise

1/4 **cup** lime juice

1 clove garlic, minced

2 **Tbsp** minced cilantro leaves

2 green onions, minced

Nonstick cooking spray

Exchanges/Choices

1 Carbohydrate
3 Lean Meat
1/2 Fat

Basic Nutritional Values

Calories 240
  Calories from Fat 65
Total Fat . . . . 7.0 g
  Saturated Fat . . . . 0.6 g
  Trans Fat . . . . 0.0 g
Cholesterol . . . . 55 mg
Sodium . . . . 185 mg
Total Carbohydrate . . . 17 g
  Dietary Fiber . . . . 1 g
  Sugars . . . . 15 g
Protein . . . . 22 g

1. Slice the chicken breasts across the grain into 1/2-inch-thick strips (about 30 strips). In a large bowl, toss the chicken with the Splenda, cilantro, chipotle chili, chili powder, garlic powder, and 1/4 tsp pepper. Cover tightly with plastic wrap and refrigerate until the flavors blend, about 30 minutes.

2. In a separate bowl, stir together all remaining ingredients. Cover with plastic wrap and let stand at room temperature until the flavors blend, about 30 minutes. If using wooden skewers, soak them in cold water.

3. Preheat the broiler. Line the bottom of a broiler pan with foil. Spray the slotted grill with nonstick cooking spray. Weave each piece of chicken onto individual skewers; lay half of the skewers on the broiler grill and cover the skewer ends with foil, making sure not to cover the chicken. Broil until the meat is lightly browned and cooked through, 5–8 minutes, flipping the skewers over halfway through. Transfer the skewers to a serving platter and serve immediately with half of the dipping sauce. While eating, cook the remaining skewers and serve with the other half of the dipping sauce.

Corn and Zucchini Combo

Serves 4   Serving size: 1/4 recipe

- **1 tsp** Smart Balance Light Spread
- **1/2 cup** onion, diced
- **1 cup** zucchini squash, sliced 1/8-inch thick
- **1 cup** frozen whole-kernel corn
- **1/4 tsp** basil leaves
- **1/8 tsp** oregano leaves
- **1/8 tsp** pepper

Melt margarine in a frying pan over low heat. Add onion and cook for 2 minutes. Add zucchini, cover, and cook for 5 minutes, stirring occasionally. Add all remaining ingredients. Cover and cook over low heat for about 5 minutes or until corn is done.

Exchanges/Choices

1/2 Starch
1 Vegetable

Basic Nutritional Values

Calories	50
Calories from Fat	5
Total Fat	0.5 g
Saturated Fat	0.2 g
Trans Fat	0.0 g
Cholesterol	0 mg
Sodium	15 mg
Total Carbohydrate	11 g
Dietary Fiber	2 g
Sugars	2 g
Protein	2 g

Waldorf Salad

Serves 4   Serving size: 1/4 recipe

- 1 (8-oz) can light pineapple chunks, juice reserved
- 1 envelope unflavored gelatin
- 1/2 **cup** Red Delicious apples, unpeeled and cubed
- 2 **Tbsp** thinly sliced celery
- 2 **Tbsp** pecans or almonds, coarsely chopped
- 1 **cup** orange juice
- 1 **Tbsp** Splenda
- 1 1/2 **tsp** cornstarch
- 1 1/2 **tsp** lemon juice
- 1 1/2 **tsp** Smart Balance Light margarine
- 1/4 **cup** fat-free whipped topping

  Romaine lettuce leaves

Exchanges/Choices

1 Fruit
1 Fat

Basic Nutritional Values

Calories	115
Calories from Fat	30
Total Fat	3.5 g
Saturated Fat	0.4 g
Trans Fat	0.0 g
Cholesterol	0 mg
Sodium	25 mg
Total Carbohydrate	20 g
Dietary Fiber	2 g
Sugars	14 g
Protein	3 g

1. Add enough water to reserved pineapple juice to measure 1 cup and set aside.

2. In a medium saucepan, soften gelatin in remaining 1/2 cup orange juice for about 1 minute. Stir over medium heat until gelatin dissolves, about 1 minute. Remove from heat and add reserved pineapple juice. Chill until it reaches the consistency of unbeaten egg whites. Fold in pineapple chunks, apples, celery, and pecans or almonds. Pour into a bowl and chill about 3 hours.

3. In a small saucepan, combine 1/2 cup orange juice, Splenda, cornstarch, lemon juice, and margarine. Heat, stirring constantly, until thickened; allow to cool. Add whipped topping and mix together. Allow to chill.

4. When ready to serve, combine the contents of both saucepans in a large bowl until thoroughly mixed. Serve portions over a small bed of lettuce leaves.

Bran Muffins
Serves 4   Serving size: 3 muffins

Nonstick cooking spray
3/4 **cup** whole-wheat flour
2 **tsp** baking powder
1 1/2 **Tbsp** Splenda

2/3 **cup** all-bran cereal
2/3 **cup** nonfat milk
1/4 **cup** egg substitute
1/4 **cup** unsweetened applesauce

Exchanges/Choices
1/2 Starch

Basic Nutritional Values
Calories 45
 Calories from Fat 0
Total Fat . . . . 0.0 g
 Saturated Fat . . . . 0.1 g
 Trans Fat . . . . 0.0 g
Cholesterol . . . . 0 mg
Sodium . . . . 85 mg
Total Carbohydrate . . . 10 g
 Dietary Fiber . . . . 2 g
 Sugars . . . . 2 g
Protein . . . . 2 g

Spray twelve 2-inch muffin-pan cups with nonstick cooking spray; set aside. Stir together flour, baking powder, and Splenda; set aside. Add cereal and milk to a large mixing bowl. Stir to combine and then allow it to stand until cereal is softened, 1–2 minutes. Add egg substitute and applesauce; beat well. Add flour mixture and stir only enough to combine. Divide batter evenly among prepared muffin cups. Bake at 400°F for 25 minutes or until lightly browned.

Peach and Apple Crisp
Serves 4   Serving size: 1/4 recipe

2 **cups** sliced peaches (fresh, frozen, or canned light)
1 1/2 **cups** apples, peeled and sliced
3 1/2 **Tbsp** Splenda
2 **Tbsp** + **2 tsp** whole-wheat flour

1 **tsp** ground cinnamon
1 **tsp** ground nutmeg
3 **Tbsp** old-fashioned oats
2 **Tbsp** Smart Balance Light margarine, melted

Exchanges/Choices
1 1/2 Carbohydrate
1/2 Fat

Basic Nutritional Values
Calories 130
 Calories from Fat 40
Total Fat . . . . 4.5 g
 Saturated Fat . . . . 1.3 g
 Trans Fat . . . . 0.0 g
Cholesterol . . . . 0 mg
Sodium . . . . 40 mg
Total Carbohydrate . . . 22 g
 Dietary Fiber . . . . 3 g
 Sugars . . . . 14 g
Protein . . . . 2 g

Preheat oven to 400°F. Place peaches and apples in a large bowl. In a small bowl, mix 2 Tbsp Splenda, 2 tsp flour, 1/2 tsp cinnamon, and 1/2 tsp nutmeg. Sprinkle over fruit and toss until fruit is evenly coated; mound mixture in a 1-quart casserole. In a small bowl, mix oats, 2 Tbsp flour, 1 1/2 Tbsp Splenda, 1/2 tsp cinnamon, and 1/2 tsp nutmeg. Stir in margarine until mixture is evenly moistened. Spoon over fruit. Bake in lower third of the oven for 30 minutes or until juices are bubbly and topping is browned. Serve warm.

Southwestern Black-Eyed Pea Salad

Serves 4   Serving size: 1/4 recipe

1/4 **cup** green bell pepper, diced

1/4 **cup** onion, diced

1 **Tbsp** jalapeño pepper, finely chopped

1 **Tbsp** red wine vinegar

1 **Tbsp** Smart Balance Omega oil

1 **Tbsp** water

1 medium clove garlic, minced

2 **cups** black-eyed peas

In a bowl, stir together all of the ingredients, except the black-eyed peas. Drain and rinse the peas and add to bowl. Mix and chill at least 2 hours before serving.

Exchanges/Choices

1 Starch
1 Lean Meat

Basic Nutritional Values

Calories 140
  Calories from Fat 35
Total Fat . . . . 4.0 g
  Saturated Fat . . . . 0.3 g
  Trans Fat . . . . 0.0 g
Cholesterol . . . . 0 mg
Sodium . . . . 140 mg
Total Carbohydrate . . . 20 g
  Dietary Fiber . . . . 6 g
  Sugars . . . . 4 g
Protein . . . . 7 g

Citrus Halibut Steak

Serves 4   Serving size: 1/4 recipe

1 **Tbsp** Smart Balance margarine

2 **Tbsp** whole-wheat flour

1 **tsp** pepper

1 **tsp** ginger, ground

4 **oz** frozen orange juice concentrate

1 **lb** halibut steaks

1 **tsp** paprika

1 medium grapefruit, sectioned

Melt the margarine in a skillet. Stir in flour, pepper, and ginger; cook for 1 minute, stirring occasionally. Stir in orange juice, increase heat, and stir until slightly thickened. Brush fillets with half of the sauce mixture. Sprinkle paprika on fillets and broil. Place grapefruit sections on fillets and brush with remaining sauce 3 minutes before fish is done. Fish is done when it flakes easily with a fork.

Exchanges/Choices

1 1/2 Fruit
3 Lean Meat

Basic Nutritional Values

Calories 240
  Calories from Fat 45
Total Fat . . . . 5.0 g
  Saturated Fat . . . . 1.0 g
  Trans Fat . . . . 0.0 g
Cholesterol . . . . 35 mg
Sodium . . . . 85 mg
Total Carbohydrate . . . 24 g
  Dietary Fiber . . . . 2 g
  Sugars . . . . 18 g
Protein . . . . 26 g

Parmesan Potatoes

Serves 4   Serving size: 1/4 recipe

2 **Tbsp** Smart Balance Light margarine, melted

12 reduced-fat butter-flavored crackers, crushed

3 **Tbsp** reduced-fat grated Parmesan cheese

1 **tsp** garlic powder

1 **tsp** paprika

1 **tsp** pepper

2 **cups** potatoes, unpeeled and thinly sliced

Combine melted margarine, crushed crackers, cheese, garlic powder, paprika, and pepper in a medium bowl; add potato slices, tossing gently to coat. Arrange coated potato slices in a 9-inch microwave-safe pie plate, sprinkle with remaining crumb mixture. Cover with wax paper and microwave on high power for 7–8 minutes or until potatoes are tender, rotating pie plate a half-turn after 2 minutes.

Exchanges/Choices

2 Starch
1/2 Fat

Basic Nutritional Values

Calories 160
  Calories from Fat 45
Total Fat . . . . 5.0 g
  Saturated Fat . . . . 1.3 g
  Trans Fat . . . . 0.0 g
Cholesterol . . . . 5 mg
Sodium . . . . 235 mg
Total Carbohydrate . . . 26 g
  Dietary Fiber . . . . 2 g
  Sugars . . . . 1 g
Protein . . . . 4 g

Tuna Melt Muffin

Serves 4   Serving size: 1/4 recipe

- 1 (**6-oz**) can tuna, packed in water, drained
- 1 (**7-oz**) jar roasted red peppers, drained and sliced
- 1 clove garlic, minced
- 1 **Tbsp** red wine vinegar
- 1 **Tbsp** chopped marjoram (or 1 tsp dried)
- 1/2 **tsp** black pepper
- 4 whole-wheat English muffins, split and lightly toasted
- 1 large tomato, thinly sliced
- 1 small red onion, thinly sliced
- 2 **oz** shredded fat-free mozzarella cheese

  Marjoram sprigs (optional)

Combine the tuna, roasted peppers, garlic, vinegar, marjoram, and pepper. Stir gently to mix. Let the filling stand 10 minutes at room temperature. Preheat the broiler. Spoon the filling onto the toasted English muffin halves. Add tomato and onion slices and then sprinkle with the cheese. Broil about 4 inches from heat source until the cheese melts and the filling becomes warm, 1–2 minutes. Garnish with a marjoram sprig, if desired.

Exchanges/Choices

2 Starch
1 Vegetable
1 Lean Meat

Basic Nutritional Values

Calories 220
  Calories from Fat 20
Total Fat . . . . 2.0 g
  Saturated Fat . . . . 0.3 g
  Trans Fat . . . . 0.0 g
Cholesterol . . . . 15 mg
Sodium . . . . 600 mg
Total Carbohydrate . . . 36 g
  Dietary Fiber . . . . 6 g
  Sugars . . . . 9 g
Protein . . . . 17 g

Texas Marinated Flank Steak

Serves 4   Serving size: 1/4 recipe

- 1 **lb** beef flank steak (trimmed of fat), tenderized and pounded
- 3/4 **cup** light Italian salad dressing
- 1/2 lemon, juiced

In a large resealable plastic bag, combine beef, Italian salad dressing, and lemon juice. Marinate in the refrigerator for at least 3 hours or overnight. Grill until desired doneness is reached.

Exchanges/Choices

3 Lean Meat
1/2 Fat

Basic Nutritional Values

Calories 170
  Calories from Fat 65
Total Fat . . . . 7.0 g
  Saturated Fat . . . . 2.6 g
  Trans Fat . . . . 0.0 g
Cholesterol . . . . 40 mg
Sodium . . . . 225 mg
Total Carbohydrate . . . 3 g
  Dietary Fiber . . . . 0 g
  Sugars . . . . 2 g
Protein . . . . 23 g

Blackberry Cobbler

Serves 4   Serving size: 1/4 recipe

Nonstick cooking spray

1/2 **cup** Splenda

1 **Tbsp** cornstarch

2 **cups** sliced blackberries, fresh or frozen

2 **Tbsp** water

1 **cup** biscuit mix

1/4 **cup** nonfat milk

Preheat oven to 425°F. Spray a round casserole dish with nonstick cooking spray. Mix 1/2 cup Splenda and cornstarch in saucepan, stir in blackberries and water. Heat to boiling, stirring constantly. Boil and stir 1 minute. Pour mixture into casserole dish. Mix biscuit mix according to package directions and drop dough by the spoonful onto the hot blackberry mixture. Bake until golden brown, about 20 minutes. Serve with milk.

Exchanges/Choices

2 Carbohydrate
1 Fat

Basic Nutritional Values

Calories 195
  Calories from Fat 40
Total Fat. . . . . 4.5 g
  Saturated Fat . . . . 1.2 g
  Trans Fat. . . . . 1.2 g
Cholesterol . . . . 0 mg
Sodium. . . . . 410 mg
Total Carbohydrate . . . 34 g
  Dietary Fiber. . . . . 5 g
  Sugars . . . . 9 g
Protein . . . . 5 g

Fruit Salad Medley

Serves 4   Serving size: 1/4 recipe

1/2 **cup** strawberries, sliced	1/2 **cup** blackberries (or canned light)
1/4 **cup** Splenda	
1/2 **cup** blueberries (or canned light)	1/2 **cup** pineapple (fresh, frozen, or canned light chunks)
1 banana, sliced	1/2 **cup** orange juice
3 **tsp** lemon juice	Sprig mint leaves
2 oranges, peeled and sliced crosswise	

In a medium bowl, stir together half of the strawberries and half of the Splenda; set aside. In a 2-quart serving bowl, add blueberries and layer bananas on top; sprinkle with lemon juice. Add a layer of strawberries with remaining Splenda, then oranges and blackberries. Arrange pineapple tidbits around outer edge. Layer remaining strawberry slices around pineapple tidbits. Pour orange juice over all the fruit. Cover and chill for 1 hour. Just before serving, top with mint leaves.

Exchanges/Choices

2 Fruit

Basic Nutritional Values

Calories 120
 Calories from Fat 5
Total Fat . . . . 0.5 g
 Saturated Fat . . . . 0.1 g
 Trans Fat . . . . 0.0 g
Cholesterol . . . . 0 mg
Sodium . . . . 0 mg
Total Carbohydrate . . . 29 g
 Dietary Fiber . . . . 5 g
 Sugars . . . . 21 g
Protein . . . . 2 g

Low-Fat Corn Bread

Serves 8   Serving size: 1/8 recipe

1/2 **cup** egg substitute	1 1/2 **cup** whole-wheat flour
1/2 **cup** Splenda	2/3 **cup** cornmeal
3/4 **cup** nonfat milk	1 **Tbsp** baking powder
1/2 **cup** unsweetened applesauce	Nonstick cooking spray

Beat together the egg substitute, Splenda, milk, and applesauce; set aside. In a separate bowl, sift and combine flour, cornmeal, and baking powder. Stir into egg mixture using as few strokes as possible. Spray an 8 × 8-inch baking pan with nonstick cooking spray. Bake at 400°F for 25–30 minutes or until a toothpick inserted near the middle comes out clean.

Exchanges/Choices

2 Starch

Basic Nutritional Values

Calories 150
 Calories from Fat 5
Total Fat . . . . 0.5 g
 Saturated Fat . . . . 0.1 g
 Trans Fat . . . . 0.0 g
Cholesterol . . . . 0 mg
Sodium . . . . 180 mg
Total Carbohydrate . . . 30 g
 Dietary Fiber . . . . 4 g
 Sugars . . . . 4 g
Protein . . . . 6 g

Grilled Portobello on Whole-Wheat Bread

Serves 4   Serving size: 1 sandwich

2 **Tbsp** canola mayonnaise

2 **Tbsp** plain fat-free yogurt

1 **Tbsp** chopped rosemary
(or 1 tsp dried)

2 1/2 **Tbsp** Smart Balance
Omega oil

2 **tsp** lemon juice

1/2 **cup** grated lemon peel

2 cloves garlic, minced

3/4 **lb** Portobello mushrooms,
wiped clean

8 **slices** whole-wheat bread
Pepper, to taste

1 **Tbsp** balsamic vinegar

4 tomato slices

Exchanges/Choices

1 1/2 Starch
1 Vegetable
2 1/2 Fat

Basic Nutritional Values

Calories 280
 Calories from Fat 115
Total Fat. . . . . .13.0 g
 Saturated Fat . . . . .1.1 g
 Trans Fat. . . . . .0.0 g
Cholesterol. . . . . .0 mg
Sodium. . . . . .320 mg
Total Carbohydrate . . .32 g
 Dietary Fiber. . . . . .6 g
 Sugars . . . . .6 g
Protein . . . . .11 g

1. Stir together the mayonnaise, yogurt, and rosemary in a small bowl. Cover and refrigerate until needed. In another small bowl, combine the oil, lemon juice, lemon peel, and garlic. Prepare a medium barbecue fire or preheat a gas grill or broiler.

2. Brush or rub all sides of the mushrooms with the flavored oil. Grill, turning once, until tender, about 8 minutes. Cut the mushrooms on the diagonal into 1/4-inch slices. Set the bread at the edge of the grill to lightly toast on one side, about 30 seconds.

3. Spread the untoasted sides of the bread with the flavored mayonnaise. Heap the mushrooms on half of the bread. Sprinkle with pepper and vinegar. Add 1 tomato slice and then top with the remaining bread, untoasted side down.

Sweet and Sour Red Cabbage

Serves 4   Serving size: 1/4 recipe

2 medium tart apples

1/2 **cup** water

6 **Tbsp** chopped onions

2 **Tbsp** Splenda Brown
Sugar Blend

1 **Tbsp** vinegar

1/4 **tsp** ground cloves

1/2 medium head red cabbage
(about 2 lb), wedged, cored,
and thinly sliced

Peel and slice apples 1/4 inch thick. In a 5-quart Dutch oven over medium heat, combine apples, water, onions, Splenda, vinegar, and cloves. Stir cabbage into apple mixture. Bring to a boil; reduce heat to low, cover, and simmer for 1 hour or until cabbage is tender. Uncover and boil for about 5 minutes more to reduce liquid, stirring occasionally.

Exchanges/Choices

1 1/2 Carbohydrate

Basic Nutritional Values

Calories 95
  Calories from Fat 0
Total Fat . . . . 0.0 g
  Saturated Fat . . . . 0.0 g
  Trans Fat . . . . 0.0 g
Cholesterol . . . . 0 mg
Sodium . . . . 15 mg
Total Carbohydrate . . . 23 g
  Dietary Fiber . . . . 3 g
  Sugars . . . . 19 g
Protein . . . . 2 g

Baked Chicken and Pineapple

Serves 4   Serving size: 1/4 recipe

1 **(20-oz)** can no-sugar-added
pineapple

1/2 **cup** raisins

1/2 **cup** green onions, sliced

2 **tsp** gingerroot, finely chopped
(or 1/2 tsp ground ginger)

1/8 **tsp** garlic powder (or 1 garlic
clove, finely chopped)

3 **cups** cooked brown rice

1 **lb** boneless, skinless chicken
breasts, cooked and cut
in small pieces

Drain the pineapple, reserving half of the juice and the pineapple chunks. Heat half of the juice over medium heat in a skillet. Add the raisins, green onions, ginger, and garlic; cook and stir for 3 minutes or until onions are tender. Stir in the pineapple chunks, brown rice, chicken, and remaining pineapple juice. Cover; turn the heat to low and cook for 5 minutes or until heated through. If desired, garnish the dish with grape tomatoes and additional green onions.

Exchanges/Choices

2 Starch
2 Fruit
3 Lean Meat

Basic Nutritional Values

Calories 420
  Calories from Fat 40
Total Fat . . . . 4.5 g
  Saturated Fat . . . . 1.1 g
  Trans Fat . . . . 0.0 g
Cholesterol . . . . 65 mg
Sodium . . . . 70 mg
Total Carbohydrate . . . 67 g
  Dietary Fiber . . . . 5 g
  Sugars . . . . 29 g
Protein . . . . 29 g

Vegetable Salad

Serves 4   Serving size: 1/4 recipe

1/2 **cup** broccoli, diced	1/2 **cup** raw carrot, diced
1/2 **cup** cauliflower, diced	10 small grape tomatoes
1/2 **cup** bell pepper, diced	1/2 **cup** light Italian salad
1/2 **cup** cucumber, diced	dressing

Break broccoli and cauliflower into florets; cut green pepper into 1-inch pieces; slice cucumber; and pare and slice carrots. Combine vegetables; toss with dressing. Cover and refrigerate overnight.

Exchanges/Choices

2 Vegetable

Basic Nutritional Values

Calories 55
 Calories from Fat 20
Total Fat . . . . 2.0 g
 Saturated Fat . . . . 0.2 g
 Trans Fat . . . . 0.0 g
Cholesterol . . . . 0 mg
Sodium . . . . 370 mg
Total Carbohydrate . . . 8 g
 Dietary Fiber . . . . 2 g
 Sugars . . . . 6 g
Protein . . . . 1 g

Apple Oatmeal Squares
Serves 6   Serving Size: 1/6 recipe

1/2 **cup** nonfat milk

1/4 **cup** Splenda

2 **Tbsp** Smart Balance margarine

1 1/2 **cup** dry oats

2 1/2 **cup** unsweetened applesauce

1 **tsp** cinnamon

1/2 **cup** raisins

Nonstick cooking spray

Heat the milk, Splenda, and margarine to a boil, stirring constantly so they don't burn. Stir in the oats, applesauce, cinnamon, and raisins. Heat without stirring until bubbles appear at the edges. Remove from heat and spread evenly in a pan lightly sprayed with nonstick cooking spray. Bake at 350°F for 30 minutes. Cut into 2-inch squares.

Exchanges/Choices

1 Starch
1 Fruit
1/2 Fat

Basic Nutritional Values

Calories 160
  Calories from Fat 40
Total Fat . . . . 4.5 g
  Saturated Fat . . . . 1.1 g
  Trans Fat . . . . 0.0 g
Cholesterol . . . . 0 mg
Sodium . . . . 45 mg
Total Carbohydrate . . . 27 g
  Dietary Fiber . . . . 3 g
  Sugars . . . . 12 g
Protein . . . . 4 g

Chicken Soft Tacos
Serves 4   Serving size: 1 taco

1/2 **lb** cooked boneless, skinless chicken breasts (trimmed of fat), diced

2 small onions, peeled and diced

2 **cups** romaine lettuce leaves, shredded

1/2 **cup** fat-free sour cream

4 **(6-inch)** flour tortillas

Place all ingredients into the tortillas and fold like a taco to serve.

Exchanges/Choices

1 Starch
1 Vegetable
3 Lean Meat

Basic Nutritional Values

Calories 235
  Calories from Fat 40
Total Fat . . . . 4.5 g
  Saturated Fat . . . . 1.2 g
  Trans Fat . . . . 0.0 g
Cholesterol . . . . 50 mg
Sodium . . . . 250 mg
Total Carbohydrate . . . 22 g
  Dietary Fiber . . . . 2 g
  Sugars . . . . 4 g
Protein . . . . 23 g

Dijon Pork Cutlets

Serves 4   Serving size: 1/4 recipe

3/4 **lb** boneless sirloin pork chops (trimmed of fat)	1 **Tbsp** sodium-free chicken bouillon
1/2 **cup** whole-wheat flour	1 **cup** water
1 **Tbsp** Smart Balance margarine	1 **cup** fat-free sour cream
2 **Tbsp** vinegar	2 **Tbsp** Dijon mustard
	2 **Tbsp** green peppercorns

Place each loin slice between two pieces of plastic wrap and flatten them to 1/8 inch thickness with mallet. Coat the cutlets with flour and discard remaining flour. Heat margarine in a large skillet over medium-high heat. Brown cutlets quickly, about 2–3 minutes on each side. Remove from pan and keep warm. Drain away any fat left in pan and add vinegar, bouillon, and water to skillet; stir and bring to boil. Lower heat, stir in sour cream and mustard; whisk until smooth. Add peppercorns, simmer, and stir gently until sauce thickens slightly. Pour sauce over cutlets and serve.

Exchanges/Choices

1 Carbohydrate
3 Lean Meat

Basic Nutritional Values

Calories 190
  Calories from Fat 40
Total Fat . . . . .4.5 g
  Saturated Fat . . . . .1.0 g
  Trans Fat . . . . .0.0 g
Cholesterol . . . . .45 mg
Sodium . . . . .445 mg
Total Carbohydrate . . .11 g
  Dietary Fiber . . . . .1 g
  Sugars . . . . .3 g
Protein . . . . .21 g

Three Bean Salad

Serves 4   Serving size: 1/4 recipe

1/2 **cup** green beans, drained (if using canned)	1/2 **cup** onions, diced
1/2 **cup** kidney beans, rinsed and drained	2 **Tbsp** Smart Balance Omega oil
1/4 **cup** garbanzo beans, rinsed and drained	1/2 **cup** cider vinegar
1/4 **cup** green pepper, diced	1/4 **cup** Splenda
	Pepper, to taste

In a bowl, gently mix together the beans, pepper, and onions. Pour the liquids and other seasonings over the beans. Mix well and chill before serving.

Exchanges/Choices

1/2 Starch
1 Vegetable
1 1/2 Fat

Basic Nutritional Values

Calories 130
  Calories from Fat 65
Total Fat . . . . .7.0 g
  Saturated Fat . . . . .0.5 g
  Trans Fat . . . . .0.0 g
Cholesterol . . . . .0 mg
Sodium . . . . .55 mg
Total Carbohydrate . . .13 g
  Dietary Fiber . . . . .3 g
  Sugars . . . . .4 g
Protein . . . . .3 g

Grilled Marinated Pineapple

Serves 4   Serving size: 1/4 recipe

1 **Tbsp** honey

1 **Tbsp** Smart balance Omega oil

2 **Tbsp** lime juice

1 **tsp** ground cinnamon

1/2 **tsp** ground cloves

1 pineapple

4 wooden skewers, soaked in water for 30 minutes

1 **Tbsp** grated lime zest

Exchanges/Choices

1 Fruit
1 Fat

Basic Nutritional Values

Calories	105
Calories from Fat	30
Total Fat	3.5 g
Saturated Fat	0.3 g
Trans Fat	0.0 g
Cholesterol	0 mg
Sodium	0 mg
Total Carbohydrate	20 g
Dietary Fiber	2 g
Sugars	15 g
Protein	1 g

1. Combine the honey, oil, lime juice, cinnamon, and cloves and whisk to blend; set aside.

2. Carefully cut the skin off the pineapple and remove the eyes from the center. Cut the pineapple in half lengthwise and then into small wedges. Place about three slices on each skewer.

3. Brush the pineapple with the marinade. Grill or broil the pineapple for about 5 minutes on each side. Remove the pineapple from the skewers and sprinkle the gated lime zest on them.

Chicken Macaroni Salad

Serves 4   Serving size: 1/4 recipe

1 **lb** boneless, skinless chicken breast (trimmed of fat)

4 **oz** macaroni, elbows or shells

1/4 **cup** fat-free cheddar cheese slices, cut into small squares

1/4 **cup** reduced-fat shredded cheddar cheese

3 **Tbsp** minced onion

1/2 **cup** plain fat-free yogurt

Exchanges/Choices

1 1/2 Starch
4 Lean Meat

Basic Nutritional Values

Calories	290
Calories from Fat	45
Total Fat	5.0 g
Saturated Fat	1.9 g
Trans Fat	0.0 g
Cholesterol	75 mg
Sodium	240 mg
Total Carbohydrate	25 g
Dietary Fiber	1 g
Sugars	3 g
Protein	33 g

Place chicken breasts in boiling water and thoroughly cook. Put chicken in the refrigerator to cool while preparing the other ingredients. Cook the macaroni according to package directions. Drain and rinse in cold water. When chicken has cooled to the touch, cut into small cubes. Combine macaroni, cheese, chicken, and onion in a large bowl. Stir together with yogurt and season to taste. Cover and chill 3 hours before serving.

Sliced Tomato Salad
Serves 4   Serving size: 1/4 recipe

2 **cups** tomatoes

1/4 **cup** Smart Balance Omega oil

2 **oz** wine vinegar

1 **Tbsp** oregano

1/4 **tsp** dry mustard

1 clove garlic, crushed Pepper, to taste

4 romaine lettuce leaves

1/2 **cup** minced onion

1/4 **cup** parsley

Arrange tomatoes in a baking dish. In a tightly covered jar, shake together the oil, vinegar, oregano, mustard, garlic, and pepper. Pour over tomatoes and chill 3 hours, spooning the dressing over the tomatoes occasionally. Just before serving, arrange the tomatoes on a few leaves of lettuce; sprinkle with onions and parsley. Pour remaining dressing over the top.

Exchanges/Choices

1 Vegetable
3 Fat

Basic Nutritional Values

Calories	155
Calories from Fat	125
Total Fat	14.0 g
Saturated Fat	1.1 g
Trans Fat	0.0 g
Cholesterol	0 mg
Sodium	10 mg
Total Carbohydrate	7 g
Dietary Fiber	2 g
Sugars	4 g
Protein	1 g

Spicy Chicken and Brown Rice
Serves 4   Serving size: 1/4 recipe

1 **lb** boneless, skinless chicken breast (trimmed of fat)

1 **cup** brown rice, uncooked

1/2 **cup** raisins

2 **cups** boiling water

1/2 **tsp** cinnamon

1/4 **tsp** ground cloves

1 small onion, diced

1 **Tbsp** sodium-free chicken bouillon

2 **Tbsp** whole-wheat flour

12 **oz** cubed pineapple (or peaches)

Heat oven to 350°F. Mix all ingredients except pineapple in a small roasting pan. Cover and bake about 1 1/2 hours. In a small skillet, heat the pineapple cubes until warmed. Cover chicken and rice with warm pineapple and serve.

Exchanges/Choices

2 1/2 Starch
1 1/2 Fruit
3 Lean Meat

Basic Nutritional Values

Calories	425
Calories from Fat	40
Total Fat	4.5 g
Saturated Fat	1.1 g
Trans Fat	0.0 g
Cholesterol	65 mg
Sodium	75 mg
Total Carbohydrate	68 g
Dietary Fiber	6 g
Sugars	22 g
Protein	30 g

Oven-Roasted Tomatoes

Serves 6   Serving size: 1 tomato

1 Tbsp Smart Balance
Omega oil

6 medium tomatoes,
sliced crosswise,
1/2- to 3/4-inch thick

2 Tbsp Splenda
Dash pepper

Preheat oven to 300°F. Line a baking sheet with aluminum foil; rub with oil. Arrange tomato slices in a single layer on the baking sheet. Sprinkle with Splenda and pepper. Roast until the tomatoes shrivel, the edges start to turn brown, and most of the liquid around the tomatoes has caramelized, about 1 hour. Roasted tomatoes will keep for 4–5 days in the refrigerator.

Exchanges/Choices

1 Vegetable
1/2 Fat

Basic Nutritional Values

Calories 45
   Calories from Fat 20
Total Fat . . . . 2.5 g
   Saturated Fat . . . . 0.2 g
   Trans Fat . . . . 0.0 g
Cholesterol . . . . 0 mg
Sodium . . . . 5 mg
Total Carbohydrate . . . 5 g
   Dietary Fiber . . . . 1 g
   Sugars . . . . 4 g
Protein . . . . 1 g

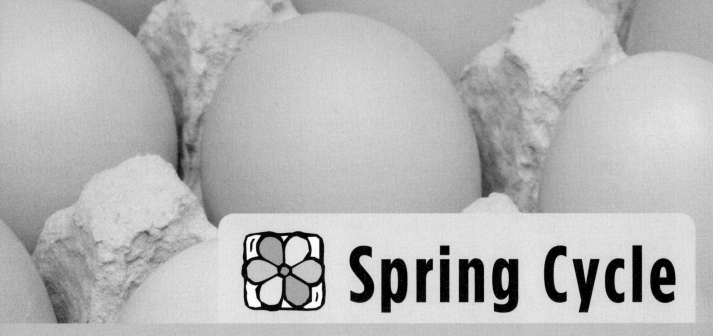

Spring Cycle

FEATURED RECIPES

Whole-Grain Pancakes or Waffles*

Beef Burgundy

Broccoli Floret Salad*

Broiled Ocean Perch

Colorful Coleslaw

Low-Fat Corn Bread*

Tuna Salad Wrap

Barbecued Chicken

Baked Squash

Oatmeal and Apple Muffins*

Grilled Colby Jack Sandwich

Baked Swiss Steak

Mashed Potatoes

Dilled Cucumber Salad*

Cold Meatloaf Sandwich

Potato Salad

Baked Fish Wrapped in Lettuce

Rice Pilaf

Whole-Wheat Cornmeal Muffin*

Chicken Fajitas

Red Cabbage Coleslaw

Turkey Meatloaf

Oven-Baked Potatoes

Zucchini Carrot Muffins*

Western Omelet

Hawaiian Dessert

Scallops, Spaghetti, and Vegetables

Southwest Tomato Salad*

Bulgur Turkey Meatball Sandwich

Far East Cabbage Salad

Pepper Steak

Sautéed Zucchini and Red Peppers*

*Indicates that the recipe has been used previously.

1500 calorie MEAL PLAN SPRING WEEK 3

	Sunday	Monday	Tuesday	Wednesday	Thursday	Friday	Saturday
Breakfast	**Whole-Grain Pancakes or Waffles*** 1/4 cup sugar-free maple syrup 1/4 cup canned plums in juice 1 cup nonfat milk 1 tsp margarine	1/2 whole-grain bagel 1 Tbsp jam 1 cup nonfat milk 1 tsp margarine	**Oatmeal and Apple Muffins*** 1 cup nonfat milk 2 tsp margarine	1 cup oatmeal 3 dried plums 1 cup nonfat milk 1 tsp margarine	**Whole-Wheat Cornmeal Muffin*** 1/2 cup Kashi cereal 1 small banana 1 cup nonfat milk 1 tsp margarine	**Zucchini Carrot Muffins*** 1/2 large grapefruit 1/2 cup nonfat milk 1/4 cup fat-free cottage cheese 1/2 tsp margarine	1 cup shredded wheat 2 Tbsp dried cranberries 1 cup nonfat milk 6 pecans
Lunch	**Beef Burgundy Broccoli Floret Salad*** 2/3 cup cooked whole-wheat pasta 1 slice whole-wheat bread 1 cup honeydew melon	**Tuna Salad Wrap** 3/4 cup pretzels 1/2 cup lentils 1/2 cup fruit packed in its own juice 1 cup raw tomatoes	**Grilled Colby Jack Sandwich** 1 cup tomato soup 2/3 cup lima beans 1 small banana	**Cold Meatloaf Sandwich Potato Salad*** 6 cherries 1 cup green bell pepper slices	**Chicken Fajitas Red Cabbage Coleslaw** 3/4 cup pineapple 1/2 cup cooked broccoli 3 almonds	**Western Omelet Hawaiian Dessert** 1 slice whole-grain bread 3/4 cup boiled potatoes 1 oz Canadian bacon 1 tsp margarine	**Bulgur Turkey Meat-ball Sandwich Far East Cabbage Salad** 8 small grapes
Snack A							
Snack B							
Dinner	**Broiled Ocean Perch Colorful Coleslaw Low-Fat Corn Bread*** 1/2 cup unsweetened peaches 1 cup nonfat milk	**Barbecued Chicken Baked Squash** 1/3 cup cooked brown rice 1 small apple 1 cup nonfat milk 2 cups romaine lettuce salad 2 Tbsp light salad dressing	**Baked Swiss Steak Mashed Potatoes Dilled Cucumber Salad*** 1 slice oatmeal bread 1/2 cup unsweetened pears 1 cup nonfat milk	**Baked Fish Wrapped in Lettuce Rice Pilaf** 1/2 cup cubed cantaloupe 1/2 cup nonfat milk 1/2 cup steamed collard greens	**Turkey Meatloaf** (1/2 serving) **Oven-Baked Potatoes** 3/4 cup blueberries 1/2 cup nonfat milk 1 cup green beans 1 1/2 tsp margarine	**Scallops, Spaghetti, and Vegetables Southwest Tomato Salad*** 1/2 cup steamed zucchini 1 1/2 tsp margarine	**Pepper Steak Sautéed Zucchini and Red Peppers*** 1/2 cup fruit cocktail in light syrup 3/4 cup nonfat milk

*Indicates that the recipe has been used previously.

	Sunday	Monday	Tuesday	Wednesday	Thursday	Friday	Saturday
Breakfast	Whole-Grain Pancakes or Waffles* 1/4 cup sugar-free maple syrup 1/4 cup canned plums in juice 1 cup nonfat milk 1 1/2 tsp margarine	1/2 whole-grain bagel 1 Tbsp jam 1 cup nonfat milk 1 oz Canadian bacon 2 tsp margarine	Oatmeal and Apple Muffins* 1 cup nonfat milk 1 oz lean beef sausage 2 tsp margarine	1 cup oatmeal 3 dried plums 1 cup nonfat milk 2 egg whites, scrambled 2 tsp margarine	Whole-Wheat Cornmeal Muffin* 1/2 cup Kashi cereal 1 small banana 1 cup nonfat milk 1 tsp margarine	Zucchini Carrot Muffins* 1/2 large grapefruit 1/2 cup nonfat milk 1/4 cup fat-free cottage cheese 1/2 tsp margarine	1 cup shredded wheat 2 Tbsp dried cranberries 1 cup nonfat milk 8 pecans
Lunch	Beef Burgundy Broccoli Floret Salad* 2/3 cup cooked whole-wheat pasta 1 slice whole-wheat bread 1 cup honeydew melon 1/2 tsp margarine	Tuna Salad Wrap 3/4 cup pretzels 1/2 cup lentils 1/2 cup fruit packed in its own juice 1 cup raw tomatoes	Grilled Colby Jack Sandwich 1 cup tomato soup 2/3 cup lima beans 1 small banana 1 tsp margarine	Cold Meatloaf Sandwich Potato Salad* 6 cherries 1 cup green bell pepper slices	Chicken Fajitas Red Cabbage Coleslaw 3/4 cup pineapple 1/2 cup cooked broccoli 9 almonds	Western Omelet Hawaiian Dessert 1 slice whole-grain bread 3/4 cup boiled potatoes 1 oz Canadian bacon 1 tsp margarine	Bulgur Turkey Meatball Sandwich Far East Cabbage Salad 8 small grapes 5 peanuts
Snack A	4 walnut halves 17 small grapes	4 walnut halves 1/2 large grapefruit	16 pistachios 8 dried apricots	1 Tbsp sunflower seeds 3/4 cup blackberries	10 peanuts 2 Tbsp raisins	16 pistachios 1 1/4 cup watermelon	2 Brazil nuts 4 dried apple rings
Snack B	1 cup nonfat milk	1 cup nonfat milk	1 cup nonfat milk	1 cup nonfat milk	3/4 cup fat-free yogurt	1 cup nonfat milk	6 oz fat-free yogurt
Dinner	Broiled Ocean Perch Colorful Coleslaw Low-Fat Corn Bread* 1/2 cup unsweetened peaches 1 cup nonfat milk	Barbecued Chicken Baked Squash 1/3 cup cooked brown rice 1 small apple 1 cup nonfat milk 2 cups romaine lettuce salad 2 Tbsp light salad dressing	Baked Swiss Steak Mashed Potatoes Dilled Cucumber Salad* 1 slice oatmeal bread 1/2 cup unsweetened pears 1 cup nonfat milk	Baked Fish Wrapped in Lettuce Rice Pilaf 1/2 cup cubed cantaloupe 1/2 cup nonfat milk 1/2 cup steamed collard greens	Turkey Meatloaf Oven-Baked Potatoes (1/2 serving) 3/4 cup nonfat milk 1 cup green beans 1 1/2 tsp margarine	Scallops, Spaghetti, and Vegetables Southwest Tomato Salad* 1/2 cup steamed zucchini 1 oz reduced-fat cheese 1 1/2 tsp margarine	Pepper Steak Sautéed Zucchini with Red Peppers* 1/2 cup fruit cocktail in light syrup 3/4 cup nonfat milk

*Indicates that the recipe has been used previously.

	Sunday	Monday	Tuesday	Wednesday	Thursday	Friday	Saturday
Breakfast	Whole-Grain Pancakes or Waffles* 1/4 cup sugar-free maple syrup 1/4 cup canned plums in juice 1 cup nonfat milk 1 1/2 tsp margarine	1/2 whole-grain bagel 1 Tbsp jam 1 cup nonfat milk 1 oz Canadian bacon 2 tsp margarine	Oatmeal and Apple Muffins* 1 cup nonfat milk 1 oz lean beef sausage 2 tsp margarine	1 cup oatmeal 3 dried plums 1 cup nonfat milk 2 egg whites, scrambled 2 tsp margarine	Whole-Wheat Cornmeal Muffin* 1/2 cup Kashi cereal 1 small banana 1 cup nonfat milk 1 tsp margarine	Zucchini Carrot Muffins* 1/2 large grapefruit 1/2 cup nonfat milk 1/4 cup fat-free cottage cheese 1/2 tsp margarine	1 cup shredded wheat 2 Tbsp dried cranberries 1 cup nonfat milk 8 pecans
Lunch	Beef Burgundy Broccoli Floret Salad* 2/3 cup cooked whole-wheat pasta 1 slice whole-wheat bread 2 cups honeydew melon 1/2 tsp margarine	Tuna Salad Wrap 3/4 cup pretzels 1/2 cup lentils 1 cup fruit packed in its own juice 1 cup raw tomatoes 1 cup salad greens	Grilled Colby Jack Sandwich 1 cup tomato soup 2/3 cup lima beans 1 small banana 1 tsp margarine	Cold Meatloaf Sandwich Potato Salad* 18 cherries 1 cup green bell pepper slices 1 cup sliced tomatoes	Chicken Fajitas Red Cabbage Coleslaw 3/4 cup pineapple 1 1/4 cup strawberries 1 cup cooked broccoli 9 almonds	Western Omelet Hawaiian Dessert 1 slice whole-grain bread 3/4 cup boiled potatoes 1 small apple 1 oz Canadian bacon 1 tsp margarine	Bulgur Turkey Meat-ball Sandwich Far East Cabbage Salad 25 small grapes 1 cup tomato slices 5 peanuts
Snack A	1 cup raw carrots 4 walnut halves 17 small grapes	1 cup raw vegetable sticks 4 walnut halves 1/2 large grapefruit	1 cup water chestnuts 16 pistachios 8 dried apricots	1 cup mixed raw vegetables 1 Tbsp sunflower seeds 3/4 cup blackberries	1 cup celery sticks 10 peanuts 2 Tbsp raisins	1/2 cup steamed green beans 16 pistachios 1 1/4 cup watermelon	1 cup raw mixed vegetables 2 Brazil nuts 4 dried apple rings
Snack B	1 cup vegetable beef soup 10 peanuts 1 cup nonfat milk	24 oyster crackers 6 cashews 1 cup nonfat milk	1 cup oven-baked French fries 1 cup nonfat milk	2 small sandwich cookies 1 cup nonfat milk	3 graham cracker squares 3/4 cup fat-free yogurt	2 rice cakes 1 1/2 tsp almond butter 1 cup nonfat milk	1 medium muffin 1/2 tsp margarine 6 oz fat-free yogurt
Dinner	Broiled Ocean Perch Colorful Coleslaw Low-Fat Corn Bread* 1/2 cup unsweetened peaches 1 cup nonfat milk	Barbecued Chicken Baked Squash 1/3 cup cooked brown rice 1 small apple 1 cup nonfat milk 2 cups romaine lettuce salad 2 Tbsp light salad dressing	Baked Swiss Steak Mashed Potatoes Dilled Cucumber Salad* 1 slice oatmeal bread 1/2 cup unsweetened pears 1 cup nonfat milk	Baked Fish Wrapped in Lettuce Rice Pilaf 1/2 cup cubed cantaloupe 1/2 cup nonfat milk 1/2 cup steamed collard greens	Turkey Meatloaf Oven-Baked Potatoes (1/2 serving) 3/4 cup nonfat milk 1 cup green beans 1 1/2 tsp margarine	Scallops, Spaghetti, and Vegetables Southwest Tomato Salad* 1/2 cup steamed zucchini 1 oz reduced-fat cheese 1 1/2 tsp margarine	Pepper Steak Sautéed Zucchini with Red Peppers* 1/2 cup fruit cocktail in light syrup 3/4 cup nonfat milk

*Indicates that the recipe has been used previously.

	Sunday	Monday	Tuesday	Wednesday	Thursday	Friday	Saturday
Breakfast	Whole-Grain Pancakes or Waffles* 1/4 cup sugar-free maple syrup 1/4 cup canned plums in juice 1 cup nonfat milk 1/4 cup egg substitute, scrambled 1 1/2 tsp margarine	1/2 whole-grain bagel 1 Tbsp jam 1 cup nonfat milk 1 oz Canadian bacon 2 tsp margarine	Oatmeal and Apple Muffins* 1 cup nonfat milk 2 oz lean beef sausage 2 tsp margarine	1 cup oatmeal 3 dried plums 1 cup nonfat milk 4 egg whites, scrambled 2 tsp margarine	Whole-Wheat Cornmeal Muffin* 1/2 cup Kashi cereal 1 small banana 1 cup nonfat milk 1 oz lean turkey sausage 1 tsp margarine	Zucchini Carrot Muffins* 1/2 large grapefruit 1/2 cup nonfat milk 1/2 cup fat-free cottage cheese 1/2 tsp margarine	1 cup shredded wheat 2 Tbsp dried cranberries 1 cup nonfat milk 1 oz reduced-fat cheese 8 pecans
Lunch	Beef Burgundy Broccoli Floret Salad* 2/3 cup cooked whole-wheat pasta 1 slice whole-wheat bread 2 cups honeydew melon 1/2 tsp margarine	Tuna Salad Wrap 3/4 cup pretzels 1/2 cup lentils 1 cup fruit packed in its own juice 1 cup raw tomatoes 1 cup salad greens	Grilled Colby Jack Sandwich 1 cup tomato soup 2/3 cup lima beans 1/2 cup corn 1 small banana 1 tsp margarine	Cold Meatloaf Sandwich Potato Salad* 18 cherries 1 cup green bell pepper slices 1 cup sliced tomatoes	Chicken Fajitas Red Cabbage Coleslaw 3/4 cup pineapple 1 1/4 cup strawberries 1 cup cooked broccoli 9 almonds	Western Omelet Hawaiian Dessert 1 slice whole-grain bread 3/4 cup boiled potatoes 1 small apple 1 oz Canadian bacon 1 tsp margarine	Bulgur Turkey Meat-ball Sandwich Far East Cabbage Salad 25 small grapes 1 cup tomato slices 5 peanuts
Snack A	1 cup raw carrots 4 walnut halves 17 small grapes	1 cup raw vegetable sticks 4 walnut halves 1/2 large grapefruit	1 cup water chestnuts 16 pistachios 8 dried apricots	1 cup mixed raw vegetables 1 Tbsp sunflower seeds 3/4 cup blackberries	1 cup celery sticks 10 peanuts 2 Tbsp raisins	1/2 cup steamed green beans 16 pistachios 1 1/4 cup watermelon	1 cup raw mixed vegetables 2 Brazil nuts 4 dried apple rings
Snack B	1 cup vegetable beef soup 10 peanuts 1 cup nonfat milk	24 oyster crackers 6 cashews 1 cup nonfat milk	1 cup oven-baked French fries 1 cup nonfat milk	2 small sandwich cookies 1 cup nonfat milk	3 graham cracker squares 3/4 cup fat-free yogurt	2 rice cakes 1 1/2 tsp almond butter 1 cup nonfat milk	1 medium muffin 1/2 tsp margarine 6 oz fat-free yogurt
Dinner	Broiled Ocean Perch Colorful Coleslaw Low-Fat Corn Bread* 3 oz baked potato 1/2 cup unsweetened peaches 1 cup nonfat milk	Barbecued Chicken Baked Squash 2/3 cup cooked brown rice 1 small apple 1 cup nonfat milk 2 cups romaine lettuce salad 2 Tbsp light salad dressing	Baked Swiss Steak Mashed Potatoes Dilled Cucumber Salad* 2 slices oatmeal bread 1/2 cup unsweetened pears 1 cup nonfat milk	Baked Fish Wrapped in Lettuce Rice Pilaf 1 slice whole-wheat bread 1/2 cup cubed cantaloupe 1/2 cup nonfat milk 1/2 cup steamed collard greens	Turkey Meatloaf (1/2 serving) Oven-Baked Potatoes 1/2 cup nonfat milk 1 cup green beans 1 1/2 tsp margarine	Scallops, Spaghetti, and Vegetables Southwest Tomato Salad* 1 cup raspberries 1/2 cup steamed zucchini 1 oz reduced-fat cheese 1 1/2 tsp margarine	Pepper Steak Sautéed Zucchini with Red Peppers* 1 small dinner roll 1/2 cup fruit cocktail in light syrup 3/4 cup nonfat milk

*Indicates that the recipe has been used previously.

SHOPPING LIST SPRING WEEK 3

VEGETABLES

_____ bell peppers, green
_____ bell peppers, red
_____ broccoli
_____ cabbage, purple, green, and red
_____ carrots
_____ celery
_____ collard greens
_____ cucumbers
_____ garlic
_____ green beans
_____ lettuce, romaine
_____ mushrooms
_____ onion, purple
_____ onion, red
_____ onions, yellow or white
_____ onions, green (scallions)
_____ pepper, jalapeño
_____ potatoes
_____ spinach
_____ squash
_____ tomatoes
_____ winter squash
_____ zucchini

MEATS

_____ bacon, Canadian
_____ beef round steaks
_____ beef sausage, lean
_____ beef steak, top round or sirloin
_____ beef, ground, 96% lean
_____ chicken breasts, boneless, skinless
_____ fish, any white
_____ fish, ocean perch
_____ ham, extra-lean, lower-sodium
_____ scallops, bay
_____ turkey breast, lean, ground

FRUITS

_____ apples
_____ bananas
_____ cantaloupe
_____ cherries
_____ cranberries, dried
_____ grapefruit
_____ grapes
_____ honeydew
_____ peaches
_____ pears, unsweetened
_____ pineapple
_____ plums, dried
_____ raisins
_____ strawberries

DAIRY

_____ egg substitute
_____ eggs
_____ milk, nonfat
_____ Smart Balance Light margarine
_____ sour cream, fat-free
_____ yogurt, fat-free, plain

CHEESE

_____ Colby jack, shredded, reduced-fat
_____ cottage cheese, fat-free
_____ mozzarella, shredded, fat-free

BREAD, GRAINS, & PASTA

_____ bagel, whole-grain
_____ bread, oatmeal
_____ bread, whole-wheat, whole-grain
_____ bulgur
_____ hoagie/sandwich buns, whole-grain
_____ pasta, any kind, whole-wheat
_____ rice, brown, whole-grain
_____ spaghetti, whole-wheat

BEANS

_____ lentils
_____ lima beans

NUTS

_____ almonds

_____ peanuts

_____ pecans

CONDIMENTS

_____ canola mayonnaise

_____ catsup, no-salt

_____ mustard, Dijon

_____ pickle relish

_____ Worcestershire sauce, reduced-sodium

SPICES & HERBS

_____ basil

_____ caraway seeds

_____ chili powder, no-added-salt

_____ cilantro

_____ cinnamon

_____ dill weed

_____ marjoram

_____ mint

_____ mustard, dry

_____ nutmeg

_____ onion powder

_____ paprika

_____ parsley

_____ pepper

_____ sage, dried

_____ thyme

OTHER

_____ applesauce, unsweetened

_____ beets, pickled, 16-oz jar

_____ cereal, Kashi

_____ cereal, shredded wheat

_____ fruit cocktail, light syrup

_____ hot pepper sauce

_____ jam

_____ mandarin orange segments, no-added-sugar

_____ maple syrup, sugar-free

_____ marshmallows, miniature

_____ plums, can, packed in juice

_____ pretzels

_____ salad dressing, Italian, light

_____ salsa

_____ seasoned croutons

_____ soup, tomato

_____ spaghetti sauce, light

_____ tomato paste, no-added-salt

_____ tomato sauce, no-added-salt

_____ tomatoes, peeled, no-added-salt, 10-oz can

_____ tomatoes, stewed, no-added-salt, 14-oz can

_____ tortillas, corn

_____ tortillas, flour, 6-inch

_____ tuna, packed in water, 6-oz can

_____ wheat germ

_____ wine, burgundy, cooking

_____ wine, white, dry

STAPLES

_____ baking powder

_____ bouillon, beef, sodium-free

_____ bouillon, chicken, sodium-free

_____ cornmeal, yellow

_____ flour, whole-wheat

_____ juice, lemon

_____ nonstick cooking spray

_____ oats, old-fashioned

_____ Smart Balance Omega oil

_____ Splenda

_____ Splenda Brown Sugar Blend

_____ juice, lime

_____ vinegar, cider

Whole-Wheat Pancakes or Waffles

Serves 4   Serving size: 2 pancakes or waffles

1/2 **cup** rolled oats	3/4 **cup** nonfat milk
1/2 **cup** whole-wheat flour, sifted	2 **Tbsp** Smart Balance Omega oil
2 **tsp** baking powder	Nonstick cooking spray
2 **Tbsp** Splenda	
1/2 **cup** egg substitute, beaten well	

Stir together dry ingredients. Combine egg substitute, milk, and oil; stir into flour mixture. Cook on a griddle lightly coated with nonstick spray until golden brown, then turn. Can also be made in a waffle iron.

Exchanges/Choices

1 1/2 Starch
1 1/2 Fat

Basic Nutritional Values

Calories 185
 Calories from Fat 70
Total Fat. . . . . 8.0 g
 Saturated Fat . . . . 0.7 g
 Trans Fat. . . . . 0.0 g
Cholesterol . . . . 0 mg
Sodium. . . . . 265 mg
Total Carbohydrate . . . 22 g
 Dietary Fiber. . . . . 3 g
 Sugars . . . . 3 g
Protein . . . . 8 g

Beef Burgundy

Serves 4   Serving size: 1/4 recipe

1 **lb** top round or sirloin steak (trimmed of fat)	1/2 **cup** mushrooms
2 medium clove garlic, minced	1 **(14-oz)** can no-added-salt stewed tomatoes
1/2 **tsp** ground thyme	8 **oz** no-added-salt tomato sauce
2 **tsp** Smart Balance Omega oil	3/4 **cup** burgundy cooking wine

Slice beef very thinly. Sauté meat, garlic, and thyme in hot oil for 3 minutes. Add mushrooms and cook 1 minute. Add tomatoes, tomato sauce, and wine. Cook uncovered over medium heat for 15 minutes, stirring occasionally. Garnish with chopped parsley, if desired.

Exchanges/Choices

2 Vegetable
3 Lean Meat
1 Fat

Basic Nutritional Values

Calories 235
 Calories from Fat 70
Total Fat. . . . . 8.0 g
 Saturated Fat . . . . 2.1 g
 Trans Fat. . . . . 0.1 g
Cholesterol . . . . 75 mg
Sodium. . . . . 70 mg
Total Carbohydrate . . . 11 g
 Dietary Fiber. . . . . 2 g
 Sugars . . . . 6 g
Protein . . . . 26 g

Broccoli Floret Salad

Serves 4   Serving size: 1/4 recipe

- **2 cups** fresh or frozen broccoli florets, cut small
- **2 Tbsp** chopped parsley
- **1 Tbsp** fresh basil
- **1** medium red pepper, thinly sliced
- Black pepper, to taste
- **1** small purple onion, diced
- **2/3 cup** light Italian salad dressing

Combine all ingredients (except dressing) in a large bowl. Add dressing. Stir well and chill for 2 hours before serving.

Exchanges/Choices

1/2 Carbohydrate
1 Vegetable
1/2 Fat

Basic Nutritional Values

Calories 80
  Calories from Fat 25
Total Fat . . . . .3.0 g
  Saturated Fat . . . . .0.3 g
  Trans Fat . . . . .0.0 g
Cholesterol . . . . .0 mg
Sodium . . . . .480 mg
Total Carbohydrate . . .12 g
  Dietary Fiber . . . . .2 g
  Sugars . . . . .9 g
Protein . . . . .2 g

Broiled Ocean Perch

Serves 4   Serving size: 1/4 recipe

- **1 Tbsp** lemon juice
- **2 tsp** reduced-sodium Worcestershire sauce
- **1 tsp** paprika
- **1 tsp** chopped thyme
- **1/2 tsp** hot pepper sauce
- **1/2 tsp** onion powder
- **1 Tbsp** Smart Balance Omega oil
- **1 lb** ocean perch

Preheat the broiler. Combine all ingredients except fish in a small bowl. Place fish on a baking sheet and coat each fillet with the seasoning mixture. Broil for about 9 minutes or until fish flakes easily when tested with a fork.

Exchanges

3 Lean Meat

Basic Nutritional Values

Calories 145
  Calories from Fat 55
Total Fat . . . . .6.0 g
  Saturated Fat . . . . .0.5 g
  Trans Fat . . . . .0.0 g
Cholesterol . . . . .50 mg
Sodium . . . . .105 mg
Total Carbohydrate . . .1 g
  Dietary Fiber . . . . .0 g
  Sugars . . . . .1 g
Protein . . . . .22 g

Colorful Coleslaw

Serves 4   Serving size: 1/4 recipe

1 **cup** green cabbage, finely chopped

1 **cup** purple cabbage, finely chopped

1/2 **cup** diced red pepper

1/2 **cup** shredded carrots

1/2 **cup** diced onions

1/2 **cup** diced celery

1/4 **cup** cider vinegar

2 **Tbsp** water

3 **Tbsp** Splenda

1/4 **cup** Smart Balance Omega oil

Combine the vegetables in a large bowl. In a separate bowl, mix the vinegar, water, Splenda, and oil. Then toss together and chill before serving.

Exchanges/Choices

2 Vegetable
2 1/2 Fat

Basic Nutritional Values

Calories 160
 Calories from Fat 125
Total Fat. . . . . 14.0 g
 Saturated Fat . . . . 1.0 g
 Trans Fat. . . . . 0.0 g
Cholesterol . . . . 0 mg
Sodium. . . . . 30 mg
Total Carbohydrate . . . 8 g
 Dietary Fiber . . . . 2 g
 Sugars . . . . 5 g
Protein . . . . 1 g

Low-Fat Corn Bread

Serves 8   Serving size: 1/8 recipe

1/2 **cup** egg substitute

1/2 **cup** Splenda

3/4 **cup** nonfat milk

1/2 **cup** unsweetened applesauce

1 1/2 **cup** whole-wheat flour

2/3 **cup** cornmeal

1 **Tbsp** baking powder

Nonstick cooking spray

Beat together the egg substitute, Splenda, milk, and applesauce; set aside. In a separate bowl, sift and combine flour, cornmeal, and baking powder. Stir into egg mixture using as few strokes as possible. Spray an 8 × 8-inch baking pan with nonstick cooking spray. Bake at 400°F for 25–30 minutes or until a toothpick inserted near the middle comes out clean.

Exchanges/Choices

2 Starch

Basic Nutritional Values

Calories 150
 Calories from Fat 5
Total Fat. . . . . 0.5 g
 Saturated Fat . . . . 0.1 g
 Trans Fat. . . . . 0.0 g
Cholesterol . . . . 0 mg
Sodium. . . . . 180 mg
Total Carbohydrate . . . 30 g
 Dietary Fiber . . . . 4 g
 Sugars . . . . 4 g
Protein . . . . 6 g

Tuna Salad Wrap
Serves 4   Serving size: 1 sandwich

- 1 **(6-oz)** can tuna, packed in water, drained
- 1/4 **cup** pickle relish
- 1/4 **cup** diced celery
- 1/4 **cup** diced onion
- 1/2 **cup** canola mayonnaise
- 4 corn tortillas

Combine the tuna, relish, celery, onion, and mayonnaise until mixed well. Chill before serving. When ready to serve, place an equal amount on each tortilla. Fold in both sides of the tortilla and then roll up the tortilla like a burrito.

Exchanges/Choices

1 Starch
1 Lean Meat
2 Fat

Basic Nutritional Values

Calories 220
  Calories from Fat 90
Total Fat. . . . . .10.0 g
  Saturated Fat . . . . .0.2 g
  Trans Fat. . . . . .0.0 g
Cholesterol . . . . .10 mg
Sodium. . . . . .440 mg
Total Carbohydrate . . .19 g
  Dietary Fiber. . . . . . . .2 g
  Sugars . . . . .7 g
Protein . . . . .11 g

Barbecued Chicken
Serves 4   Serving size: 1/4 recipe

- 1 **cup** water
- 6 **oz** no-added-salt tomato paste
- 1/2 **cup** no-salt catsup
- 1/4 **cup** Splenda Brown Sugar Blend
- 1 **Tbsp** no-added-salt chili powder
- 1 **Tbsp** lemon juice
- 1 **Tbsp** cider vinegar
- 1 **Tbsp** Smart Balance Omega oil
- 1 **tsp** dry mustard
- 1 **tsp** paprika
- 1 clove garlic, minced
  Pepper, to taste
- 1 **lb** boneless, skinless chicken breasts (trimmed of fat)

In a large saucepan, whisk together all ingredients except chicken. Bring to a boil over high heat and then reduce heat and simmer for about 20 minutes. Place the chicken on a cooking sheet and coat with the sauce. Broil and turn until cooked thoroughly.

This recipe is high in sodium.

Exchanges/Choices

1/2 Carbohydrate
3 Lean Meat

Basic Nutritional Values

Calories 180
  Calories from Fat 45
Total Fat. . . . . .5.0 g
  Saturated Fat . . . . .1.5 g
  Trans Fat. . . . . .0.0 g
Cholesterol . . . . .65 mg
Sodium. . . . . .725 mg
Total Carbohydrate . . .8 g
  Dietary Fiber. . . . . . . .0 g
  Sugars . . . . .6 g
Protein . . . . .21 g

Baked Squash

Serves 4   Serving size: 1/4 recipe

1 winter squash (about 1 1/4 lb)	**1/8 tsp** black pepper
2 Tbsp Smart Balance margarine, melted	

Cut squash in half, clean out seeds, brush cut surfaces with melted margarine, and bake cut side down on a cookie sheet at 350°F for 30 minutes. Turn squash cut side up and continue baking until squash is tender when pierced with a pointed knife. Baking time ranges from 45 minutes to 1 hour. Cut through skin into serving-size pieces and season to taste with pepper. Any kind of winter squash can be used, such as acorn, Hubbard, butternut, or buttercup.

Exchanges/Choices

1/2 Starch
1 Fat

Basic Nutritional Values

Calories	75
Calories from Fat	45
Total Fat	5.0 g
Saturated Fat	1.4 g
Trans Fat	0.0 g
Cholesterol	0 mg
Sodium	45 mg
Total Carbohydrate	8 g
Dietary Fiber	3 g
Sugars	3 g
Protein	1 g

Oatmeal and Apple Muffins

Serves 8   Serving size: 1 muffin

1/4 **cup** egg substitute

2/3 **cup** whole-wheat flour

2 **tsp** baking powder

2 **tsp** cinnamon

1 **tsp** nutmeg

1/2 **cup** nonfat milk

1 **cup** raisins

1 apple, peeled, cored, and chopped

1/4 **cup** natural unsweetened applesauce

2/3 **cup** rolled oats

4 **Tbsp** Splenda Brown Sugar Blend

Preheat oven to 400°F. Beat egg substitute. Sift together flour, baking powder, cinnamon, and nutmeg. Combine all ingredients, mixing just to moisten. Spoon batter into muffin cups until 3/4 full. Bake for 15–20 minutes.

Exchanges/Choices

3 Carbohydrate

Basic Nutritional Values

Calories 190
 Calories from Fat 10
Total Fat . . . . 1.0 g
 Saturated Fat . . . . 0.2 g
 Trans Fat . . . . 0.0 g
Cholesterol . . . . 0 mg
Sodium . . . . 120 mg
Total Carbohydrate . . . 44 g
 Dietary Fiber . . . . 3 g
 Sugars . . . . 28 g
Protein . . . . 4 g

Grilled Colby Jack Sandwich

Serves 4   Serving size: 1 sandwich

4 **Tbsp** fat-free margarine

8 slices whole-grain bread

4 **oz** shredded reduced-fat Colby jack cheese

2 medium green bell peppers, sliced

2 medium tomatoes, sliced

Spread 1 Tbsp margarine on each sandwich (1 slice of bread). Place the cheese and pepper and tomato slices between the bread slices and then place under the broiler or in a frying pan. Heat until cheese is melted and bread is toasted to golden brown.

Exchanges/Choices

1 Starch
1 Vegetable
1 Medium-Fat Meat
1/2 Fat

Basic Nutritional Values

Calories 195
 Calories from Fat 70
Total Fat . . . . 8.0 g
 Saturated Fat . . . . 2.5 g
 Trans Fat . . . . 0.0 g
Cholesterol . . . . 15 mg
Sodium . . . . 470 mg
Total Carbohydrate . . . 24 g
 Dietary Fiber . . . . 5 g
 Sugars . . . . 6 g
Protein . . . . 15 g

Baked Swiss Steak

Serves 4   Serving size: 1/4 recipe

- **1 lb** beef round steaks, cut into 1/2-inch-thick slices (trimmed of fat)
- **2 Tbsp** whole-wheat flour
- **2 Tbsp** Smart Balance Omega oil
- **1/2** large onion, chopped
- **1/2** large green bell pepper, chopped
- **1/2 cup** chopped celery
- **1 lb** tomatoes, diced
- **1/2 cup** water

Preheat oven to 350°F. Cut meat into serving-size pieces and dust with 1 Tbsp flour. Put oil in a heavy skillet and sauté meat over high heat until brown. Transfer to a 3-quart baking dish. Cover and bake for 2 hours. Add vegetables and bake for 1 hour or until meat is very tender. Place the meat in a serving dish; keep warm. Put vegetables back in the skillet. Mix 1 Tbsp whole-wheat flour and water and add to vegetables to form gravy. Stir and cook 3 to 4 minutes. Pour over meat.

Exchanges/Choices

2 Vegetable
3 Lean Meat
1 Fat

Basic Nutritional Values

Calories 240
 Calories from Fat 100
Total Fat . . . . 11.0 g
 Saturated Fat . . . . 1.7 g
 Trans Fat . . . . 0.0 g
Cholesterol . . . . 60 mg
Sodium . . . . 50 mg
Total Carbohydrate . . . 11 g
 Dietary Fiber . . . . 3 g
 Sugars . . . . 5 g
Protein . . . . 26 g

Mashed Potatoes

Serves 4   Serving size: 1/4 recipe

- **2 cups** peeled, diced potatoes
- **1/4 cup** nonfat milk
- **5 tsp** Smart Balance margarine
- Pepper, to taste

Peel the potatoes and cut into cubes; place in a large pan. Cover with water, bring to a boil, and then simmer for approximately 45 minutes, until potatoes are tender. Mash potatoes until no lumps remain, slowly adding milk and margarine to make potatoes smoother and fluffy. Season with pepper and serve.

Exchanges/Choices

1 Starch
1/2 Fat

Basic Nutritional Values

Calories 85
 Calories from Fat 35
Total Fat . . . . 4.0 g
 Saturated Fat . . . . 1.1 g
 Trans Fat . . . . 0.0 g
Cholesterol . . . . 0 mg
Sodium . . . . 50 mg
Total Carbohydrate . . . 12 g
 Dietary Fiber . . . . 1 g
 Sugars . . . . 2 g
Protein . . . . 1 g

Dilled Cucumber Salad

Serves 4   Serving size: 1/4 recipe

1/4 **cup** fat-free sour cream	1 1/2 **Tbsp** dill weed
1 **Tbsp** canola mayonnaise	Black pepper, to taste
1/4 **cup** plain fat-free yogurt	1 1/2 medium cucumber
1 1/2 **Tbsp** lime juice	

In a bowl, whisk together sour cream, mayonnaise, yogurt, lime juice, dill, and pepper. Peel the cucumbers and cut crosswise into 1/8-inch-thick slices. Stir them into the dressing. Serve chilled.

Exchanges/Choices

1 Vegetable

Basic Nutritional Values

Calories 40
  Calories from Fat 15
Total Fat . . . . 1.5 g
  Saturated Fat . . . . 0.0 g
  Trans Fat . . . . 0.0 g
Cholesterol . . . . 5 mg
Sodium . . . . 45 mg
Total Carbohydrate . . . 4 g
  Dietary Fiber . . . . 1 g
  Sugars . . . . 3 g
Protein . . . . 2 g

Cold Meatloaf Sandwich

Serves 4   Serving size: 1 sandwich

- **1 Tbsp** sodium-free beef bouillon
- **1/4 cup** water
- **3/4 lb** 96% lean ground beef
- **1/2 cup** quick-cooking oats
- **1/4 cup** egg substitute
- **1/3 cup** finely chopped onions
- **8** slices whole-grain bread

In a large bowl, combine bouillon and water until a broth forms. Add beef, oats, egg substitute, and onions and combine. Firmly shape the mixture into a loaf. Bake at 350°F for about 1 1/4 hours. After cooking, place in the refrigerator to cool. Slice meatloaf in thin slices and place between slices of whole-grain bread. If desired, top with catsup.

Exchanges/Choices

2 Starch
3 Lean Meat

Basic Nutritional Values

Calories 310
 Calories from Fat 65
Total Fat . . . . 7.0 g
 Saturated Fat . . . . 2.5 g
 Trans Fat . . . . 0.1 g
Cholesterol . . . . 50 mg
Sodium . . . . 345 mg
Total Carbohydrate . . . 33 g
 Dietary Fiber . . . . 5 g
 Sugars . . . . 5 g
Protein . . . . 27 g

Potato Salad

Serves 4   Serving size: 1/4 recipe

- **2 cups** potatoes, peeled, boiled, and cubed
- **1/4 cup** onion, chopped and diced
- **1/4 cup** light Italian salad dressing
- **1/2 cup** canola mayonnaise
- **2** eggs, hard boiled and chopped

Wash and peel potatoes. Cook potatoes in boiling water for about 30 minutes. Drain and slice into small cubes. In a large bowl, combine the potatoes with all other ingredients and mix well. Serve chilled.

Exchanges/Choices

1 1/2 Starch
2 Fat

Basic Nutritional Values

Calories 215
 Calories from Fat 115
Total Fat . . . . 13.0 g
 Saturated Fat . . . . 0.9 g
 Trans Fat . . . . 0.0 g
Cholesterol . . . . 105 mg
Sodium . . . . 395 mg
Total Carbohydrate . . . 20 g
 Dietary Fiber . . . . 2 g
 Sugars . . . . 5 g
Protein . . . . 5 g

Baked Fish Wrapped in Lettuce

Serves 4   Serving size: 1/4 recipe

4 large romaine lettuce leaves

1 **lb** white fish

1 zucchini, diced

1 small squash, diced

1 carrot, shredded

4 **tsp** Smart Balance margarine

1 **Tbsp** marjoram

Dash pepper

Preheat oven to 400°F. Place lettuce leaves in hot water and let stand until wilted and then drain. Place the fish on the lettuce. Mound a portion of the zucchini, squash, and carrots on the fillet along with a small amount of margarine. Season with marjoram and pepper. Then fold the leaf around the fish and place seam side down in a large baking dish and place in oven. Bake for approximately 25–30 minutes, until fish flakes easily with a fork.

Exchanges/Choices

1 Vegetable
3 Lean Meat
1 Fat

Basic Nutritional Values

Calories 210
  Calories from Fat 90
Total Fat. . . . . .10.0 g
  Saturated Fat . . . . .2.0 g
  Trans Fat. . . . . .0.0 g
Cholesterol. . . . . .70 mg
Sodium. . . . . .110 mg
Total Carbohydrate . . .5 g
  Dietary Fiber. . . . . .2 g
  Sugars . . . . .3 g
Protein . . . . .24 g

Rice Pilaf

Serves 4   Serving size: 1/4 recipe

1/2 **cup** finely chopped onion

2 **Tbsp** Smart Balance margarine

1 **cup** whole-grain brown rice, uncooked

2 **cups** water

1 **Tbsp** sodium-free chicken bouillon

Pepper, to taste

Sauté onions in margarine until soft and tender; do not brown. Add rice and cook, stirring frequently for 5 minutes. Add water, bouillon, and pepper. Cook covered for 20–25 minutes. Bell peppers, carrots, green onions, or celery can also be added.

Exchanges/Choices

2 1/2 Starch
1 Fat

Basic Nutritional Values

Calories 225
  Calories from Fat 55
Total Fat. . . . . .6.0 g
  Saturated Fat . . . . .1.5 g
  Trans Fat. . . . . .0.0 g
Cholesterol. . . . . .0 mg
Sodium. . . . . .55 mg
Total Carbohydrate . . .39 g
  Dietary Fiber. . . . . .2 g
  Sugars . . . . .2 g
Protein . . . . .4 g

THURSDAY

Whole-Wheat Cornmeal Muffin

Serves 8   Serving size: 1 muffin

2/3	**cup** yellow cornmeal		**2/3**	**cup** nonfat milk
2/3	**cup** whole-wheat flour		**1/4**	**cup** egg substitute
1	**Tbsp** Splenda		**2**	**Tbsp** Smart Balance Omega oil
2	**tsp** baking powder			

Preheat oven to 400°F. Place paper liners in muffin trays. Thoroughly mix dry ingredients. Combine milk, egg substitute, and oil; add to dry ingredients. Stir until dry ingredients are just moistened. Batter will be lumpy. Fill muffin tins 2/3 full. Bake until slightly browned, about 20 minutes.

Exchanges/Choices

1 Carbohydrate
1 Fat

Basic Nutritional Values

Calories 120
  Calories from Fat 35
Total Fat . . . . 4.0 g
  Saturated Fat . . . . 0.3 g
  Trans Fat . . . . 0.0 g
Cholesterol . . . . 0 mg
Sodium . . . . 115 mg
Total Carbohydrate . . . 18 g
  Dietary Fiber . . . . 2 g
  Sugars . . . . 1 g
Protein . . . . 4 g

Chicken Fajitas

Serves 4   Serving size: 1 fajita

3/4 **lb** boneless, skinless chicken breasts (trimmed of fat)

1 **Tbsp** Worcestershire sauce

2 **Tbsp** lemon juice

1 **Tbsp** Smart Balance Omega oil

1 medium clove garlic, minced

1/8 **tsp** black pepper

1 medium onion

1 large green bell pepper

4 (**6-inch**) flour tortillas

Exchanges/Choices

1 Starch
1 Vegetable
3 Lean Meat

Basic Nutritional Values

Calories 230
 Calories from Fat 55
Total Fat . . . . .6.0 g
 Saturated Fat . . . . .0.9 g
 Trans Fat . . . . .0.0 g
Cholesterol . . . . .50 mg
Sodium . . . . .315 mg
Total Carbohydrate . . .23 g
 Dietary Fiber . . . . .2 g
 Sugars . . . . .4 g
Protein . . . . .22 g

1. Cut the chicken lengthwise into 3-inch strips. In a large bowl, stir together the Worcestershire sauce, lemon juice, oil, garlic, and pepper to form a marinade. Add the chicken to the marinade. Stir and coat evenly, cover, and refrigerate for about 20 minutes.

2. Cut the onion and bell pepper into 1/8-inch strips.

3. Place the tortillas in foil and place them in the oven at 350°F for about 10 minutes.

4. Heat a large nonstick skillet over medium-high heat. Place the chicken and the marinade in the skillet and cook for about 4 minutes. Add the onion and pepper slices and cook, stirring constantly, for another 5 minutes, until the onion is lightly browned and the chicken is no longer pink in the center.

5. To serve, place equal amounts of the chicken-vegetable mixture on each tortilla and then roll the tortilla around the mixture.

Red Cabbage Coleslaw

Serves 4   Serving size: 1/4 recipe

2 **cups** finely chopped red cabbage

1 **(16-oz)** jar pickled beets, diced and drained

1/2 **cup** red onion, diced

1/4 **cup** cider vinegar

2 **Tbsp** Splenda Brown Sugar Blend

1 **Tbsp** Smart Balance Omega oil

1/2 **tsp** caraway seeds

Pepper, to taste

In a large bowl, combine the cabbage, beets, and red onion. In a small saucepan, mix the vinegar, Splenda, oil, caraway seeds, and pepper. Over medium heat, bring to a boil and pour over the cabbage mixture. Toss well. Cover and chill at least 4 hours before serving.

Exchanges/Choices

1 Carbohydrate
2 Vegetable
1/2 Fat

Basic Nutritional Values

Calories	125
Calories from Fat	30
Total Fat	3.5 g
Saturated Fat	0.3 g
Trans Fat	0.0 g
Cholesterol	0 mg
Sodium	260 mg
Total Carbohydrate	23 g
Dietary Fiber	3 g
Sugars	17 g
Protein	1 g

Turkey Meatloaf

Serves 4   Serving size: 1/4 recipe

1 **cup** oats

1/4 **cup** nonfat milk

1 **lb** ground lean turkey

1/2 **cup** egg substitute, slightly beaten

1/4 **cup** chopped onions

1 **tsp** black pepper

1 **tsp** dried sage

1/4 **cup** Splenda Brown Sugar Blend

1/2 **cup** salsa

1/4 **tsp** nutmeg

1 **tsp** Dijon mustard

Combine oats, milk, turkey, egg substitute, onions, pepper, and sage. Spoon into a loaf pan and press to make even. In a small bowl, combine Splenda, salsa, nutmeg, and mustard; set aside. Bake loaf at 350°F for 1 hour. Remove from oven and spread sauce over loaf; bake for an additional 15 minutes.

Exchanges/Choices

1 Starch
1 Carbohydrate
3 Lean Meat

Basic Nutritional Values

Calories	280
Calories from Fat	20
Total Fat	2.0 g
Saturated Fat	0.5 g
Trans Fat	0.0 g
Cholesterol	75 mg
Sodium	330 mg
Total Carbohydrate	30 g
Dietary Fiber	3 g
Sugars	14 g
Protein	34 g

Oven-Baked Potatoes

Serves 4   Serving size: 1/4 recipe

4 medium potatoes

1/4 cup Smart Balance Light margarine

1/8 tsp black pepper

Wash potatoes and cut into small cubes, leaving the skins on. Place margarine on top of potatoes and bake at 350°F for about 1 hour. Check frequently and spoon the melted margarine over the potatoes. Season with pepper.

Exchanges/Choices

2 1/2 Starch
1/2 Fat

Basic Nutritional Values

Calories 205
  Calories from Fat 45
Total Fat . . . . 5.0 g
  Saturated Fat . . . . 1.6 g
  Trans Fat . . . . 0.0 g
Cholesterol . . . . 0 mg
Sodium . . . . 100 mg
Total Carbohydrate . . . 37 g
  Dietary Fiber . . . . 4 g
  Sugars . . . . 2 g
Protein . . . . 4 g

Zucchini Carrot Muffins

Serves 8   Serving size: 1 muffin

3/4	**cup** rolled oats	2	**tsp** ground nutmeg
2 1/2	**cups** whole-wheat flour	3	**Tbsp** Smart Balance Omega oil
2/3	**cup** nonfat milk	3	egg whites, beaten
1/2	**cup** wheat germ, toasted	1	**cup** carrots, finely shredded
3	**tsp** baking powder	1/2	**cup** zucchini, stemmed and grated
3/4	**cup** Splenda		
1	**Tbsp** ground cinnamon		

Preheat oven to 350°F. Combine all ingredients and mix well; pour into muffin liners in muffin pans. Bake for about 1 hour. Let cool for about 30 minutes before removing.

Exchanges/Choices

2 1/2 Carbohydrate
1 1/2 Fat

Basic Nutritional Values

Calories 260
  Calories from Fat 65
Total Fat . . . . 7.0 g
  Saturated Fat . . . . 0.9 g
  Trans Fat . . . . 0.0 g
Cholesterol . . . . 0 mg
Sodium . . . . 180 mg
Total Carbohydrate . . . 42 g
  Dietary Fiber . . . . 7 g
  Sugars . . . . 5 g
Protein . . . . 11 g

Western Omelet

Serves 4   Serving size: 1/4 recipe

1	**cup** egg substitute	1/2	**cup** diced onion
2	**Tbsp** Smart Balance Light margarine	1/2	**cup** diced bell pepper
4	**oz** extra-lean, lower-sodium ham, cooked, sliced, and diced		

Make each omelet individually. Mix egg substitute until blended. Place margarine in a skillet and melt. When it just begins to brown, the skillet is the right temperature. Pour a single portion of egg into the skillet and cook quickly. Fold the ham, onions, and peppers into the omelet and cover. Repeat for additional omelets.

Exchanges/Choices

1 Vegetable
1 Lean Meat
1/2 Fat

Basic Nutritional Values

Calories 95
  Calories from Fat 25
Total Fat . . . . 3.0 g
  Saturated Fat . . . . 1.0 g
  Trans Fat . . . . 0.0 g
Cholesterol . . . . 15 mg
Sodium . . . . 390 mg
Total Carbohydrate . . . 5 g
  Dietary Fiber . . . . 1 g
  Sugars . . . . 3 g
Protein . . . . 11 g

Hawaiian Dessert

Serves 4   Serving size: 1/4 recipe

8 **oz** fat-free plain yogurt

1/2 **cup** miniature marshmallows

1 **cup** pineapple chunks

8 **oz** no-added-sugar mandarin orange segments

Mix all ingredients until well blended. Chill 3 hours before serving.

Exchanges/Choices

1 1/2 Carbohydrate

Basic Nutritional Values

Calories 95
  Calories from Fat 0
Total Fat . . . . 0.0 g
  Saturated Fat . . . . 0.1 g
  Trans Fat . . . . 0.0 g
Cholesterol . . . . 5 mg
Sodium . . . . 45 mg
Total Carbohydrate . . . 21 g
  Dietary Fiber . . . . 1 g
  Sugars . . . . 20 g
Protein . . . . 4 g

Scallops, Spaghetti, and Vegetables

Serves 4   Serving size: 1/4 recipe

8 **oz** spaghetti

2 **Tbsp** sodium-free chicken bouillon

1 **cup** water

1/2 **cup** dry white wine

2 **Tbsp** lemon juice

2 cloves garlic, minced

1 **tsp** dill

1/2 **tsp** ground black pepper

1 **cup** sliced celery

2 **cups** sliced carrots

4 scallions, sliced

3/4 **lb** bay scallops

2 **cups** chopped spinach leaves

1. Cook spaghetti according to package instructions.

2. Bring bouillon and water to a boil in a large skillet over medium heat. Add wine, lemon juice, garlic, dill, pepper, celery, carrots, and scallions. Reduce heat, cover, and simmer for 10 minutes. Add scallops and spinach and simmer for 5 minutes. Serve pasta topped with scallop-vegetable sauce.

Exchanges/Choices

3 Starch
2 Vegetable
2 Lean Meat

Basic Nutritional Values

Calories 355
  Calories from Fat 20
Total Fat . . . . 2.5 g
  Saturated Fat . . . . 0.3 g
  Trans Fat . . . . 0.0 g
Cholesterol . . . . 35 mg
Sodium . . . . 255 mg
Total Carbohydrate . . . 56 g
  Dietary Fiber . . . . 6 g
  Sugars . . . . 8 g
Protein . . . . 24 g

Southwest Tomato Salad

Serves 4   Serving size: 1/4 recipe

2 cups diced tomatoes (about 4 medium tomatoes)

1/2 cup diced green bell pepper

1/2 cup chopped, peeled cucumber

1/2 cup finely chopped red onion

1 Tbsp minced jalapeño

1/2 cup seasoned croutons

1/4 cup light Italian salad dressing

In a large bowl, combine tomatoes, green bell pepper, cucumber, onion, and jalapeño. Add croutons and dressing; toss thoroughly to combine.

Exchanges/Choices

2 Vegetable
1/2 Fat

Basic Nutritional Values

Calories 70
  Calories from Fat 20
Total Fat . . . . 2.0 g
  Saturated Fat . . . . 0.4 g
  Trans Fat . . . . 0.0 g
Cholesterol . . . . 0 mg
Sodium . . . . 245 mg
Total Carbohydrate . . . 12 g
  Dietary Fiber . . . . 2 g
  Sugars . . . . 6 g
Protein . . . . 2 g

Bulgur Turkey Meatball Sandwich

Serves 4   Serving size: 1 sandwich

1 **cup** water	1/8 **tsp** ground black pepper
1/2 **cup** bulgur	1 **cup** light spaghetti sauce
3/4 **lb** ground turkey breast	4 small whole-grain hoagie/ sandwich buns
1 medium onion, minced	
2 **Tbsp** minced parsley	4 **oz** fat-free shredded mozzarella
1/2 **tsp** dried mint	

1. Bring water to a boil. Stir in bulgur, cover, and let stand 15 minutes, until bulgur is just tender.

2. Preheat oven to 375°F. Drain excess liquid from bulgur and add turkey, onion, parsley, mint, and pepper. Mix well. Form balls 1 1/4 inches in diameter. Place meatballs in a nonstick baking dish and bake until lightly browned, about 15 minutes.

3. Place the meatballs in the hoagie buns and cover with spaghetti sauce and mozzarella cheese. Place back in the oven for 5 minutes, until sauce is warmed and cheese is melted.

This recipe is high in sodium.

Exchanges/Choices

3 1/2 Starch
3 Lean Meat

Basic Nutritional Values

Calories 395
 Calories from Fat 30
Total Fat . . . . 3.5 g
 Saturated Fat . . . . 0.7 g
 Trans Fat . . . . 0.0 g
Cholesterol . . . . 45 mg
Sodium . . . . 860 mg
Total Carbohydrate . . . 60 g
 Dietary Fiber . . . . 10 g
 Sugars . . . . 12 g
Protein . . . . 32 g

Far East Cabbage Salad

Serves 4   Serving size: 1/4 recipe

2 **Tbsp** lemon juice	4 **Tbsp** diced mint leaves
2 **tsp** Splenda	4 **Tbsp** chopped cilantro
4 **cups** cabbage, shredded	2 **Tbsp** Smart Balance Omega oil
2/3 medium onion red, diced	

In a bowl, stir together the lemon juice and Splenda until dissolved. Add all other ingredients and toss well until mixed.

Exchanges/Choices

1 Vegetable
1 1/2 Fat

Basic Nutritional Values

Calories 90
 Calories from Fat 65
Total Fat . . . . 7.0 g
 Saturated Fat . . . . 0.5 g
 Trans Fat . . . . 0.0 g
Cholesterol . . . . 0 mg
Sodium . . . . 15 mg
Total Carbohydrate . . . 7 g
 Dietary Fiber . . . . 2 g
 Sugars . . . . 4 g
Protein . . . . 1 g

Pepper Steak

Serves 4   Serving size: 1/4 recipe

1 lb lean round steak (trimmed of fat)

2 Tbsp Smart Balance margarine

2 Tbsp whole-wheat flour

1 (10-oz) can no-added-salt peeled tomatoes

1 Tbsp sodium-free beef bouillon

1 medium onion

2 cups whole-grain rice, uncooked

1 medium green pepper

Cut steak into 1-inch thin strips and brown in a skillet with the margarine. Stir in flour. Drain tomatoes and reserve the liquid. Add water to the tomato liquid to make 4 cups total. Add the bouillon. Chop onion. Add onion and bouillon mixture to skillet; stir. Cover and cook over low heat for 1 hour or until meat is tender. Stir occasionally. Cook the rice according to package directions. Cut green pepper into thin strips. When meat is almost done, add peeled tomatoes and pepper strips to the skillet. Cover and heat for 5 more minutes. Serve over brown rice.

Exchanges/Choices

2 Starch
1 Vegetable
3 Lean Meat
1 Fat

Basic Nutritional Values

Calories	360
Calories from Fat	100
Total Fat	11.0 g
Saturated Fat	3.4 g
Trans Fat	0.1 g
Cholesterol	75 mg
Sodium	115 mg
Total Carbohydrate	35 g
Dietary Fiber	4 g
Sugars	6 g
Protein	29 g

Sautéed Zucchini and Red Peppers

Serves 4   Serving size: 1/4 recipe

2 medium red bell peppers, seeded and cut into 1/2-inch strips

2 medium zucchini, cut into 1/2-inch strips

1 clove garlic, minced

2 Tbsp Smart Balance Omega oil

Black pepper, to taste

2 Tbsp minced parsley

In a large skillet over medium heat, sauté peppers, zucchini, and garlic in oil until zucchini is golden. Season with pepper and parsley. Serve hot.

Exchanges/Choices

2 Vegetable
1 Fat

Basic Nutritional Values

Calories	95
Calories from Fat	65
Total Fat	7.0 g
Saturated Fat	0.6 g
Trans Fat	0.0 g
Cholesterol	0 mg
Sodium	15 mg
Total Carbohydrate	8 g
Dietary Fiber	3 g
Sugars	5 g
Protein	2 g

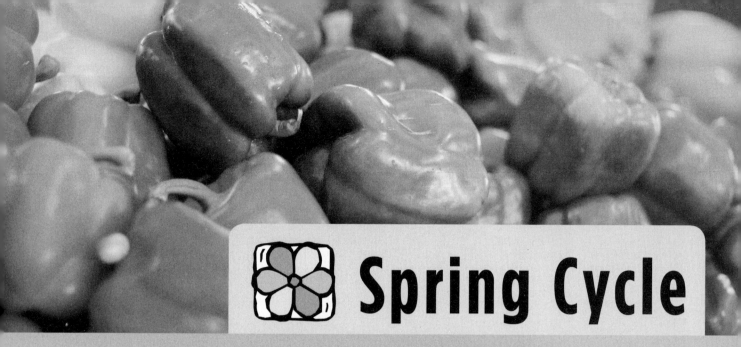

Spring Cycle

WEEK 4

FEATURED RECIPES

Whole-Wheat Pancakes or Waffles*

Frozen Pumpkin Dessert

Country-Fried Steak

Mashed Potatoes*

Scalloped Potatoes*

Turkey Chili con Carne

Marinated Turkey Fillets

Poppy Seed Fruit Salad*

Multigrain Rice Pilaf*

Whole-Wheat Blueberry Muffins*

Pita Tuna Melts

Potato Salad*

Blackened Pork Cutlet

Green Beans and Red Peppers

Deli Ham Sandwich

Carrot Slaw*

Baked Fillet of Sole

Cucumber Salad

Lemon Parsley Carrots*

Bran Muffins*

Whole-Wheat Pasta Salad*

Mexican Coleslaw

Asian Chicken

Fruit Medley*

Pumpkin Spice Muffins*

Whole-Grain Burger

Turkey Cutlet Parmesan

Carrot-Raisin Salad

Chilled Cauliflower Salad*

Peach Cobbler*

Tuna Salad

Chicken Burritos

Corn and Zucchini Combo*

Ambrosia Salad*

*Indicates that the recipe has been used previously.

	Sunday	Monday	Tuesday	Wednesday	Thursday	Friday	Saturday
Breakfast	Whole-Wheat Pancakes or Waffles* 1/4 cup sugar-free maple syrup 1/2 cup unsweetened applesauce 1 cup nonfat milk 1/2 tsp margarine	Scalloped Potatoes* 1/2 whole-wheat English muffin 3/4 cup blackberries 1/2 cup nonfat milk 1 oz Canadian bacon 2 tsp margarine	Whole-Wheat Blueberry Muffin* 1/2 cup Cheerios 1 medium banana 1 cup nonfat milk 1/4 cup egg substitute, scrambled 1 tsp margarine	1/2 cup Fiber One cereal 1 slice multigrain bread 1 kiwi fruit 1 cup nonfat milk 1 Tbsp peanut butter	Bran Muffins* 1/2 cup oatmeal 1 1/4 cup strawberries 1 cup nonfat milk	Pumpkin Spice Muffins* 1/2 Tbsp jam 1/2 cup unsweetened applesauce 1 cup nonfat milk 1 oz reduced-sodium ham 1/2 tsp margarine	Peach Cobbler* 1/2 English muffin 1/2 cup nonfat milk 1 oz lean beef sausage 1 1/2 tsp margarine
Lunch	Frozen Pumpkin Dessert 1/2 cup sweet potatoes 1 small dinner roll 1/2 cup steamed green beans 2 oz baked turkey breast 1 tsp margarine	Turkey Chili con Carne 1 small dinner roll 1 cup honeydew melon	Pita Tuna Melts Potato Salad* (1/2 cup) 1 small orange 1 cup raw celery	Deli Ham Sandwich Carrot Slaw* 2 cups mixed corn, peas, and pasta	Whole-Wheat Pasta Salad* Mexican Coleslaw 1/2 large pear 2 oz pork tenderloin	Whole-Grain Burger 2 slices whole-wheat bread 2 tangerines 1 cup raw vegetable sticks 1 oz reduced-fat cheese 1/2 Tbsp light salad dressing	Tuna Salad 3 rice cakes 3/4 oz baked potato chips 3/4 cup blueberries 1 cup salad greens 1/4 cup fat-free cottage cheese
Snack A							
Snack B							
Dinner	Country-Fried Steak Mashed Potatoes* 1 slice whole-wheat bread 1/2 cup mango 1 cup nonfat milk 1 cup cooked turnip greens 1/2 tsp margarine	Marinated Turkey Fillets Poppy Seed Fruit Salad* Multigrain Rice Pilaf* 1 cup mixed vegetables 2 tsp margarine	Blackened Pork Cutlet Green Beans and Red Peppers 1 small baked potato 1/2 cup fruit cocktail in light syrup 1 cup nonfat milk 2 tsp margarine	Baked Fillet of Sole Cucumber Salad Lemon Parsley Carrots* 1 1/2 slices multigrain bread 1/2 cup unsweetened plums 1 cup nonfat milk 1/2 cup steamed, mixed nonstarchy vegetables 1/2 tsp margarine	Asian Chicken Fruit Medley* 1 oz angel food cake 1/2 cup blackberries 1 cup nonfat milk 1/2 cup steamed broccoli 1 tsp margarine	Turkey Cutlet Parmesan Carrot-Raisin Salad Chilled Cauliflower Salad* 1/2 cup steamed green beans	Chicken Burritos Corn and Zucchini Combo* Ambrosia Salad (1/2 serving)* 1/2 cup nonfat milk 1 oz reduced-fat cheese 4 pecans

*Indicates that the recipe has been used previously.

	Sunday	Monday	Tuesday	Wednesday	Thursday	Friday	Saturday
Breakfast	Whole-Wheat Pancakes or Waffles* 1/4 cup sugar-free maple syrup 1/2 cup unsweetened applesauce 1 cup nonfat milk 1 oz lean turkey sausage 1/2 tsp margarine	Scalloped Potatoes* 1/2 whole-wheat English muffin 3/4 cup blackberries 1/2 cup nonfat milk 1 oz Canadian bacon 2 tsp margarine	Whole-Wheat Blueberry Muffin* 1/2 cup Cheerios 1 medium banana 1 cup nonfat milk 1/4 cup egg substitute, scrambled 1 tsp margarine	1/2 cup Fiber One cereal 1 slice multigrain bread 1 kiwi fruit 1 cup nonfat milk 1 oz low-fat turkey pastrami 1 Tbsp peanut butter	Bran Muffins* 1/2 cup oatmeal 1 1/4 cup strawberries 1 cup nonfat milk 1/4 cup egg substitute, scrambled 1 tsp margarine	Pumpkin Spice Muffins* 1/2 Tbsp jam 1/2 cup unsweetened applesauce 1 cup nonfat milk 1 oz reduced-sodium ham 1/2 tsp margarine	Peach Cobbler* 1/2 English muffin 1/2 cup nonfat milk 1 oz lean beef sausage 2 tsp margarine
Lunch	Frozen Pumpkin Dessert 1/2 cup sweet potatoes 1 small dinner roll 1/2 cup steamed green beans 2 oz baked turkey breast 2 tsp margarine	Turkey Chili con Carne 1 small dinner roll 1 cup honeydew melon 1 tsp margarine	Pita Tuna Melts Potato Salad* (1/2 cup) 1 small orange 1 cup raw celery 1 1/2 Tbsp low-fat cream cheese	Deli Ham Sandwich Carrot Slaw* 2 cups mixed corn, peas, and pasta 1 tsp margarine	Whole-Wheat Pasta Salad* Mexican Coleslaw 1/2 large pear 2 oz pork tenderloin	Whole-Grain Burger 2 slices whole-wheat bread 2 tangerines 1 cup raw vegetable sticks 1 oz reduced-fat cheese 1 1/2 Tbsp light salad dressing	Tuna Salad 3 rice cakes 3/4 oz baked potato chips 3/4 cup blueberries 1 cup salad greens 1/4 cup fat-free cottage cheese
Snack A	1 Tbsp sunflower seeds 2 small tangerines	1 1/2 tsp peanut butter 1 small apple	6 almonds 3/4 cup mandarin oranges packed in juice	5 hazelnuts 1 cup papaya	2 Brazil nuts 1 1/4 cup watermelon	3 macadamia nuts 1 medium banana	4 walnut halves 4 apricots
Snack B	1 cup nonfat milk	1 cup nonfat milk	1 cup nonfat milk	1 cup nonfat milk	1 cup nonfat milk	6 oz fat-free yogurt	1 cup nonfat milk
Dinner	Country-Fried Steak Mashed Potatoes* 1 slice whole-wheat bread 1/2 cup mango 1 cup nonfat milk 1 cup cooked turnip greens 1/2 tsp margarine	Marinated Turkey Fillets Poppy Seed Fruit Salad* Multigrain Rice Pilaf* 1 cup mixed vegetables 2 tsp margarine	Blackened Pork Cutlet Green Beans and Red Peppers 1 small baked potato 1/2 cup fruit cocktail in light syrup 1 cup nonfat milk 1 oz reduced-fat cheese 2 tsp margarine	Baked Fillet of Sole Cucumber Salad Lemon Parsley Carrots* 1 1/2 slices multigrain bread 1/2 cup unsweetened plums 1 cup nonfat milk 1/2 cup steamed, mixed nonstarchy vegetables 1/2 tsp margarine	Asian Chicken Fruit Medley* 1 oz angel food cake 1/2 cup blackberries 1 cup nonfat milk 1/2 cup steamed broccoli 1 tsp margarine	Turkey Cutlet Parmesan Carrot-Raisin Salad Chilled Cauliflower Salad* 1/2 cup steamed green beans	Chicken Burritos Corn and Zucchini Combo* Ambrosia Salad (1/2 serving)* 1/2 cup nonfat milk 2 oz reduced-fat cheese 4 pecans

*Indicates that the recipe has been used previously.

2000 calorie MEAL PLAN SPRING WEEK 4

	Sunday	Monday	Tuesday	Wednesday	Thursday	Friday	Saturday
Breakfast	Whole-Wheat Pancakes or Waffles* 1/4 cup sugar-free maple syrup 1/2 cup unsweetened applesauce 1 cup nonfat milk 1 oz lean turkey sausage 1/2 tsp margarine	Scalloped Potatoes* 1/2 whole-wheat English muffin 3/4 cup blackberries 1/2 cup nonfat milk 1 oz Canadian bacon 2 tsp margarine	1/2 cup Cheerios 1 medium banana 1 cup nonfat milk 1/4 cup egg substitute, scrambled 1 tsp margarine	1/2 cup Fiber One cereal 1 slice multigrain bread 1 kiwi fruit 1 cup nonfat milk 1 oz low-fat turkey pastrami 1 Tbsp peanut butter	Bran Muffins* 1/2 cup oatmeal 1 1/4 cup strawberries 1 cup nonfat milk 1/4 cup egg substitute, scrambled 1 tsp margarine	Pumpkin Spice Muffins* 1/2 Tbsp jam 1/2 cup unsweetened applesauce 1 cup nonfat milk 1 oz reduced-sodium ham 1/2 tsp margarine	Peach Cobbler* 1/2 English muffin 1/2 cup nonfat milk 1 oz lean beef sausage 2 tsp margarine
Lunch	Frozen Pumpkin Dessert 1/2 cup sweet potatoes 1 small dinner roll 1/8 cup cranberry sauce 1 cup steamed green beans 2 oz baked turkey breast 2 tsp margarine	Turkey Chili con Carne 1 small dinner roll 2 cups honeydew melon 1/2 cup steamed asparagus 1 tsp margarine	Pita Tuna Melts Potato Salad* (1/2 cup) 1 medium orange 2 cups raw celery 1 1/2 low-fat cream cheese	Deli Ham Sandwich Carrot Slaw* 2 cups mixed corn, peas, and pasta 3 dates 1 tsp margarine	Whole-Wheat Pasta Salad* **Mexican Coleslaw** 1 large pear 1/2 cup carrots 2 oz pork tenderloin	Whole-Grain Burger 2 slices whole-wheat bread 2 tangerines 1/2 cup no-added-sugar canned pears 2 cups raw vegetable sticks 1 oz reduced-fat cheese 1 1/2 Tbsp light salad dressing	Tuna Salad 3 rice cakes 3/4 oz baked potato chips 1 1/2 cup blueberries 2 cups salad greens 1/4 cup fat-free cottage cheese 1 1/2 tsp olive oil and vinegar salad dressing
Snack A	1 cup cucumber sticks 1 Tbsp sunflower seeds 2 small tangerines	1 cup raw broccoli 1 1/2 tsp peanut butter 1 small apple	1 cup water chestnuts 6 almonds 3/4 cup mandarin oranges packed in juice	1 cup raw vegetable sticks 5 hazelnuts 1 cup papaya	1 cup raw carrots 2 Brazil nuts 6 almonds	1 cup mixed vegetable sticks 3 macadamia nuts 1 medium banana	1 cup raw cucumbers 4 walnut halves 4 apricots
Snack B	1 1/2 low-fat corn bread 1 tsp margarine 1 cup nonfat milk	5 oz corn on the cob 1 tsp margarine 1 cup nonfat milk	1 slice wheat bread 1 1/2 tsp cashew butter 1 cup nonfat milk	1/2 English muffin 1 tsp margarine 1 cup nonfat milk	2 oz oven-baked French fries 1 1/4 cup watermelon 1 cup nonfat milk	3 ginger snaps 1/2 tsp cashew butter 6 oz fat-free yogurt	1 small muffin (1 oz) 1/2 tsp margarine 1 cup nonfat milk
Dinner	Country-Fried Steak Mashed Potatoes* 1 slice whole-wheat bread 1/2 cup mango 1 cup nonfat milk 1 cup cooked turnip greens 1/2 tsp margarine	Marinated Turkey Fillets Poppy Seed Fruit Salad* Multigrain Rice Pilaf* 1 cup mixed vegetables 2 tsp margarine	Blackened Pork Cutlet Green Beans and Red Peppers 1 small baked potato 1/2 cup fruit cocktail in light syrup 1 cup nonfat milk 1 oz reduced-fat cheese 2 tsp margarine	Baked Fillet of Sole Cucumber Salad Lemon Parsley Carrots* 1 1/2 slices multigrain bread 1/2 cup unsweetened plums 1 cup nonfat milk 1/2 cup steamed, mixed nonstarchy vegetables 1/2 tsp margarine	Asian Chicken Fruit Medley* 1 oz angel food cake 1/2 cup blackberries 1 cup nonfat milk 1/2 cup steamed broccoli 1 tsp margarine	Turkey Cutlet Parmesan Carrot-Raisin Salad Chilled Cauliflower Salad* 1/2 cup steamed green beans	Chicken Burritos Corn and Zucchini Combo* Ambrosia Salad (1/2 serving)* 1/2 cup nonfat milk 2 oz reduced-fat cheese 4 pecans

*Indicates that the recipe has been used previously.

	Sunday	Monday	Tuesday	Wednesday	Thursday	Friday	Saturday
Breakfast	Whole-Wheat Pancakes or Waffles* 1/4 cup sugar-free maple syrup 1/2 cup unsweetened applesauce 1 oz lean turkey sausage 1 cup nonfat milk 1/2 tsp margarine	Scalloped Potatoes* 1/2 whole-wheat English muffin 3/4 cup blackberries 1/2 cup nonfat milk 2 oz Canadian bacon 2 tsp margarine	Whole-Wheat Blueberry Muffin* 1/2 cup Cheerios 1 medium banana 1 cup nonfat milk 1/2 cup egg substitute, scrambled 1 tsp margarine	1/2 cup Fiber One cereal 1 slice multigrain bread 1 kiwi fruit 1 cup nonfat milk 2 oz low-fat turkey pastrami 1 Tbsp peanut butter	Bran Muffins* 1/2 cup oatmeal 1 1/4 cup strawberries 1 cup nonfat milk 1/4 cup egg substitute, scrambled 1 tsp margarine	Pumpkin Spice Muffins* 1/2 Tbsp jam 1/2 cup unsweetened applesauce 1 cup nonfat milk 2 oz reduced-sodium ham 1/2 tsp margarine	Peach Cobbler* 1/2 English muffin 1/2 cup nonfat milk 2 oz lean beef sausage 2 tsp margarine
Lunch	Frozen Pumpkin Dessert 1/2 cup sweet potatoes 1 small dinner roll 1/8 cup cranberry sauce 1 cup steamed green beans 2 oz baked turkey breast 2 tsp margarine	Turkey Chili con Carne 1 small dinner roll 2 cups honeydew melon 1/2 cup steamed asparagus 1 tsp margarine	Pita Tuna Melts Potato Salad* (1/2 cup) 1 medium orange 2 cups raw celery 1 1/2 Tbsp low-fat cream cheese	Deli Ham Sandwich Carrot Slaw* 2 cups mixed corn, peas, and pasta 3 dates 1 tsp margarine	Whole-Wheat Pasta Salad* Mexican Coleslaw 1 large pear 1/2 cup carrots 2 oz pork tenderloin	Whole-Grain Burger 2 slices whole-wheat bread 2 tangerines 1/2 cup no-added-sugar canned pears 2 cups raw vegetable sticks 1 oz reduced-fat cheese 1 1/2 Tbsp light salad dressing	Tuna Salad 3 rice cakes 3/4 oz baked potato chips 1 1/2 cup blueberries 2 cups salad greens 1/4 cup fat-free cottage cheese 1 1/2 tsp olive oil and vinegar salad dressing
Snack A	1 cup cucumber sticks 1 Tbsp sunflower seeds 2 small tangerines	1 cup raw broccoli 1 1/2 tsp peanut butter 1 small apple	1 cup water chestnuts 6 almonds 3/4 cup mandarin oranges packed in juice	1 cup raw vegetable sticks 5 hazelnuts 1 cup papaya	1 cup raw carrots 2 Brazil nuts 6 almonds	1 cup mixed vegetable sticks 3 macadamia nuts 1 medium banana	1 cup raw cucumbers 4 walnut halves 4 apricots
Snack B	1 1/2 low-fat corn bread 1 tsp margarine 1 cup nonfat milk	5 oz corn on the cob 1 tsp margarine 1 cup nonfat milk	1 slice wheat bread 1 1/2 tsp cashew butter 1 cup nonfat milk	1/2 English muffin 1 tsp margarine 1 cup nonfat milk	2 oz oven-baked French fries 1 1/4 cup watermelon 1 cup nonfat milk	3 ginger snaps 1/2 tsp cashew butter 6 oz fat-free yogurt	1 small muffin (1 oz) 1/2 tsp margarine 1 cup nonfat milk
Dinner	Country-Fried Steak Mashed Potatoes* 5 small wheat dinner rolls 1/2 cup mango 1 cup nonfat milk 1 cup cooked turnip greens 1/2 tsp margarine	Marinated Turkey Fillets Poppy Seed Fruit Salad* Multigrain Rice Pilaf* 1 dinner roll 1 cup mixed vegetables 2 tsp margarine	Blackened Pork Cutlet Green Beans and Red Peppers 1 small baked potato 1 slice whole-wheat bread 1/2 cup fruit cocktail in light syrup 1 cup nonfat milk 1 oz reduced-fat cheese 2 tsp margarine	Baked Fillet of Sole Cucumber Salad Lemon Parsley Carrots* 1 1/2 slices multigrain bread 1/2 cup unsweetened plums 1 cup nonfat milk 1/2 cup steamed, mixed nonstarchy vegetables 1/2 tsp margarine	Asian Chicken Fruit Medley* 3 oz angel food cake 1/2 cup blackberries 1 cup nonfat milk 1/2 cup steamed broccoli 1 tsp margarine	Turkey Cutlet Parmesan Carrot-Raisin Salad Chilled Cauliflower Salad* 1 small wheat dinner roll 1/2 cup steamed green beans	Chicken Burritos Corn and Zucchini Combo* Ambrosia Salad (1/2 serving)* 1/3 cup baked beans 1/2 cup nonfat milk 1 oz reduced-fat cheese 4 pecans

*Indicates that the recipe has been used previously.

SHOPPING LIST

VEGETABLES

____ asparagus
____ bell peppers, green
____ bell peppers, red
____ broccoli
____ cabbage, green
____ carrots
____ cauliflower
____ celery
____ corn, whole-kernel, frozen
____ cucumbers
____ garlic
____ green beans
____ jalapeño pepper
____ lettuce, iceberg
____ lettuce, romaine
____ mushrooms
____ olives, black, pitted
____ onions, yellow or white
____ onions, green
____ peapods, snow, frozen
____ potatoes, russet
____ potatoes, sweet
____ tomatoes
____ turnip greens
____ zucchini squash

MEATS

____ bacon, Canadian
____ beef patties, ground, 96% lean
____ beef sausage, lean
____ chicken breasts, boneless, skinless
____ ham, light/reduced-sodium
____ pork chops, boneless sirloin
____ pork tenderloin
____ sole fillets
____ turkey breast strips, boneless, skinless
____ turkey breast, baked
____ turkey breast, ground
____ turkey cutlets, lean, boneless
____ turkey pastrami, low-fat
____ turkey sausage, lean

FRUITS

____ bananas
____ blackberries
____ blueberries
____ cantaloupe
____ grapefruit
____ grapes, seedless
____ kiwi fruit
____ lemon
____ mango
____ melon, honeydew
____ oranges
____ peaches
____ pears, no-added-sugar can
____ pineapple, crushed, no-added-sugar can
____ plums, unsweetened
____ raisins
____ strawberries
____ tangerines

DAIRY

____ egg substitute
____ eggs
____ ice cream, fat-free, vanilla
____ milk, nonfat
____ Smart Balance Light margarine
____ Smart Balance Light spread
____ sour cream, fat-free
____ whipped topping, fat-free
____ yogurt, fat-free, plain

CHEESE

____ cheddar, shredded, fat-free
____ cottage cheese, fat-free
____ cream cheese, fat-free
____ cream cheese, low-fat
____ Parmesan, reduced-fat
____ Swiss, reduced-fat

BREAD, GRAINS, & PASTA

____ barley, pearl
____ bread, whole-wheat, whole-grain
____ dinner rolls
____ English muffins, whole-wheat
____ pita breads, 6-inch
____ ice, brown, short-grain
____ rice, wild
____ shell or elbow pasta, whole-wheat

BEANS

____ kidney, 16-oz can
____ refried beans, fat-free

NUTS

____ dates
____ pecans

CONDIMENTS

_____ canola mayonnaise
_____ catsup, no-salt
_____ mustard, Dijon
_____ mustard, yellow
_____ pickle relish
_____ Worcestershire sauce

SPICES & HERBS

_____ basil
_____ bay leaves
_____ black pepper
_____ cayenne pepper
_____ chili powder
_____ cilantro
_____ cinnamon, ground
_____ coriander, ground
_____ cumin, ground
_____ dill weed
_____ garlic powder
_____ gingerroot
_____ Italian seasoning, no-salt
_____ marjoram
_____ mint sprigs
_____ nutmeg, ground
_____ oregano
_____ paprika
_____ parsley
_____ poppy seeds
_____ pumpkin pie spice
_____ red pepper flakes
_____ thyme, ground
_____ turmeric, ground

OTHER

_____ angel food cake
_____ applesauce, unsweetened
_____ biscuit mix
_____ cereal, all-bran
_____ cereal, Cheerios
_____ cereal, Fiber One
_____ cranberry sauce
_____ fruit cocktail in light syrup
_____ graham crackers
_____ honey
_____ jam, any kind
_____ maple syrup, sugar-free
_____ peanut butter
_____ potato chips, baked
_____ pumpkin, canned
_____ rice cakes
_____ salad dressing, Italian, light
_____ salsa, no-added-salt
_____ tomatoes, whole, no-added-salt, 16-oz can
_____ tortillas, 8-inch, fat-free
_____ tuna, white albacore, packed in water, 6.5-oz can

STAPLES

_____ baking powder
_____ bouillon, beef, sodium-free
_____ bouillon, chicken, sodium-free
_____ cornstarch
_____ flour, whole-wheat
_____ juice, lemon
_____ juice, lime
_____ juice, orange concentrate, frozen
_____ nonstick cooking spray
_____ oats, rolled, old-fashioned
_____ olive oil
_____ Smart Balance Omega oil
_____ Splenda
_____ vinegar, rice
_____ vinegar, white
_____ vinegar, white balsamic
_____ vinegar, white wine

Whole-Wheat Pancakes or Waffles

Serves 4   Serving size: 2 pancakes or waffles

1/2 **cup** rolled oats

1/2 **cup** whole-wheat flour, sifted

2 **tsp** baking powder

2 **Tbsp** Splenda

1/2 **cup** egg substitute, beaten well

3/4 **cup** nonfat milk

2 **Tbsp** Smart Balance Omega oil

Nonstick cooking spray

Stir together dry ingredients. Combine egg substitute, milk, and oil; stir into flour mixture. Cook on a griddle lightly coated with nonstick spray until golden brown, then turn. Can also be made in a waffle iron.

Exchanges/Choices

1 1/2 Starch
1 1/2 Fat

Basic Nutritional Values

Calories 185
  Calories from Fat 70
Total Fat . . . . 8.0 g
  Saturated Fat . . . . 0.7 g
  Trans Fat . . . . 0.0 g
Cholesterol . . . . 0 mg
Sodium . . . . 265 mg
Total Carbohydrate . . . 22 g
  Dietary Fiber . . . . 3 g
  Sugars . . . . 3 g
Protein . . . . 8 g

Frozen Pumpkin Dessert

Serves 4   Serving size: 1/4 recipe

Nonstick cooking spray

1/4 **cup** graham cracker crumbs

1 **tsp** Smart Balance Light Spread, melted

1/2 **cup** canned pumpkin

1/4 **cup** Splenda

1 **tsp** pumpkin pie spice

2 **cups** fat-free vanilla ice cream, softened

Lightly coat an 8-inch square baking dish with nonstick cooking spray. Mix the crumbs with the margarine. Evenly pat the crumbs into the bottom of the dish. In a medium bowl, stir together the pumpkin, Splenda, and pumpkin pie spice until well blended. In a large bowl, stir ice cream until smooth but not melted. Add the pumpkin mixture to the ice cream and mix until just well blended. Carefully pour into the baking dish. Cover dish with foil or plastic wrap. Freeze for at least 4 hours. To serve, cut into squares using a sharp knife.

Exchanges/Choices

2 Carbohydrate

Basic Nutritional Values

Calories 135
  Calories from Fat 10
Total Fat . . . . 1.0 g
  Saturated Fat . . . . 0.3 g
  Trans Fat . . . . 0.0 g
Cholesterol . . . . 0 mg
Sodium . . . . 95 mg
Total Carbohydrate . . . 30 g
  Dietary Fiber . . . . 5 g
  Sugars . . . . 17 g
Protein . . . . 4 g

Country-Fried Steak

Serves 4 Serving size: 1/4 recipe

1 **lb** 96% lean ground beef patties

1/8 **cup** nonfat milk

1/4 **cup** whole-wheat flour

Pepper, to taste

Paprika, to taste

1 **Tbsp** Smart Balance Omega oil

1/4 **cup** mushrooms, sliced

Dip the beef patties in nonfat milk and then in flour, pepper, and paprika. Discard excess flour. Coat a skillet with oil and brown the meat. Cover with the mushrooms and cook until done.

Exchanges/Choices

1/2 Starch
3 Lean Meat
1 Fat

Basic Nutritional Values

Calories 235
Calories from Fat 115
Total Fat . . . . 13.0 g
Saturated Fat . . . . 3.9 g
Trans Fat . . . . 0.6 g
Cholesterol . . . . 70 mg
Sodium . . . . 70 mg
Total Carbohydrate . . . 6 g
Dietary Fiber . . . . 1 g
Sugars . . . . 0 g
Protein . . . . 23 g

Mashed Potatoes

Serves 4 Serving size: 1/4 recipe

2 **cups** peeled, diced potatoes

1/4 **cup** nonfat milk

5 **tsp** Smart Balance margarine

Pepper, to taste

Peel the potatoes and cut into cubes; place in a large pan. Cover with water, bring to a boil, and then simmer for approximately 45 minutes, until potatoes are tender. Mash potatoes until no lumps remain, slowly adding milk and margarine to make potatoes smoother and fluffy. Season with pepper and serve.

Exchanges/Choices

1 Starch
1/2 Fat

Basic Nutritional Values

Calories 85
Calories from Fat 35
Total Fat . . . . 4.0 g
Saturated Fat . . . . 1.1 g
Trans Fat . . . . 0.0 g
Cholesterol . . . . 0 mg
Sodium . . . . 50 mg
Total Carbohydrate . . . 12 g
Dietary Fiber . . . . 1 g
Sugars . . . . 2 g
Protein . . . . 1 g

Scalloped Potatoes

Serves 4   Serving size: 1/4 recipe

1 medium onion, chopped	1 **cup** nonfat milk
1 **tsp** Smart Balance Omega oil	2 bay leaves
1 **tsp** minced garlic	2 **Tbsp** cornstarch
1 **tsp** minced thyme	1 **Tbsp** water
1/4 **tsp** ground black pepper	3 **Tbsp** fat-free cream cheese
2 **cups** russet potatoes, peeled and sliced 1/8-inch thick	2 **Tbsp** reduced-fat Parmesan cheese

Exchanges

1 Starch
1/2 Fat-Free Milk
1 Vegetable

Basic Nutritional Values

Calories 160
 Calories from Fat 20
Total Fat . . . . .2.0 g
 Saturated Fat . . . . .0.5 g
 Trans Fat . . . . .0.0 g
Cholesterol . . . . .5 mg
Sodium . . . . 185 mg
Total Carbohydrate . . .29 g
 Dietary Fiber . . . . .2 g
 Sugars . . . . .6 g
Protein . . . . .6 g

1. Adjust an oven rack to the middle position and preheat the oven to 450°F. Combine the onion and oil in a large pot. Cover and cook over medium-low heat, stirring occasionally, until the onion is softened, 8–10 minutes. Stir in the garlic, thyme, and pepper; cook until fragrant, about 1 minute.

2. Add the potatoes, milk, and bay leaves and bring to a simmer. Cover, reduce heat to low, and simmer until partially tender, about 10 minutes. Discard the bay leaves. Whisk the cornstarch and water together and add to the pot; bring to a simmer. Remove from heat and stir in the cream cheese and 1 Tbsp Parmesan cheese, being careful not to break up the potatoes.

3. Transfer the mixture to an 8-inch square baking dish and sprinkle with the remaining Parmesan. Cover the dish with foil and bake for 20 minutes. Uncover and continue to bake until the potatoes are completely tender. Let cool for 10 minutes before serving.

Turkey Chili Con Carne

Serves 4   Serving size: 1/4 recipe

1/2 **lb** ground turkey breast

2 **Tbsp** Smart Balance Omega oil

1 large onion, chopped

1 clove garlic, minced

1 green bell pepper, chopped

1 **(16-oz)** can kidney beans

1 **(16-oz)** can no-added-salt whole tomatoes, coarsely chopped

1/4 **cup** no-salt catsup

2 **Tbsp** chili powder

1/2 **tsp** dried oregano

2 **Tbsp** sodium-free beef bouillon

2 **cups** water

In a skillet, cook the turkey breast until just done; set aside. In a Dutch oven or large skillet, heat oil over medium heat; add onion and garlic and sauté for 5 minutes, stirring constantly. Add green pepper, stir, and cook for another 5 minutes. Stir in beans, cooked turkey, tomatoes, catsup, chili powder, oregano, bouillon, and water. Simmer, uncovered, for 30 minutes, adding more liquid as necessary. Stir occasionally.

Exchanges/Choices

1 Starch
4 Vegetable
2 Lean Meat
1 Fat

Basic Nutritional Values

Calories 330
  Calories from Fat 80
Total Fat . . . . 9.0 g
  Saturated Fat . . . . 0.7 g
  Trans Fat . . . . 0.0 g
Cholesterol . . . . 45 mg
Sodium . . . . 515 mg
Total Carbohydrate . . . 40 g
  Dietary Fiber . . . . 9 g
  Sugars . . . . 16 g
Protein . . . . 25 g

Marinated Turkey Fillets

Serves 4   Serving size: 1/4 recipe

3 **Tbsp** Smart Balance Omega oil

1/3 **cup** white balsamic vinegar

1/4 **cup** reduced-fat grated Parmesan cheese

1 **tsp** no-salt Italian seasoning

1/2 **tsp** coarse ground black pepper

1 **lb** boneless, skinless turkey breast strips

In a small bowl, combine the oil, vinegar, cheese, Italian seasoning, and pepper. Pour marinade into a plastic resealable bag. Add turkey, close bag, and work marinade around turkey. Refrigerate for 1 hour. Heat broiler or prepare an outdoor grill for direct-heat cooking. Cook 18–20 minutes, turning once or twice, until turkey reaches an internal temperature of 170°F.

Exchanges/Choices

4 Lean Meat

Basic Nutritional Values

Calories 190
  Calories from Fat 65
Total Fat. . . . . 7.0 g
  Saturated Fat . . . . 1.0 g
  Trans Fat. . . . . 0.0 g
Cholesterol. . . . . 80 mg
Sodium. . . . . 105 mg
Total Carbohydrate . . . 4 g
  Dietary Fiber. . . . . 0 g
  Sugars . . . . 1 g
Protein . . . . 28 g

Poppy Seed Fruit Salad

Serves 4   Serving size: 1/4 recipe

2 large oranges

1 1/2 **cup** cantaloupe cubes

1 **cup** fat-free yogurt (any flavor)

1/2 **tsp** poppy seeds

4 mint sprigs (for garnish)

Cut each orange in half; then remove the flesh of the orange from each of the halves, taking care not to damage them. Dice the orange pulp. Retain the empty orange peels (they should look like little bowls). Remove the skin and seeds from the cantaloupe; dice into very small pieces. Place diced oranges and cantaloupe into the orange peel bowls, letting any extra spill over onto the plate. In a small bowl, whisk together the yogurt and poppy seeds; then pour over the fruit. Top each orange peel bowl with a sprig of mint.

Exchanges/Choices

1 Fruit
1/2 Fat-Free Milk

Basic Nutritional Values

Calories 105
  Calories from Fat 0
Total Fat. . . . . 0.0 g
  Saturated Fat . . . . 0.1 g
  Trans Fat. . . . . 0.0 g
Cholesterol. . . . . 0 mg
Sodium. . . . . 35 mg
Total Carbohydrate . . . 23 g
  Dietary Fiber. . . . . 3 g
  Sugars . . . . 18 g
Protein . . . . 3 g

Multigrain Rice Pilaf

Serves 6   Serving size: 1/6 recipe

- 1/2 **cup** pearl barley
- 1/2 **cup** parsley
- 1/2 **cup** wild rice, uncooked
- 1/2 **cup** brown rice, uncooked
- 2 **Tbsp** Smart Balance Light margarine
- 1/2 **cup** diced onion
- 1/4 **cup** diced celery
- 1 **Tbsp** sodium-free chicken bouillon
- 1 **cup** water
- 1/2 **tsp** ground thyme
- 1/2 **tsp** pepper

Rinse the pearl barley. Chop the parsley. Bring a large pot of water to a full boil and add the wild rice first. Let it cook for about 10 minutes and then add the barley and the brown rice (wild rice takes longer to cook). Reduce heat; simmer until tender. Drain and rinse under cold water. Melt margarine in a large skillet over medium heat. Add onions and celery; cook until tender, about 4 minutes. In a small bowl, combine the bouillon and water to create a broth. Add cooked rice mixture, broth, thyme, and pepper to the skillet; cook, stirring occasionally, until heated through, about 5 minutes. Add parsley just before serving.

Exchanges/Choices

2 1/2 Starch

Basic Nutritional Values

Calories 190
 Calories from Fat 20
Total Fat . . . . .2.5 g
 Saturated Fat . . . . .0.7 g
 Trans Fat . . . . .0.0 g
Cholesterol . . . . .0 mg
Sodium . . . . .40 mg
Total Carbohydrate . . .38 g
 Dietary Fiber . . . . .4 g
 Sugars . . . . .2 g
Protein . . . . .4 g

Whole-Wheat Blueberry Muffins
Serves 12   Serving size: 1 muffin

1 cup whole-wheat flour	**3 Tbsp** Smart Balance margarine
5 1/2 Tbsp Splenda	**1/2 cup** egg substitute
1 tsp baking powder	**1/2 cup** blueberries
6 Tbsp nonfat milk	

Preheat oven to 400°F. In a medium bowl, combine flour, Splenda, and baking powder. In a small bowl, beat milk, margarine, and egg substitute; stir into dry ingredients until just moist. Fold in blueberries and spoon batter into 12 paper-lined muffin cups. Bake for 20–25 minutes or until golden brown. Serve immediately.

Exchanges/Choices
1/2 Starch
1/2 Fat

Basic Nutritional Values
Calories	70
Calories from Fat	20
Total Fat	2.5 g
Saturated Fat	0.7 g
Trans Fat	0.0 g
Cholesterol	0 mg
Sodium	75 mg
Total Carbohydrate	9 g
Dietary Fiber	1 g
Sugars	2 g
Protein	3 g

Pita Tuna Melts
Serves 4   Serving size: 1 melt

2 (6-inch) pita breads, cut in half	**1 Tbsp** sweet pickle relish
1 (6.5-oz) can white albacore tuna, packed in water and drained	**1/4 tsp** dried dill weed
	1 medium tomato, cut into 12 wedges
1 Tbsp canola mayonnaise	**1/4 cup** fat-free shredded cheddar cheese

Preheat oven to 400°F. Place pita breads in a single layer on a nonstick baking sheet and bake for about 5 minutes or until lightly toasted. While the pita breads are toasting, combine tuna, mayonnaise, relish, and dill weed in a small bowl. Spread the tuna mixture equally on each pita. Arrange tomato wedges on the pitas and sprinkle with cheese. Bake for 5 more minutes or until cheese melts.

Exchanges/Choices
1 Starch
2 Lean Meat

Basic Nutritional Values
Calories	165
Calories from Fat	20
Total Fat	2.0 g
Saturated Fat	0.1 g
Trans Fat	0.0 g
Cholesterol	15 mg
Sodium	425 mg
Total Carbohydrate	20 g
Dietary Fiber	1 g
Sugars	3 g
Protein	16 g

Potato Salad

Serves 4   Serving size: 1/4 recipe

2 cups potatoes, peeled, boiled, and cubed

1/4 cup onion, chopped and diced

1/4 cup light Italian salad dressing

1/2 cup canola mayonnaise

2 eggs, hard boiled and chopped

Wash and peel potatoes. Cook potatoes in boiling water for about 30 minutes. Drain and slice into small cubes. In a large bowl, combine the potatoes with all other ingredients and mix well. Serve chilled.

Exchanges/Choices

1 1/2 Starch
2 Fat

Basic Nutritional Values

Calories 215
  Calories from Fat 115
Total Fat . . . . .13.0 g
  Saturated Fat . . . . .0.9 g
  Trans Fat . . . . .0.0 g
Cholesterol . . . . .105 mg
Sodium . . . . .395 mg
Total Carbohydrate . . .20 g
  Dietary Fiber . . . . .2 g
  Sugars . . . . .5 g
Protein . . . . .5 g

Blackened Pork Cutlet

Serves 4   Serving size: 1/4 recipe

- **1 cup** chopped pineapple
- **1** medium red or green bell pepper, chopped
- **1 Tbsp** finely chopped onion
- **1 Tbsp** lime juice
- **3 tsp** chili powder
- **1/2** jalapeño pepper, finely chopped
- **1/8 tsp** cayenne pepper
- **1/2 tsp** black pepper
- **1 tsp** ground coriander
- **1/2 tsp** ground cumin
- **1/2 tsp** paprika
- **3/4 lb** boneless sirloin pork chops (trimmed of fat)
- **1 tsp** Smart Balance Omega oil

Exchanges/Choices

1/2 Carbohydrate
2 Lean Meat

Basic Nutritional Values

Calories 135
  Calories from Fat 35
Total Fat . . . . .4.0 g
  Saturated Fat . . . . .0.5 g
  Trans Fat . . . . .0.0 g
Cholesterol . . . . .40 mg
Sodium . . . . .230 mg
Total Carbohydrate . . . 10 g
  Dietary Fiber . . . . .2 g
  Sugars . . . . .6 g
Protein . . . . .16 g

1. Prepare the salsa: in a medium bowl, combine pineapple, bell pepper, onion, lime juice, 1 tsp chili powder, jalapeño pepper, a dash of cumin, and cayenne. Season to taste with black pepper; set aside.

2. In a small bowl, combine 2 tsp chili powder, coriander, 1/2 tsp cumin, paprika, and 1/2 tsp black pepper. Stir in oil.

3. Rub the mixture over the cutlets. Heat a large heavy skillet over medium-high heat. Cook cutlets for 5–6 minutes, turning occasionally, until evenly browned on both sides and cutlets are fully cooked. Pour salsa over chops before serving.

Green Beans and Red Peppers

Serves 4   Serving size: 1/4 recipe

1/2 medium red bell pepper

1/2 **cup** water

1 **Tbsp** sodium-free chicken bouillon

16 **oz** frozen green beans

1/2 **Tbsp** Smart Balance Light margarine

1/4 **tsp** garlic powder

Cut bell pepper into strips. In a medium saucepan, combine water and bouillon to make a broth; bring to a boil. Add green beans. Cover and cook over medium heat for 8–12 minutes or until beans are crisp-tender. Drain. Meanwhile, melt margarine in a small skillet. Add pepper strips and cook until just tender. In a serving bowl, combine green beans, pepper strips, and garlic powder; toss gently.

Exchanges/Choices

2 Vegetable

Basic Nutritional Values

Calories 45
  Calories from Fat 10
Total Fat . . . . 1.0 g
  Saturated Fat . . . . 0.2 g
  Trans Fat . . . . 0.0 g
Cholesterol . . . . 0 mg
Sodium . . . . 20 mg
Total Carbohydrate . . . 9 g
  Dietary Fiber . . . . 3 g
  Sugars . . . . 4 g
Protein . . . . 2 g

Deli Ham Sandwich

Serves 4   Serving size: 1 sandwich

- **4 oz** light ham
- **4** slices reduced-fat Swiss cheese
- **4** romaine lettuce leaves
- **4** tomato slices
- **1 Tbsp** yellow mustard
- **8** slices whole-wheat bread

Divide ingredients among four sandwiches and serve.

Exchanges/Choices

1 Starch
1 Vegetable
2 Lean Meat

Basic Nutritional Values

Calories	195
Calories from Fat	55
Total Fat	6.0 g
Saturated Fat	2.4 g
Trans Fat	0.0 g
Cholesterol	25 mg
Sodium	485 mg
Total Carbohydrate	23 g
Dietary Fiber	4 g
Sugars	5 g
Protein	19 g

Carrot Slaw

Serves 4   Serving size: 1/4 recipe

- **1/2 cup** crushed pineapple (or can of no-added-sugar crushed pineapple)
- **1 tsp** honey
- **1 tsp** lemon juice
- **1/4 tsp** nutmeg
- **1/2 cup** fat-free sour cream
- **2 cups** carrot, grated

Drain pineapple. In a medium bowl, mix honey, lemon juice, and nutmeg. Blend in sour cream. Add carrots and pineapple. Serve chilled.

Exchanges/Choices

1/2 Carbohydrate
1 Vegetable

Basic Nutritional Values

Calories	65
Calories from Fat	0
Total Fat	0.0 g
Saturated Fat	0.1 g
Trans Fat	0.0 g
Cholesterol	5 mg
Sodium	55 mg
Total Carbohydrate	11 g
Dietary Fiber	2 g
Sugars	8 g
Protein	3 g

Baked Fillet of Sole

Serves 4   Serving size: 1/4 recipe

- 1 **lb** sole fillets (about 6)
- 2 **Tbsp** lemon juice
- 1/4 **tsp** black pepper, freshly ground
- 2 **Tbsp** Smart Balance margarine
- 2/3 medium garlic head, cloves peeled and finely chopped
- 1 **tsp** gingerroot, finely chopped
- 1/2 **cup** onions, finely chopped
- 1/16 **tsp** red pepper flakes
- 1/2 **tsp** ground turmeric
- 2/3 **tsp** dill weed

Season one side of the fillets with lemon juice and pepper. In a heavy 7- or 8-inch skillet, heat margarine over medium-high heat and add all remaining ingredients. Fry, stirring occasionally with a wooden spoon, until the onions are limp and slightly golden, about 5–7 minutes. Remove from heat and spread equal portions of stuffing on top of each fillet. Starting at the narrow end, roll up each fillet to enclose the stuffing and fasten each with a toothpick. Place the rolled fillets seam side down in a baking dish. Spoon any remaining stuffing or lemon juice over the top. Bake for 12 minutes at 350°F or until the rolls are firm when pressed lightly with a fork. Remove from the oven. Place the fish rolls on a warm platter using a pancake turner, remove toothpicks, and pour the pan drippings over the fish.

Exchanges/Choices

3 Lean Meat
1/2 Fat

Basic Nutritional Values

Calories 155
  Calories from Fat 55
Total Fat . . . . 6.0 g
  Saturated Fat . . . . 1.6 g
  Trans Fat . . . . 0.0 g
Cholesterol . . . . 60 mg
Sodium . . . . 140 mg
Total Carbohydrate . . . 3 g
  Dietary Fiber . . . . 0 g
  Sugars . . . . 1 g
Protein . . . . 22 g

Cucumber Salad

Serves 4   Serving size: 1/4 recipe

2 medium cucumbers, peeled and thinly sliced

1 cup white vinegar

1/2 cup Splenda

Pepper, to taste

1 Tbsp chopped parsley

Rinse sliced cucumbers, drain, and place in a serving dish. Combine vinegar, Splenda, and pepper. Let stand 5 minutes. Pour over cucumbers; sprinkle with parsley. Chill 2 hours. Before serving, drain off about 3/4 of the vinegar.

Exchanges/Choices

1/2 Carbohydrate

Basic Nutritional Values

Calories 40
  Calories from Fat 0
Total Fat . . . . 0.0 g
  Saturated Fat . . . . 0.0 g
  Trans Fat . . . . 0.0 g
Cholesterol . . . . 0 mg
Sodium . . . . 0 mg
Total Carbohydrate . . . 9 g
  Dietary Fiber . . . . 1 g
  Sugars . . . . 8 g
Protein . . . . 1 g

Lemon Parsley Carrots

Serves 4   Serving size: 1/4 recipe

2 cups carrots, sliced 1/4-inch thick

2 Tbsp water

2 Tbsp Smart Balance margarine

1 Tbsp Splenda

1 Tbsp fresh parsley, chopped

1/2 tsp lemon peels, grated

1 Tbsp lemon juice

Place carrots and water in a 2-quart covered glass casserole. Microwave, covered, at 100% power (700 watts) for 8–9 minutes until crisp-tender, stirring once after 5 minutes. Drain. Stir in margarine, Splenda, parsley, lemon peels, and lemon juice. Microwave again, covered, at 100% power for 1–2 minutes, until heated through.

Exchanges/Choices

1 Vegetable
1 Fat

Basic Nutritional Values

Calories 70
  Calories from Fat 40
Total Fat . . . . 4.5 g
  Saturated Fat . . . . 1.3 g
  Trans Fat . . . . 0.0 g
Cholesterol . . . . 0 mg
Sodium . . . . 90 mg
Total Carbohydrate . . . 7 g
  Dietary Fiber . . . . 2 g
  Sugars . . . . 3 g
Protein . . . . 1 g

Bran Muffins

Serves 4   Serving size: 3 muffins

Nonstick cooking spray

3/4 **cup** whole-wheat flour

2 **tsp** baking powder

1 1/2 **Tbsp** Splenda

2/3 **cup** all-bran cereal

2/3 **cup** nonfat milk

1/4 **cup** egg substitute

1/4 **cup** unsweetened applesauce

Spray twelve 2-inch muffin-pan cups with nonstick cooking spray; set aside. Stir together flour, baking powder, and Splenda; set aside. Add cereal and milk to a large mixing bowl. Stir to combine and then allow it to stand until cereal is softened, 1–2 minutes. Add egg substitute and applesauce; beat well. Add flour mixture and stir only enough to combine. Divide batter evenly among prepared muffin cups. Bake at 400°F for 25 minutes or until lightly browned.

Exchanges/Choices

1/2 Starch

Basic Nutritional Values

Calories 45
 Calories from Fat 0
Total Fat. . . . . 0.0 g
 Saturated Fat . . . . 0.1 g
 Trans Fat. . . . . 0.0 g
Cholesterol . . . . 0 mg
Sodium. . . . . 85 mg
Total Carbohydrate . . . 10 g
 Dietary Fiber . . . . 2 g
 Sugars . . . . 2 g
Protein . . . . 2 g

Whole-Wheat Pasta Salad

Serves 4   Serving size: 1/4 recipe

8 **oz** whole-wheat pasta, shells or elbows

1/2 **cup** canola mayonnaise

1/2 **cup** celery, diced

1/2 **cup** onion, diced

2 **Tbsp** Dijon mustard

1 **tsp** dill weed

1/2 **tsp** marjoram

1/4 **tsp** black pepper

Cook pasta according to package directions. Drain. In a medium bowl, stir together all of the remaining ingredients until well blended. Stir in cooked pasta; gently toss until well coated. Cover and chill at least 2 hours before serving.

Exchanges/Choices

3 Starch
1 1/2 Fat

Basic Nutritional Values

Calories 305
 Calories from Fat 90
Total Fat. . . . . 10.0 g
 Saturated Fat . . . . 0.2 g
 Trans Fat. . . . . 0.0 g
Cholesterol . . . . 0 mg
Sodium. . . . . 380 mg
Total Carbohydrate . . . 46 g
 Dietary Fiber . . . . 5 g
 Sugars . . . . 4 g
Protein . . . . 9 g

Mexican Coleslaw

Serves 4   Serving size: 1/4 recipe

4 **cups** thinly sliced
green cabbage

1 **cup** grated carrots

1 **Tbsp** cilantro

1/4 **cup** rice vinegar

2 **Tbsp** Smart Balance
Omega oil

Place cabbage and carrots in a colander; rinse with cold water. Allow to drain for 5 minutes. Meanwhile, whisk together cilantro, vinegar, and oil in a large bowl. Add cabbage; toss well to coat. Toss again just before serving.

Exchanges/Choices

1 Vegetable
1 1/2 Fat

Basic Nutritional Values

Calories 90
  Calories from Fat 65
Total Fat . . . . 7.0 g
  Saturated Fat . . . . 0.5 g
  Trans Fat . . . . 0.0 g
Cholesterol . . . . 0 mg
Sodium . . . . 35 mg
Total Carbohydrate . . . 7 g
  Dietary Fiber . . . . 2 g
  Sugars . . . . 4 g
Protein . . . . 1 g

Asian Chicken

Serves 4   Serving size: 1/4 recipe

2 **Tbsp** Smart Balance Omega oil

2/3 **cup** sliced carrots

4 **oz** frozen snow pea pods, thawed

1/3 **cup** chopped green onion

1 **lb** boneless, skinless chicken breasts (trimmed of fat)

1 medium garlic clove, crushed

1 **oz** gingerroot, finely chopped

2 **Tbsp** water

1 **Tbsp** cornstarch

1 **cup** orange juice

2 **Tbsp** grated orange peel

2 **cups** cooked brown rice

Exchanges/Choices

1 1/2 Starch
1/2 Fruit
1 Vegetable
3 Lean Meat
1 Fat

Basic Nutritional Values

Calories 365
  Calories from Fat 100
Total Fat . . . . 11.0 g
  Saturated Fat . . . . 1.5 g
  Trans Fat . . . . 0.0 g
Cholesterol . . . . 65 mg
Sodium . . . . 80 mg
Total Carbohydrate . . . 37 g
  Dietary Fiber . . . . 4 g
  Sugars . . . . 9 g
Protein . . . . 28 g

1. In a skillet over medium heat, heat 1 Tbsp oil; add carrots; cook 2 minutes, stirring frequently. Add pea pods and green onions; cook and stir for 2 minutes, until vegetables are crisp-tender. Transfer vegetables to a bowl.

2. Add chicken breasts to skillet; cook 3 minutes on each side until lightly browned and cooked through. Transfer breasts to a serving platter; keep warm.

3. Add garlic and ginger to the drippings in the skillet; cook and stir over medium-high heat, 1–2 minutes until soft.

4. In a small bowl, stir water into cornstarch to blend and add to skillet. Add orange juice and grated orange peel. Bring to a boil, stirring constantly. Reduce heat to medium low. Cook 2–3 minutes, stirring occasionally, until sauce is slightly thickened. Return vegetables to skillet; cook 1–2 minutes more until heated through, stirring to coat with sauce. Spoon vegetables and rice around chicken on platter; spoon remaining sauce over chicken.

Fruit Medley

Serves 4   Serving size: 1/4 recipe

1 medium banana

1 cup seedless grapes

1 orange, peeled and sectioned

1 grapefruit, peeled and sectioned

1 cup canned light pineapple, juice reserved

Combine all ingredients and chill 30 minutes before serving. Be sure to cover the banana with the pineapple juice to keep it fresh.

Exchanges/Choices

2 Fruit

Basic Nutritional Values

Calories 130
  Calories from Fat 5
Total Fat . . . . 0.5 g
  Saturated Fat . . . . 0.1 g
  Trans Fat . . . . 0.0 g
Cholesterol . . . . 0 mg
Sodium . . . . 0 mg
Total Carbohydrate . . . 33 g
  Dietary Fiber . . . . 3 g
  Sugars . . . . 25 g
Protein . . . . 2 g

Pumpkin Spice Muffins

Serves 8   Serving size: 2 muffins

1 **cup** whole-wheat flour

3 **tsp** baking powder

2 **tsp** ground cinnamon

2 **tsp** ground nutmeg

1/4 **cup** egg substitute

2 **Tbsp** Splenda

1 **cup** canned pumpkin

1/2 **cup** nonfat milk

1/4 **cup** unsweetened applesauce

1/4 **cup** raisins or chopped nuts

Exchanges/Choices
1 1/2 Carbohydrate

Basic Nutritional Values
Calories	95
Calories from Fat	5
Total Fat	0.5 g
Saturated Fat	0.2 g
Trans Fat	0.0 g
Cholesterol	0 mg
Sodium	160 mg
Total Carbohydrate	20 g
Dietary Fiber	3 g
Sugars	6 g
Protein	4 g

Preheat oven to 400°F. Line sixteen muffin-pan cups with paper liners or spray with nonstick cooking spray. In a large bowl, stir together the flour, baking powder, cinnamon, and nutmeg. In a medium bowl, beat egg substitute with a whisk. Add Splenda, pumpkin, milk, and applesauce; stir until well blended. Stir in raisins. Stir into flour mixture until just blended. Fill muffin-pan cups 2/3 full. Bake 20–25 minutes until a wooden toothpick inserted in the center comes out clean. Remove muffins from muffin pans. Serve warm or at room temperature.

Whole-Grain Burger

Serves 4   Serving size: 1 burger

1 **Tbsp** Smart Balance Omega oil

1/2 **cup** minced mushrooms

1 small onion, minced

3 **Tbsp** ground oats

2 **cups** cooked short-grain brown rice

1/4 **cup** egg substitute

1 **Tbsp** reduced-fat Parmesan cheese

1 **Tbsp** Worcestershire sauce

Exchanges/Choices
2 Starch
1/2 Fat

Basic Nutritional Values
Calories	185
Calories from Fat	45
Total Fat	5.0 g
Saturated Fat	0.7 g
Trans Fat	0.0 g
Cholesterol	0 mg
Sodium	115 mg
Total Carbohydrate	30 g
Dietary Fiber	3 g
Sugars	3 g
Protein	6 g

Heat the oil in a small skillet over medium-high heat. Add the mushrooms and onions; sauté until mushrooms are dark and onions are golden, about 6–7 minutes. Combine the mushrooms and onions with the remaining ingredients. Form the mixture into four patties and grill or broil the burgers for about 7 minutes, turning once.

Turkey Cutlet Parmesan

Serves 4   Serving size: 1/4 recipe

- **1/4 cup** reduced-fat grated Parmesan cheese
- **1/4 tsp** Italian seasoning
- **1/4 tsp** ground black pepper

- Nonstick cooking spray
- **3/4 lb** lean boneless turkey breast cutlets (trimmed of fat)

Combine cheese, Italian seasoning, and pepper in small dish. Place cheese mixture on a plate and coat each cutlet. Spray a large nonstick skillet with nonstick cooking spray and heat over medium-high heat. Add cutlets and cook until no longer pink, about 2 minutes for each side. Keep cooked cutlets warm until serving.

Exchanges/Choices

3 Lean Meat

Basic Nutritional Values

Calories 120
  Calories from Fat 20
Total Fat . . . . 2.0 g
  Saturated Fat . . . . 0.9 g
  Trans Fat . . . . 0.0 g
Cholesterol . . . . 60 mg
Sodium . . . . 155 mg
Total Carbohydrate . . . 3 g
  Dietary Fiber . . . . 0 g
  Sugars . . . . 0 g
Protein . . . . 22 g

Carrot-Raisin Salad

Serves 6   Serving size: 1/6 recipe

- **1 lb** carrots, coarsely grated
- **1 cup** raisins
- **1 cup** crushed pineapple
- **1 cup** canola mayonnaise

- **2 Tbsp** frozen orange juice concentrate
- **6** iceberg lettuce leaves

In a large bowl, mix carrots, raisins, and crushed pineapple. In another bowl, combine mayonnaise and orange juice concentrate. Gently fold mayonnaise mixture in with the pineapple mixture. Chill, covered, for 2 hours. Evenly divide salad among lettuce leaves.

Exchanges/Choices

2 Fruit
1 Vegetable
2 1/2 Fat

Basic Nutritional Values

Calories 245
  Calories from Fat 110
Total Fat . . . . 12.0 g
  Saturated Fat . . . . 0.0 g
  Trans Fat . . . . 0.0 g
Cholesterol . . . . 0 mg
Sodium . . . . 290 mg
Total Carbohydrate . . . 33 g
  Dietary Fiber . . . . 3 g
  Sugars . . . . 26 g
Protein . . . . 2 g

Chilled Cauliflower Salad

Serves 4   Serving size: 1/4 recipe

- **1** medium cauliflower head, broken into florets
- **2** medium tomatoes, cut into wedges
- **2 Tbsp** Smart Balance Omega oil
- **3 Tbsp** white wine vinegar
- **3 Tbsp** black pitted olives, sliced
- **3 Tbsp** sweet pickle relish
- **1/2 tsp** Splenda
- **1 tsp** paprika
- **1/2 tsp** black pepper
- **4** lettuce leaves

1. In a covered saucepan, cook cauliflower in small amount of boiling water, 9–10 minutes or until crisp-tender. Drain. In large bowl, combine the cooked cauliflower and tomato wedges.

2. Combine the oil, vinegar, olives, relish, Splenda, paprika, and pepper. Mix well. Pour dressing over cauliflower and tomatoes. Cover and refrigerate 24 hours, stirring occasionally. To serve, lift vegetables from dressing with slotted spoon; place in a lettuce-lined bowl.

Exchanges/Choices

3 Vegetable
1 Fat

Basic Nutritional Values

Calories 125
  Calories from Fat 65
Total Fat . . . . 7.0 g
  Saturated Fat . . . . 0.5 g
  Trans Fat . . . . 0.0 g
Cholesterol . . . . 0 mg
Sodium . . . . 160 mg
Total Carbohydrate . . . 16 g
  Dietary Fiber . . . . 5 g
  Sugars . . . . 9 g
Protein . . . . 4 g

Peach Cobbler

Serves 4   Serving size: 1/4 recipe

Nonstick cooking spray

1/2 **cup** Splenda

1 **Tbsp** cornstarch

2 **cups** sliced peaches

2 **Tbsp** water

1 **cup** biscuit mix

1/4 **cup** nonfat milk

Preheat oven to 425°F. Spray a round casserole dish with nonstick cooking spray. Mix 1/2 cup Splenda and cornstarch in a saucepan; stir in peaches and water. Heat to boiling, stirring constantly. Boil and stir 1 minute. Pour mixture into casserole dish. Mix biscuit mix according to package directions and drop dough by spoonfuls onto the hot peach mixture. Bake until golden brown, about 20 minutes. Serve with nonfat milk.

Exchanges/Choices

2 1/2 Carbohydrate
1/2 Fat

Basic Nutritional Values

Calories 200
  Calories from Fat 35
Total Fat . . . . .4.0 g
  Saturated Fat . . . . .1.2 g
  Trans Fat . . . . .1.2 g
Cholesterol . . . . .0 mg
Sodium . . . . .410 mg
Total Carbohydrate . . .35 g
  Dietary Fiber . . . . .2 g
  Sugars . . . . .12 g
Protein . . . . .5 g

Tuna Salad

Serves 4   Serving size: 1/4 recipe

1 **(6-oz)** can tuna, packed
  in water, drained

1/4 **cup** pickle relish

1/4 **cup** diced celery

1/4 **cup** diced onion

1/2 **cup** canola mayonnaise

Mix all ingredients well. Chill before serving.

Exchanges/Choices

1/2 Carbohydrate
1 Lean Meat
1 1/2 Fat

Basic Nutritional Values

Calories 145
  Calories from Fat 80
Total Fat . . . . .9.0 g
  Saturated Fat . . . . .0.0 g
  Trans Fat . . . . .0.0 g
Cholesterol . . . . .10 mg
Sodium . . . . .325 mg
Total Carbohydrate . . .8 g
  Dietary Fiber . . . . .0 g
  Sugars . . . . .7 g
Protein . . . . .7 g

Chicken Burritos

Serves 4   Serving size: 1 burrito

Nonstick cooking spray

1/2 **lb** boneless, skinless chicken breasts, cut into small strips

1 **cup** diced red bell pepper

1/2 **cup** no-added-salt salsa

1 **cup** fat-free refried beans

4 **(8-inch)** fat-free flour tortillas

1. Coat a large nonstick skillet with cooking spray; heat over medium-high heat. Add chicken and pepper; sauté 3 minutes. Add 1/4 cup salsa; reduce heat to medium-low and cook 2 minutes, stirring occasionally.

2. While chicken cooks, combine refried beans and remaining salsa in a small microwave-safe bowl. Cover loosely and microwave at high power for 2 minutes or until thoroughly heated, stirring after 1 minute.

3. Wrap tortillas in paper towels. Microwave at high power for 30–45 seconds or until warm. Spread bean mixture evenly down the centers of tortillas; top evenly with chicken mixture. Roll up tortillas and serve.

Exchanges/Choices

2 Starch
1 Vegetable
1 Lean Meat

Basic Nutritional Values

Calories 230
Calories from Fat 15
Total Fat . . . . 1.5 g
Saturated Fat . . . . 0.4 g
Trans Fat . . . . 0.0 g
Cholesterol . . . . 35 mg
Sodium . . . . 625 mg
Total Carbohydrate . . . 36 g
Dietary Fiber . . . . 5 g
Sugars . . . . 4 g
Protein . . . . 20 g

Corn and Zucchini Combo

Serves 4   Serving size: 1/4 recipe

1 **tsp** Smart Balance Light Spread

1/2 **cup** onion, diced

1 **cup** zucchini squash, sliced 1/8-inch thick

1 **cup** frozen whole-kernel corn

1/4 **tsp** basil leaves

1/8 **tsp** oregano leaves

1/8 **tsp** pepper

Melt margarine in a frying pan over low heat. Add onion and cook for 2 minutes. Add zucchini, cover, and cook for 5 minutes, stirring occasionally. Add all remaining ingredients. Cover and cook over low heat for about 5 minutes or until corn is done.

Exchanges/Choices

1/2 Starch
1 Vegetable

Basic Nutritional Values

Calories 50
Calories from Fat 5
Total Fat . . . . 0.5 g
Saturated Fat . . . . 0.2 g
Trans Fat . . . . 0.0 g
Cholesterol . . . . 0 mg
Sodium . . . . 15 mg
Total Carbohydrate . . . 11 g
Dietary Fiber . . . . 2 g
Sugars . . . . 2 g
Protein . . . . 2 g

Ambrosia Salad

Serves 4   Serving size: 1/4 recipe

1 **cup** diced fresh oranges

2 fresh bananas, sliced

1 **cup** seedless green grapes

1/2 **cup** raisins

2 **Tbsp** lemon juice

1/4 **cup** canola mayonnaise

2/3 **cup** fat-free whipped topping

6 **Tbsp** nonfat milk

4 small lettuce leaves

Combine the oranges, bananas, grapes, and raisins; sprinkle with lemon juice and chill. Stir in mayonnaise and mix with remaining ingredients. Serve on lettuce.

Exchanges/Choices

3 Fruit
1 Fat

Basic Nutritional Values

Calories 235
   Calories from Fat 45
Total Fat . . . . 5.0 g
   Saturated Fat . . . . 0.2 g
   Trans Fat . . . . 0.0 g
Cholesterol . . . . 0 mg
Sodium . . . . 115 mg
Total Carbohydrate . . . 47 g
   Dietary Fiber . . . . 4 g
   Sugars . . . . 33 g
Protein . . . . 3 g

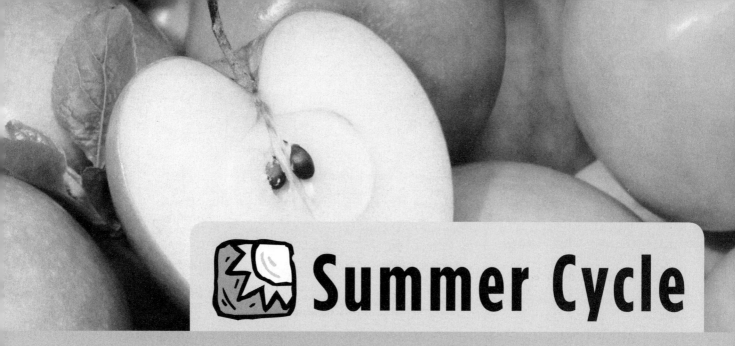

Summer Cycle

FEATURED RECIPES

Mashed Potatoes*

Prune Delight Spread

Mediterranean Ocean Perch

Rice Pilaf*

Shredded Wheat Custard*

Turkey Vegetable Soup

Chicken Piccata

Apple Salad Dijon*

Low-Fat Corn Bread*

Zucchini Bread*

Tuna and Pasta Salad

Cinnamon Red Cabbage*

Carrot Slaw*

Banana Bran Muffin*

Peanut Butter, Banana, and Jelly Sandwich

Blackened Catfish

Spinach-Orange Salad*

Strawberry Whip Parfaits*

All-Natural High-Fiber Peach Squares

Chicken Pasta Salad with

Tropical Fruit Dressing

Orange Marmalade Pork Cutlets

Baked Sweet Potato Fries*

Green Bean Sesame Salad*

Splendid Blueberry Crisp*

Baked Apples*

Carrot-Raisin Salad*

Banana Baked Chicken

Italian Zucchini

Zucchini Carrot Muffins*

Chicken, Escarole, and Rice Soup

Limed Chicken Breast

Sautéed Zucchini and Red Peppers*

Fruit Salad Medley*

Buttered Parsley Potatoes

*Indicates that the recipe has been used previously.

1500 calorie MEAL PLAN SUMMER WEEK 1

	Sunday	Monday	Tuesday	Wednesday	Thursday	Friday	Saturday
Breakfast	2 (4-inch) pancakes 1/4 cup sugar-free maple syrup 1/4 cup unsweetened applesauce 1 cup nonfat milk 2 tsp margarine	**Shredded Wheat Custard*** 1 small bagel 4 grapes 1/2 cup nonfat milk 1 Tbsp peanut butter	**Zucchini Bread*** 1/2 large grapefruit 1 cup nonfat milk 2 tsp margarine	**Banana Bran Muffin*** 1 1/2 cup puffed rice cereal 1 cup nonfat milk 1/2 tsp margarine 5 hazelnuts	**All-Natural High-Fiber Peach Squares** 1/2 cup oatmeal 1 1/4 cup strawberries 1 cup nonfat milk 1 oz lean beef sausage 1 tsp margarine	**Baked Apples*** 1 slice raisin bread 1 cup nonfat milk 1 1/2 tsp margarine	**Zucchini Carrot Muffins*** 1/2 Tbsp jam 1 cup nonfat milk 1/2 tsp margarine
Lunch	**Mashed Potatoes*** **Prune Delight Spread** 1 1/2 small dinner rolls 1/2 cup steamed green beans 2 oz lean sirloin tip roast 1/2 tsp margarine	**Turkey Vegetable Soup** (2 servings) 1 (2 oz) crusty roll 1 cup mixed melon cubes 1/2 cup steamed asparagus 1 tsp margarine	**Tuna and Pasta Salad** **Cinnamon Red Cabbage*** 1/2 cup steamed green beans 1 tsp margarine	**Peanut Butter, Banana, and Jelly Sandwich** 1 oz baked potato chips 3/4 cup blueberries 1 cup celery sticks 1 oz reduced-fat cheese	**Chicken Pasta Salad with Tropical Fruit Dressing** 1/2 oz wheat crackers 1 cup mixed broccoli and cauliflower	**Carrot-Raisin Salad** (1/2 serving)* 1 whole-wheat English muffin 1/2 cup steamed peas 1/2 cup tomatoes 2 oz reduced-fat mozzarella cheese	**Chicken, Escarole, and Rice Soup** 1 small bagel 3/4 cup pineapple cubes 1 tsp margarine
Snack A							
Snack B							
Dinner	**Mediterranean Ocean Perch Rice Pilaf*** 17 grapes 1/2 cup nonfat milk 1/2 tsp margarine	**Chicken Piccata** **Apple Salad Dijon*** **Low-Fat Corn Bread*** 1/2 cup nonfat milk 1 cup tomato slices 1/2 cup steamed spinach 1 tsp margarine	**Carrot Slaw*** 1 cup oven-baked French fries 1 slice whole-grain bread 1 cup nonfat milk 1/2 cup steamed Brussels sprouts 2 oz ground sirloin 1 tsp margarine	**Blackened Catfish** **Spinach-Orange Salad*** **Strawberry Whip Parfaits*** 1/2 cup blueberries 1 cup nonfat milk 1/2 cup cooked squash	**Orange Marmalade Pork Cutlets** **Baked Sweet Potato Fries*** **Green Bean Sesame Salad*** **Splendid Blueberry Crisp*** 1 cup nonfat milk	**Banana Baked Chicken** **Italian Zucchini** 1 cup steamed broccoli 6 walnut halves	**Limed Chicken Breast** **Sautéed Zucchini and Red Peppers*** **Fruit Salad Medley*** **Buttered Parsley Potatoes** 1 slice whole-grain bread 1/2 tsp margarine

*Indicates that the recipe has been used previously.

	Sunday	Monday	Tuesday	Wednesday	Thursday	Friday	Saturday
Breakfast	2 (4-inch) pancakes 1/4 cup sugar-free maple syrup 1/4 cup unsweetened applesauce 1 cup nonfat milk 1/4 cup egg substitute, scrambled 2 tsp margarine	Shredded Wheat Custard* 1 small bagel 4 grapes 1/2 cup nonfat milk 1 oz lean turkey sausage 1 Tbsp peanut butter	Zucchini Bread* 1/2 large grapefruit 1 cup nonfat milk 2 tsp margarine	Banana Bran Muffin* 1 1/2 cup puffed rice cereal 1 cup nonfat milk 1/4 cup egg substitute 1/2 tsp margarine 5 hazelnuts	All-Natural High-Fiber Peach Squares 1/2 cup oatmeal 1 1/4 cup strawberries 1 cup nonfat milk 1 oz lean beef sausage 1 tsp margarine	Baked Apples* 1 slice raisin bread 1 cup nonfat milk 1/4 cup egg substitute, scrambled 1 1/2 tsp margarine	Zucchini Carrot Muffins* 1/2 Tbsp jam 1 cup nonfat milk 1/4 cup low-fat cottage cheese 1/2 tsp margarine
Lunch	Mashed Potatoes* Prune Delight Spread 1 1/2 small dinner rolls 1/2 cup steamed green beans 2 oz lean sirloin tip roast 1 1/2 tsp margarine	Turkey Vegetable Soup (2 servings) 1 (2 oz) crusty roll 1 cup mixed melon cubes 1/2 cup steamed asparagus 2 tsp margarine	Tuna and Pasta Salad Cinnamon Red Cabbage* 1/2 cup steamed green beans 2 tsp margarine	Peanut Butter, Banana, and Jelly Sandwich 1 oz baked potato chips 3/4 cup blueberries 1 cup celery sticks 1 oz reduced-fat cheese 1 Tbsp sunflower seeds	Chicken Pasta Salad with Tropical Fruit Dressing 1/2 oz wheat crackers 1 cup mixed broccoli and cauliflower 2 Brazil nuts	Carrot-Raisin Salad (1/2 serving)* 1 whole-wheat English muffin 1/2 cup steamed peas 1/2 cup tomatoes 2 oz reduced-fat mozzarella cheese	Chicken, Escarole, and Rice Soup 1 small bagel 3/4 cup pineapple cubes 2 tsp margarine
Snack A	6 almonds 3/4 cup blackberries	4 pecans 1/2 cup peaches in juice	4 pecans 1 medium peach	1 1/2 tsp peanut butter 1 medium banana	2 Tbsp fat-free whipped topping 3/4 cup blackberries	6 almonds 2 Tbsp dried cherries	6 almonds 1 1/3 cup watermelon cubes
Snack B	1 cup nonfat milk	1 cup nonfat milk	1 cup nonfat milk	1 cup nonfat milk	1 cup nonfat milk	6 oz fat-free yogurt	1 cup nonfat milk
Dinner	Mediterranean Ocean Perch Rice Pilaf* 17 grapes 1/2 cup nonfat milk 1/2 tsp margarine	Chicken Piccata Apple Salad Dijon* Low-Fat Corn Bread* 1/2 cup nonfat milk 1 cup tomato slices 1/2 cup steamed spinach 1 tsp margarine	Carrot Slaw* 1 cup oven-baked French fries 1 slice whole-grain bread 1 cup nonfat milk 1/2 cup steamed Brussels sprouts 3 oz ground sirloin 1 tsp margarine	Blackened Catfish Spinach-Orange Salad* Strawberry Whip Parfaits* 1/2 cup blueberries 1 cup nonfat milk 1/2 cup cooked squash	Orange Marmalade Pork Cutlets Baked Sweet Potato Fries* Green Bean Sesame Salad* Splendid Blueberry Crisp* 1 cup nonfat milk 1 oz reduced-fat cheese	Banana Baked Chicken Italian Zucchini 1 cup steamed broccoli 6 walnut halves	Limed Chicken Breast Sautéed Zucchini and Red Peppers* Fruit Salad Medley* Buttered Parsley Potatoes 1 slice whole-grain bread 1/2 tsp margarine

*Indicates that the recipe has been used previously.

2000 calorie MEAL PLAN SUMMER WEEK 1

	Sunday	Monday	Tuesday	Wednesday	Thursday	Friday	Saturday
Breakfast	2 (4-inch) pancakes 1/4 cup sugar-free maple syrup 1/4 cup unsweetened applesauce 1 cup nonfat milk 2 tsp margarine	Shredded Wheat Custard* 1 small bagel 4 grapes 1/2 cup nonfal milk 1 oz lean turkey sausage 1 Tbsp peanut butter	Zucchini Bread* 1/2 large grapefruit 1 cup nonfat milk 2 tsp margarine	Banana Bran Muffin* 1 1/2 cup puffed rice cereal 1 cup nonfat milk 1/4 cup egg substitute, scrambled 1/2 tsp margarine 5 hazelnuts	All-Natural High-Fiber Peach Squares 1/2 cup oatmeal 1 1/4 cup strawberries 1 cup nonfat milk 1 oz lean beef sausage 1 tsp margarine	Baked Apples* 1 slice raisin bread 1 cup nonfat milk 1/4 cup egg substitute, scrambled 1 1/2 tsp margarine	Zucchini Carrot Muffins* 1/2 Tbsp jam 1 cup nonfat milk 1/4 cup low-fat cottage cheese 1/2 tsp margarine
Lunch	Mashed Potatoes* Prune Delight Spread 2 small dinner rolls 1 small tangerine 1 cup steamed green beans 2 oz lean sirloin tip roast 1 1/2 tsp margarine	Turkey Vegetable Soup (2 servings) 1 (2 oz) crusty roll 2 cups mixed melon cubes 1 cup steamed asparagus 2 tsp margarine	Tuna and Pasta Salad Cinnamon Red Cabbage* 1 cup steamed green beans 2 tsp margarine	Peanut Butter, Banana, and Jelly Sandwich 1 oz baked potato chips 1 1/2 cup blueberries 2 cups celery sticks 1 oz reduced-fat cheese 1 Tbsp sunflower seeds	Chicken Pasta Salad with Tropical Fruit Dressing 1/2 oz wheat crackers 2 Tbsp raisins 2 cups mixed broccoli and cauliflower 2 Brazil nuts	Carrot-Raisin Salad (1/2 serving)* 1 whole-wheat English muffin 1/2 cup steamed peas 17 grapes 1 1/2 cup tomatoes 2 oz reduced-fat mozzarella cheese	Chicken, Escarole, and Rice Soup 1 small bagel 1 1/2 cup pineapple cubes 1 cup salad greens 1 tsp margarine 1 Tbsp light salad dressing
Snack A	1 cup tomato wedges 6 almonds 3/4 cup blackberries	1 cup mixed vegetable sticks 4 pecans 1/2 cup peaches in juice	1 cup carrot sticks 4 pecans 1 medium peach	1 cup small grape tomatoes 1 Tbsp light salad dressing 1 medium banana	1 cup mixed raw vegetables 2 Tbsp fat-free whipped topping 3/4 cup blackberries	1 cup cucumber sticks 6 almonds 2 Tbsp dried cranberries	1 cup mixed vegetable sticks 2 Tbsp light salad dressing 1 1/3 cup watermelon cubes
Snack B	3/4 oz baked tortilla chips 1 oz avocado 1 cup nonfat milk	2-inch square unfrosted cake 1 cup nonfat milk	3 cups popcorn 1 tsp margarine 1 cup nonfat milk	3 graham cracker squares 1 1/2 tsp peanut butter 1 cup nonfat milk	3 ginger snaps 1 cup nonfat milk	4 rice crackers 1 1/2 tsp almond butter 6 oz fat-free yogurt	3/4 oz pretzels 6 almonds 1 cup nonfat milk
Dinner	Mediterranean Ocean Perch Rice Pilaf* 17 grapes 1/2 cup nonfat milk 1/2 tsp margarine	Chicken Piccata Apple Salad Dijon* Low-Fat Corn Bread* 1/2 cup nonfat milk 1 cup tomato slices 1/2 cup steamed spinach 1 tsp margarine	Carrot Slaw* 1 cup oven-baked French fries 1 slice whole-grain bread 1 cup nonfat milk 1/2 cup steamed Brussels sprouts 3 oz ground sirloin 1 tsp margarine	Blackened Catfish Spinach-Orange Salad* Strawberry Whip Parfaits* 1/2 cup blueberries 1 cup nonfat milk 1/2 cup cooked squash	Orange Marmalade Pork Cutlets Baked Sweet Potato Fries* Green Bean Sesame Salad* Splendid Blueberry Crisp* 1 cup nonfat milk 1 oz reduced-fat cheese	Banana Baked Chicken Italian Zucchini 1 cup steamed broccoli 6 walnut halves	Limed Chicken Breast Sautéed Zucchini and Red Peppers* Fruit Salad Medley* Buttered Parsley Potatoes 1 slice whole-grain bread 1 tsp margarine

*Indicates that the recipe has been used previously.

	Sunday	Monday	Tuesday	Wednesday	Thursday	Friday	Saturday
Breakfast	2 (4-inch) pancakes 1/4 cup sugar-free maple syrup 1/4 cup unsweetened applesauce 1 cup nonfat milk 1/2 cup egg substitute, scrambled 2 tsp margarine	**Shredded Wheat Custard*** 1 small bagel 4 grapes 1/2 cup nonfat milk 2 oz lean turkey sausage 1 Tbsp peanut butter	**Zucchini Bread*** 1/2 large grapefruit 1 cup nonfat milk 1 oz lean ham 2 tsp margarine	**Banana Bran Muffin*** 1 1/2 cup puffed rice cereal 1 cup nonfat milk 1/2 cup egg substitute, scrambled 1/2 tsp margarine 5 hazelnuts	**All-Natural High-Fiber Peach Squares** 1/2 cup oatmeal 1 1/4 cup strawberries 1 cup nonfat milk 2 oz lean beef sausage 1 tsp margarine	**Baked Apples*** 1 slice raisin bread 1 cup nonfat milk 1/2 cup egg substitute, scrambled 1 1/2 tsp margarine	**Zucchini Carrot Muffins*** 1/2 Tbsp jam 1 cup nonfat milk 1/2 cup low-fat cottage cheese 1/2 tsp margarine
Lunch	**Mashed Potatoes*** **Prune Delight Spread** 2 small dinner rolls 1 small tangerine 1 cup steamed green beans 2 oz lean sirloin tip roast 1 1/2 tsp margarine	**Turkey Vegetable Soup** (2 servings) 1 (2 oz) crusty roll 2 cups mixed melon cubes 1 cup steamed asparagus 2 tsp margarine	**Tuna and Pasta Salad** **Cinnamon Red Cabbage*** 1 cup steamed green beans 2 tsp margarine	**Peanut Butter, Banana, and Jelly Sandwich** 1 oz baked potato chips 1 1/2 cup blueberries 2 cups celery sticks 1 oz reduced-fat cheese 1 Tbsp sunflower seeds	**Chicken Pasta Salad with Tropical Fruit Dressing** 1/2 oz wheat crackers 2 Tbsp raisins 2 cups mixed broccoli and cauliflower 2 Brazil nuts	**Carrot-Raisin Salad** (1/2 serving)* 1 whole-wheat English muffin 1/2 cup steamed peas 17 grapes 1 1/2 cup tomatoes 2 oz reduced-fat mozzarella cheese	**Chicken, Escarole, and Rice Soup** 1 small bagel 1 1/2 cup pineapple cubes 1 cup salad greens 1 tsp margarine 1 Tbsp light salad dressing
Snack A	1 cup tomato wedges 6 almonds 3/4 cup blackberries	1 cup mixed vegetable sticks 4 pecans 1/2 cup peaches in juice	1 cup carrot sticks 4 pecans 1 medium peach	1 cup small grape tomatoes 1 Tbsp light salad dressing 1 medium banana	1 cup mixed raw vegetables 2 Tbsp fat-free whipped topping 3/4 cup blackberries	1 cup cucumber sticks 6 almonds 2 Tbsp dried cranberries	1 cup mixed vegetable sticks 2 Tbsp light salad dressing 1 1/3 cup watermelon cubes
Snack B	3/4 oz baked tortilla chips 1 oz avocado 1 cup nonfat milk	2-inch square unfrosted cake 1 cup nonfat milk	3 cups popcorn 1 tsp margarine 1 cup nonfat milk	3 graham cracker squares 1 1/2 tsp peanut butter 1 cup nonfat milk	3 ginger snaps 1 cup nonfat milk	4 rice crackers 1 1/2 tsp almond butter 6 oz fat-free yogurt	3/4 oz pretzels 6 almonds 1 cup nonfat milk
Dinner	**Mediterranean Ocean Perch Rice Pilaf*** 1 slice whole-wheat bread 17 grapes 1 cup nonfat milk 1/2 tsp margarine	**Chicken Piccata** **Apple Salad Dijon*** **Low-Fat Corn Bread*** 1 slice whole-wheat bread 1 cup nonfat milk 1 cup tomato slices 1/2 cup steamed spinach 1 tsp margarine	**Carrot Slaw*** 2 cups oven-baked French fries 1 slice whole-grain bread 1 cup nonfat milk 1/2 cup steamed Brussels sprouts 3 oz ground sirloin 1 tsp margarine	**Blackened Catfish** **Spinach-Orange Salad*** **Strawberry Whip Parfaits*** 1 slice whole-grain bread 1/2 cup blueberries 1 cup nonfat milk 1/2 cup cooked squash	**Orange Marmalade Pork Cutlets** **Baked Sweet Potato Fries*** **Green Bean Sesame Salad*** **Splendid Blueberry Crisp*** 1/2 cup unsweetened applesauce 1 cup nonfat milk 1 oz reduced-fat cheese	**Banana Baked Chicken** **Italian Zucchini** 1/3 cup brown rice 1 cup steamed broccoli 6 walnut halves	**Limed Chicken Breast** **Sautéed Zucchini and Red Peppers*** **Fruit Salad Medley*** **Buttered Parsley Potatoes** 2 slices whole-grain bread 1 tsp margarine

*Indicates that the recipe has been used previously.

SHOPPING LIST SUMMER WEEK 1

VEGETABLES
_____ asparagus
_____ bell peppers, green
_____ bell peppers, red
_____ broccoli
_____ Brussels sprouts
_____ cabbage, red
_____ carrots
_____ cauliflower
_____ celery
_____ corn, whole-kernel, no-added-salt, frozen
_____ escarole
_____ garlic
_____ green beans
_____ green peas
_____ lettuce, iceberg
_____ mushrooms
_____ onions, green
_____ onions, red
_____ onions, yellow or white
_____ potatoes
_____ potatoes, sweet
_____ spinach
_____ squash, any kind
_____ tomatoes
_____ zucchini

MEATS
_____ catfish fillets
_____ chicken breasts, boneless, skinless
_____ ground sirloin
_____ ocean perch fillets
_____ pork chops, boneless sirloin
_____ sausage, beef, lean
_____ sausage, turkey, lean
_____ sirloin tip roast, lean
_____ tuna, packed in water
_____ turkey breast

FRUITS
_____ apples
_____ apples, Granny Smith
_____ apples, tart (Jonathan, York, or Rome Beauty)
_____ bananas
_____ blackberries
_____ blueberries
_____ grapefruit
_____ grapes
_____ lemon
_____ melon, any kind
_____ oranges
_____ oranges, mandarin, packed in juice, can
_____ peaches
_____ pears
_____ pineapple cubes
_____ pineapple, chunks, light can
_____ pineapple, crushed, no-added-sugar can
_____ prunes, canned in light syrup
_____ raisins
_____ strawberries
_____ tangerines

DAIRY
_____ egg substitute
_____ eggs
_____ half and half, fat-free
_____ milk, nonfat
_____ Smart Balance Light margarine
_____ sour cream, fat-free
_____ whipped topping, fat-free
_____ yogurt, fat-free, plain

CHEESE
_____ cheese, any kind, reduced-fat
_____ cottage cheese, low-fat
_____ mozzarella, reduced-fat
_____ Parmesan, reduced-fat

BREAD, GRAINS, & PASTA
_____ bagels, whole-wheat, small
_____ bread, raisin
_____ bread, whole-wheat, whole-grain
_____ crusty bread roll
_____ dinner rolls
_____ English muffins, whole-wheat
_____ pasta, bowtie, whole-wheat
_____ pasta, fusilli
_____ rice, brown
_____ rice, white, long-grain

NUTS
_____ almonds
_____ Brazil nuts
_____ hazelnuts
_____ peanuts, dry roasted, unsalted
_____ walnuts

CONDIMENTS
_____ canola mayonnaise
_____ mustard, Dijon
_____ red hot sauce
_____ soy sauce, light
_____ Worcestershire sauce

SPICES & HERBS

_____ basil
_____ bay leaf
_____ chives
_____ cinnamon, ground
_____ cloves, ground
_____ cream of tartar
_____ cumin seeds
_____ curry powder
_____ dry mustard
_____ ginger, ground
_____ lemon pepper
_____ mint leaves
_____ nutmeg, ground
_____ onion powder
_____ oregano
_____ paprika
_____ parsley
_____ pepper, black
_____ pepper, red
_____ peppercorns
_____ pumpkin pie spice
_____ sesame seeds
_____ tarragon
_____ turmeric, ground

OTHER

_____ angel food cake
_____ applesauce, unsweetened
_____ cereal, bran
_____ cereal, puffed rice
_____ cereal, shredded wheat
_____ crackers, wheat
_____ French fries, oven-baked
_____ gelatin, unflavored
_____ honey
_____ jelly, jam, or preserves, sugar-free
_____ maple syrup, sugar-free
_____ marmalade, orange, sugar-free
_____ olives, black
_____ pancake mix
_____ peanut butter, low-sugar
_____ potato chips, baked
_____ salad dressing, light
_____ salad dressing, red wine vinaigrette
_____ salsa
_____ sunflower seeds
_____ tomatoes, diced, no-added-salt can
_____ wheat germ
_____ wine, red

STAPLES

_____ baking powder
_____ baking soda
_____ bouillon, beef, sodium-free
_____ bouillon, chicken, sodium-free
_____ cornmeal, yellow
_____ flour, whole-wheat
_____ juice, lemon
_____ juice, lime
_____ juice, orange concentrate, frozen
_____ juice, pineapple
_____ nonstick cooking spray
_____ oats, old-fashioned
_____ Smart Balance Omega oil
_____ Splenda
_____ Splenda Brown Sugar Blend
_____ vanilla extract
_____ vinegar, cider
_____ vinegar, malt
_____ vinegar, red wine

Mashed Potatoes

Serves 4   Serving size: 1/4 recipe

2 cups peeled, diced potatoes	**5 tsp** Smart Balance margarine
1/4 cup nonfat milk	Pepper, to taste

Peel the potatoes and cut into cubes; place in a large pan. Cover with water, bring to a boil, and then simmer for approximately 45 minutes, until potatoes are tender. Mash potatoes until no lumps remain, slowly adding milk and margarine to make potatoes smoother and fluffy. Season with pepper and serve.

Exchanges/Choices

1 Starch
1/2 Fat

Basic Nutritional Values

Calories 85
 Calories from Fat 35
Total Fat . . . . 4.0 g
 Saturated Fat . . . . 1.1 g
 Trans Fat . . . . 0.0 g
Cholesterol . . . . 0 mg
Sodium . . . . 50 mg
Total Carbohydrate . . . 12 g
 Dietary Fiber . . . . 1 g
 Sugars . . . . 2 g
Protein . . . . 1 g

Prune Delight Spread

Serves 4   Serving size: 1/4 recipe

1 1/2   envelopes unflavored gelatin

2   **cups** canned prunes in light syrup, drained, discard 1/2 juice

3   **Tbsp** Splenda

2/3   **tsp** pure vanilla extract

2   egg whites

1/16   **tsp** cream of tartar

1. In a small saucepan, add gelatin to 1/2 cup water; let stand for 1 minute. Cook and stir over low heat until gelatin is dissolved; set aside. Place drained prunes in a blender. Cover and blend at high speed for 30 seconds or until thickened and well blended.

2. In a large metal bowl, combine 6 Tbsp water, Splenda, vanilla, and gelatin-prune mixture. Place bowl in a larger bowl half filled with ice water. Stir mixture until syrupy. Remove bowl from water bath.

3. In a small mixer bowl at high speed, beat egg whites until foamy. Add cream of tartar and continue beating until stiff but not dry.

4. Return prune mixture to ice water bath and stir until mixture mounds slightly when dropped from a spoon. Fold in egg whites. Spoon into 6 dessert dishes. Chill for 30 minutes or until set.

Exchanges/Choices

1 1/2 Fruit

Basic Nutritional Values

Calories	95
Calories from Fat	0
Total Fat	0.0 g
Saturated Fat	0.0 g
Trans Fat	0.0 g
Cholesterol	0 mg
Sodium	60 mg
Total Carbohydrate	19 g
Dietary Fiber	1 g
Sugars	18 g
Protein	4 g

Mediterranean Ocean Perch
Serves 4 Serving size: 1/4 recipe

2 **Tbsp** Smart Balance Omega oil

1 **cup** sliced onions

1 medium clove garlic, crushed

2 medium tomatoes, diced

3 **oz** salsa

1/4 **tsp** cinnamon

1/2 **tsp** basil

1 **lb** ocean perch fillets

In 1 1/2-quart microwave-safe dish, combine oil, onion, and garlic. Cover and cook on high for 3 minutes. Stir in tomatoes, salsa, cinnamon, and basil. Top with fish. Cover and cook on high for 3–4 minutes or until fish flakes with a fork.

Exchanges/Choices

2 Vegetable
3 Lean Meat
1/2 Fat

Basic Nutritional Values

Calories 210
 Calories from Fat 80
Total Fat . . . . 9.0 g
 Saturated Fat . . . . 0.8 g
 Trans Fat . . . . 0.0 g
Cholesterol . . . . 50 mg
Sodium . . . . 220 mg
Total Carbohydrate . . . 9 g
 Dietary Fiber . . . . 2 g
 Sugars . . . . 4 g
Protein . . . . 23 g

Rice Pilaf
Serves 4 Serving size: 1/4 recipe

1/2 **cup** finely chopped onion

2 **Tbsp** Smart Balance margarine

1 **cup** brown rice, uncooked

2 **cups** water

1 **Tbsp** sodium-free chicken bouillon

Pepper, to taste

Sauté onions in margarine until soft and tender; do not brown. Add rice and cook, stirring frequently for 5 minutes. Add water, bouillon, and pepper. Cook covered for 20–25 minutes. Bell peppers, carrots, green onions, or celery can also be added.

Exchanges/Choices

2 1/2 Starch
1 Fat

Basic Nutritional Values

Calories 225
 Calories from Fat 55
Total Fat . . . . 6.0 g
 Saturated Fat . . . . 1.5 g
 Trans Fat . . . . 0.0 g
Cholesterol . . . . 0 mg
Sodium . . . . 55 mg
Total Carbohydrate . . . 39 g
 Dietary Fiber . . . . 2 g
 Sugars . . . . 2 g
Protein . . . . 4 g

Shredded Wheat Custard
Serves 4   Serving size: 1/4 recipe

1 quart nonfat milk, warm	**1 tsp** pure vanilla extract
6 shredded wheat biscuits, crushed	**1/2 cup** Splenda
4 egg whites, beaten	**3/4 cup** raisins

Combine the warm milk and crushed shredded wheat. Add egg whites, vanilla, Splenda, and raisins. Bake at 350°F for 60 minutes or until fully set (a knife inserted in the center comes out clean).

Exchanges/Choices

2 Starch
1 1/2 Fruit
1 Fat-Free Milk

Basic Nutritional Values

Calories 325
 Calories from Fat 5
Total Fat . . . . 0.5 g
 Saturated Fat . . . . 0.2 g
 Trans Fat . . . . 0.0 g
Cholesterol . . . . 5 mg
Sodium . . . . 190 mg
Total Carbohydrate . . . 67 g
 Dietary Fiber . . . . 5 g
 Sugars . . . . 33 g
Protein . . . . 17 g

Turkey Vegetable Soup
Serves 6   Serving size: 1/6 recipe

1 tsp Smart Balance margarine	**2 cups** water
1/2 cup chopped onion	**1/2 cup** frozen peas
1/4 cup diced celery	**1/2 cup** frozen no-added-salt whole-kernel corn
1 cup cooked and diced turkey breast (trimmed of fat)	**1/2 tsp** pepper
2 Tbsp sodium-free chicken bouillon	**1/4 tsp** red hot sauce

1. Heat a stockpot or Dutch oven over medium heat. Add margarine and swirl to coat bottom. Cook onion and celery for 3–4 minutes or until onion is translucent, stirring occasionally.

2. Stir in remaining ingredients (no need to thaw frozen vegetables). Simmer, covered, for 30 minutes or until vegetables are tender.

Exchanges/Choices

1/2 Starch
1 Lean Meat

Basic Nutritional Values

Calories 75
 Calories from Fat 10
Total Fat . . . . 1.0 g
 Saturated Fat . . . . 0.2 g
 Trans Fat . . . . 0.0 g
Cholesterol . . . . 20 mg
Sodium . . . . 40 mg
Total Carbohydrate . . . 8 g
 Dietary Fiber . . . . 1 g
 Sugars . . . . 3 g
Protein . . . . 8 g

Chicken Piccata

Serves 4   Serving size: 1/4 recipe

2 slices whole-wheat bread, torn into large pieces

1 **lb** boneless, skinless chicken breasts (trimmed of fat)

1/8 **tsp** black pepper

1/4 **cup** egg substitute

1 **Tbsp** nonfat milk

1 large clove garlic, crushed

2 **Tbsp** Smart Balance Light margarine

1 **cup** water

2 **Tbsp** lemon juice

1 **Tbsp** sodium-free chicken bouillon

Exchanges/Choices

1/2 Starch
3 Lean Meat

Basic Nutritional Values

Calories 185
  Calories from Fat 45
Total Fat . . . . 5.0 g
  Saturated Fat . . . . 1.6 g
  Trans Fat . . . . 0.0 g
Cholesterol . . . . 65 mg
Sodium . . . . 160 mg
Total Carbohydrate . . . 5 g
  Dietary Fiber . . . . 0 g
  Sugars . . . . 2 g
Protein . . . . 27 g

1. Preheat oven to 350°F. Place bread in a blender. Cover and blend at high speed to make soft bread crumbs (about 1/2 cup); set aside.

2. Place one chicken breast at a time between two pieces of wax paper. With a wooden mallet or a rolling pin, flatten to 1/8 inch thickness. Peel off waxed paper. Sprinkle one side of each breast with pepper.

3. In a shallow dish, beat the egg substitute and milk until blended. With tongs, dip both sides of the chicken in the egg mixture and then in bread crumbs to coat; set aside.

4. In a 10-inch skillet over medium heat, sauté garlic in margarine until brown. Sauté chicken breasts for 2–3 minutes on each side or until lightly browned; transfer to a baking dish and place in the oven to keep warm.

5. Remove skillet from heat and add water, lemon juice, and bouillon. Cook and stir over low heat to loosen particles from bottom of skillet. Simmer for 2 minutes or until slightly reduced. Pour mixture over chicken and bake for 35–45 minutes.

Apple Salad Dijon

Serves 4   Serving size: 1/4 recipe

- 8 medium celery sticks
- 2 medium Granny Smith apples
- 4 **Tbsp** canola mayonnaise
- 2 **Tbsp** Dijon mustard
- 2 **tsp** cider vinegar
- 1/2 **tsp** Splenda
- 2 **tsp** tarragon
  Black pepper, to taste

1. Cut the celery into 1 1/4-inch matchsticks and reserve celery leaves for garnish. Cut the apples into 1 1/2-inch slices.

2. In a bowl, whisk together the mayonnaise, mustard, vinegar, Splenda, tarragon, and pepper until the dressing is smooth. Add the celery and the apples. Toss the salad and serve garnished with celery leaves.

Exchanges/Choices

1 Fruit
1 Fat

Basic Nutritional Values

Calories 110
  Calories from Fat 45
Total Fat . . . . 5.0 g
  Saturated Fat . . . . 0.1 g
  Trans Fat . . . . 0.0 g
Cholesterol . . . . 0 mg
Sodium . . . . 360 mg
Total Carbohydrate . . . 16 g
  Dietary Fiber . . . . 4 g
  Sugars . . . . 11 g
Protein . . . . 1 g

Low-Fat Corn Bread

Serves 8   Serving size: 1/8 recipe

- 1/2 **cup** egg substitute
- 1/2 **cup** Splenda
- 3/4 **cup** nonfat milk
- 1/2 **cup** unsweetened applesauce
- 1 1/2 **cup** whole-wheat flour
- 2/3 **cup** cornmeal
- 1 **Tbsp** baking powder
  Nonstick cooking spray

Beat together the egg substitute, Splenda, milk, and applesauce; set aside. In a separate bowl, sift and combine flour, cornmeal, and baking powder. Stir into egg mixture using as few strokes as possible. Spray an 8 × 8-inch baking pan with nonstick cooking spray. Bake at 400°F for 25–30 minutes or until a toothpick inserted near the middle comes out clean.

Exchanges/Choices

2 Starch

Basic Nutritional Values

Calories 150
  Calories from Fat 5
Total Fat . . . . 0.5 g
  Saturated Fat . . . . 0.1 g
  Trans Fat . . . . 0.0 g
Cholesterol . . . . 0 mg
Sodium . . . . 180 mg
Total Carbohydrate . . . 30 g
  Dietary Fiber . . . . 4 g
  Sugars . . . . 4 g
Protein . . . . 6 g

Zucchini Bread

Serves 8   Serving size: 1 slice

Nonstick cooking spray

1 **cup** whole-wheat flour

1/2 **cup** Splenda Brown Sugar Blend

1 **tsp** baking powder

1 **tsp** ground cinnamon

1/4 **tsp** baking soda

1 **cup** shredded zucchini

1 **Tbsp** finely chopped walnuts

1/4 **cup** egg substitute

1 **Tbsp** Smart Balance Omega oil

1/2 **tsp** vanilla extract

1/2 **cup** pineapple juice

Exchanges/Choices

2 Carbohydrate

Basic Nutritional Values

Calories 140
  Calories from Fat 20
Total Fat. . . . . 2.5 g
  Saturated Fat . . . . 0.2 g
  Trans Fat. . . . . 0.0 g
Cholesterol. . . . . 0 mg
Sodium. . . . . 105 mg
Total Carbohydrate. . . 26 g
  Dietary Fiber . . . . 2 g
  Sugars . . . . 14 g
Protein. . . . . 3 g

Preheat the oven to 350°F. Spray a 9 × 5 × 3-inch loaf pan with nonstick cooking spray. In a large bowl, combine the flour, Splenda, baking powder, cinnamon, and baking soda. Then stir in the zucchini and walnuts. In a small bowl, combine the egg substitute with the oil, vanilla extract, and the pineapple juice. Combine ingredients from both bowls and stir until moistened. Pour the batter into the baking dish. Bake about 1 hour or until a toothpick inserted into the center of the loaf comes out clean.

Tuna and Pasta Salad

Serves 4   Serving size: 1/4 recipe

8 **oz** whole-wheat bowtie pasta	1 1/2 medium tomatoes, cut into thin wedges
2 **cups** cut green beans (or 1 lb frozen)	3/4 medium red onion, thinly sliced
1 **cup** sliced carrots	4 large black olives, pitted and sliced
1/2 **cup** red wine vinaigrette dressing	3 **Tbsp** chives
12 **oz** canned tuna, packed in water	Pepper, to taste

Fill a 5-quart saucepan two-thirds full with water; bring to a boil. Add pasta and cook according to package directions. Reduce heat to low; simmer, uncovered, for 8 minutes. Add green beans and carrots; simmer uncovered for 4 minutes, until pasta is tender and vegetables are crisp-tender. Drain well. Return pasta and vegetables to saucepan and add vinaigrette; toss well to coat. Break tuna into large pieces. Add tuna, tomato, onion, olives, chives, and pepper; toss gently but thoroughly to mix.

Exchanges/Choices

2 1/2 Starch
1/2 Carbohydrate
3 Vegetable
3 Lean Meat

Basic Nutritional Values

Calories 425
  Calories from Fat 65
Total Fat . . . . 7.0 g
  Saturated Fat . . . . 1.5 g
  Trans Fat . . . . 0.0 g
Cholesterol . . . . 25 mg
Sodium . . . . 565 mg
Total Carbohydrate . . . 64 g
  Dietary Fiber . . . . 9 g
  Sugars . . . . 14 g
Protein . . . . 30 g

Cinnamon Red Cabbage

Serves 4   Serving size: 1/4 recipe

4 **cups** red cabbage	1 **tsp** cinnamon
1 medium Granny Smith apple	1 **tsp** ground cloves
1 medium pear	3 **Tbsp** red wine vinegar
1/4 **cup** sugar-free orange marmalade	3 **Tbsp** red table wine

Thinly slice the cabbage. Peel and slice the apple. Peel and chop the pear. In a large pot, combine the cabbage, apple, pear, marmalade, cinnamon, cloves, vinegar, wine, and 1 cup water. Bring to a boil and cook the mixture, covered, over moderately low heat, stirring occasionally, for 3 hours. Serve the cabbage chilled as an accompaniment to cold sliced meats.

Exchanges/Choices

1 Fruit
1 Vegetable

Basic Nutritional Values

Calories 80
  Calories from Fat 0
Total Fat . . . . 0.0 g
  Saturated Fat . . . . 0.1 g
  Trans Fat . . . . 0.0 g
Cholesterol . . . . 0 mg
Sodium . . . . 15 mg
Total Carbohydrate . . . 22 g
  Dietary Fiber . . . . 4 g
  Sugars . . . . 14 g
Protein . . . . 1 g

Carrot Slaw

Serves 4   Serving size: 1/4 recipe

1/2 **cup** crushed pineapple
(or can of no-added-sugar
crushed pineapple)

1 **tsp** honey

1 **tsp** lemon juice

1/4 **tsp** nutmeg

1/2 **cup** fat-free sour cream

2 **cups** carrot, grated

Drain pineapple. In a medium bowl, mix honey, lemon juice, and nutmeg. Blend in sour cream. Add carrots and pineapple. Serve chilled.

Exchanges/Choices

1/2 Carbohydrate
1 Vegetable

Basic Nutritional Values

Calories	65
Calories from Fat	0
Total Fat	0.0 g
Saturated Fat	0.1 g
Trans Fat	0.0 g
Cholesterol	5 mg
Sodium	55 mg
Total Carbohydrate	11 g
Dietary Fiber	2 g
Sugars	8 g
Protein	3 g

Banana Bran Muffin

Serves 8   Serving size: 1 muffin

2/3 **cup** bran cereal	3/16 **tsp** ground nutmeg
2/3 **cup** plain fat-free yogurt	2 **cups** bananas, mashed
5/8 **cup** whole-wheat flour	1/4 **cup** unsweetened applesauce
5 **Tbsp** Splenda	1/2 **cup** egg substitute, beaten
1 **tsp** ground cinnamon	
1/2 **tsp** baking soda	

1. Preheat oven to 375°F. Place paper liners in muffin pan cups.

2. In a medium bowl, mix cereal and yogurt. Let stand for 5 minutes or until cereal is softened and breaks up.

3. Meanwhile, in a small bowl, combine the flour, Splenda, cinnamon, baking soda, and nutmeg; set aside.

4. Stir banana, applesauce, and egg substitute into cereal mixture. Stir in flour mixture until moistened. Fill muffin cups to about 2/3 full. Bake for 20–25 minutes or until muffins are lightly browned on top. Remove from pan and let cool on a wire rack before serving.

Exchanges/Choices

1 Starch
1 Fruit

Basic Nutritional Values

Calories 120
  Calories from Fat 5
Total Fat. . . . . .0.5 g
  Saturated Fat . . . . .0.2 g
  Trans Fat. . . . . .0.0 g
Cholesterol. . . . . .0 mg
Sodium. . . . . .135 mg
Total Carbohydrate. . .27 g
  Dietary Fiber. . . . . .5 g
  Sugars . . . . .11 g
Protein. . . . . .5 g

Peanut Butter, Banana, and Jelly Sandwich

Serves 8   Serving size: 1 sandwich

1 1/3 **cup** unsalted dry roasted peanuts	2 medium bananas, peeled and vertically sliced
1 **tsp** ground cinnamon	8 **Tbsp** sugar-free jelly
8 slices whole-grain bread	

Place peanuts and cinnamon in a blender or food processor. Cover and blend until spreadable. Stop several times to scrape blades, so the peanut butter is smooth. Blend about 10 minutes. Spread the peanut butter on the bread and top with banana and jelly. Cut sandwiches in half and serve.

Exchanges/Choices

1 1/2 Carbohydrate
1 High-Fat Meat

Basic Nutritional Values

Calories 205
  Calories from Fat 80
Total Fat. . . . . .9.0 g
  Saturated Fat . . . . .1.4 g
  Trans Fat. . . . . .0.0 g
Cholesterol. . . . . .0 mg
Sodium. . . . . .135 mg
Total Carbohydrate. . .27 g
  Dietary Fiber. . . . . .4 g
  Sugars . . . . .9 g
Protein. . . . . .8 g

Blackened Catfish

Serves 4   Serving size: 1/4 recipe

1 **Tbsp** parsley

1/2 **Tbsp** paprika

1/4 **tsp** onion powder

1/4 **tsp** red pepper

1 **lb** catfish fillets

1 **Tbsp** Smart Balance Omega oil

Mix parsley, paprika, onion powder, and ground red pepper. Place catfish on wax paper. Rub spice mixture on both sides of each fillet. In a nonstick 12-inch skillet over medium-high heat, heat oil and cook fillets. Turn fillets once, until golden on both sides and fish flakes easily when tested with a fork, 5–7 minutes.

Exchanges/Choices

3 Lean Meat
1 Fat

Basic Nutritional Values

Calories 190
  Calories from Fat 110
Total Fat . . . . 12.0 g
  Saturated Fat . . . . 2.1 g
  Trans Fat . . . . 0.0 g
Cholesterol . . . . 65 mg
Sodium . . . . 85 mg
Total Carbohydrate . . . 1 g
  Dietary Fiber . . . . 0 g
  Sugars . . . . 0 g
Protein . . . . 19 g

Spinach-Orange Salad

Serves 4   Serving size: 1/4 recipe

4 **cups** spinach, torn into pieces

2 medium oranges, peeled and sectioned, juice reserved (about 1/4 cup)

2/3 **cup** mushrooms, sliced

1/2 **cup** red onion, sliced

2 **Tbsp** Smart Balance Omega oil

2 **Tbsp** malt vinegar

1/2 **tsp** ginger, ground

1/4 **tsp** pepper

Place spinach in a bowl. Add orange sections, mushrooms, and onion. Toss lightly to mix. In a separate bowl, mix oil, vinegar, orange juice, ginger, and pepper. Pour over spinach. Toss to mix and chill; serve.

Exchanges/Choices

1/2 Fruit
1 Vegetable
1 1/2 Fat

Basic Nutritional Values

Calories 115
  Calories from Fat 65
Total Fat . . . . 7.0 g
  Saturated Fat . . . . 0.5 g
  Trans Fat . . . . 0.0 g
Cholesterol . . . . 0 mg
Sodium . . . . 25 mg
Total Carbohydrate . . . 13 g
  Dietary Fiber . . . . 3 g
  Sugars . . . . 8 g
Protein . . . . 2 g

Strawberry Whip Parfaits

Serves 4   Serving size: 1/4 recipe

2 cups sliced strawberries

2 cups fat-free whipped
topping

4 (1-oz) slices angel food cake

Place sliced strawberries in an electric blender. Cover and blend until smooth, stopping once to scrape the sides. Fold strawberry puree into whipped topping. Tear angel food cake into pieces and fold into strawberry mixture. Spoon into parfait glasses, cover, and serve chilled.

Exchanges/Choices

2 Carbohydrate

Basic Nutritional Values

Calories 125
  Calories from Fat 15
Total Fat . . . . 1.5 g
  Saturated Fat . . . . 0.6 g
  Trans Fat . . . . 0.0 g
Cholesterol . . . . 5 mg
Sodium . . . . 160 mg
Total Carbohydrate . . . 27 g
  Dietary Fiber . . . . 2 g
  Sugars . . . . 16 g
Protein . . . . 3 g

THURSDAY

All-Natural High-Fiber Peach Squares

Serves 9   Serving Size: 1 square

- 3/4 **cup** fresh or frozen peaches, diced
- 1 **cup** Splenda
- 3/4 **cup** + 3/4 **Tbsp** whole-wheat flour
- 3/4 **cup** warm water
- 1 **cup** old-fashioned oats
- 1/4 **cup** Smart Balance margarine
- 1 **tsp** baking soda
- 1 **tsp** pure vanilla extract

1. Prepare the filling: bring the peaches, 1/2 cup Splenda, 3/4 Tbsp flour, and 3/4 cup water to a boil in a double boiler. Stir continuously until thickened.

2. Prepare the crumb base and topping: combine oats, margarine, 1/2 cup Splenda, 3/4 cup flour, baking soda, and vanilla; halve the mixture. Place half in the bottom of a 9-inch square baking dish. Layer the thickened filling on top. Add the remaining crumb base to the top.

3. Bake at 350°F for 30 minutes.

Exchanges/Choices

1 Starch
1 Fat

Basic Nutritional Values

Calories 125
 Calories from Fat 45
Total Fat . . . . 5.0 g
 Saturated Fat . . . . 1.2 g
 Trans Fat . . . . 0.0 g
Cholesterol . . . . 0 mg
Sodium . . . . 180 mg
Total Carbohydrate . . . 18 g
 Dietary Fiber . . . . 2 g
 Sugars . . . . 4 g
Protein . . . . 3 g

Chicken Pasta Salad with Tropical Fruit Dressing

Serves 4   Serving size: 1/4 recipe

1/2 **lb** boneless, skinless chicken breasts (trimmed of fat)

6 **oz** fusilli pasta

1 **cup** canned light pineapple chunks, 1/4 cup juice reserved

1/2 **cup** canola mayonnaise

2 **tsp** Splenda Brown Sugar Blend

1 **tsp** curry powder

1 **cup** mandarin orange sections, packed in juice

1/2 **cup** chopped green bell pepper

2 green onions, chopped

Exchanges/Choices

2 Starch
1 1/2 Fruit
2 Lean Meat
1 Fat

Basic Nutritional Values

Calories 385
  Calories from Fat 100
Total Fat . . . . .11.0 g
  Saturated Fat . . . . .0.5 g
  Trans Fat . . . . .0.0 g
Cholesterol . . . . .35 mg
Sodium . . . . .215 mg
Total Carbohydrate . . .51 g
  Dietary Fiber . . . . .3 g
  Sugars . . . . .19 g
Protein . . . . .19 g

1. Cook chicken breasts for several minutes in boiling water until thoroughly cooked and then cut into thin strips.

2. Cook pasta according to package directions; drain. Pasta should be cooked through but still firm. Drain cooked pasta into a colander in the sink. Allow to cool to room temperature.

3. Combine reserved pineapple juice, mayonnaise, Splenda, and curry powder in a large bowl. Stir in pasta, pineapple chunks, mandarin oranges, chicken, bell pepper, and green onions and mix well. Chill for 1 hour before serving.

Orange Marmalade Pork Cutlets

Serves 4   Serving size: 1/4 recipe

2 **tsp** lemon pepper	2 **Tbsp** cider vinegar	
3/4 **lb** boneless sirloin pork chops (trimmed of fat)	1/4 **cup** sugar-free orange marmalade	

Heat a heavy skillet over medium-high heat. Sprinkle lemon pepper on both sides of each pork chop. Add chops to heated skillet and pan broil about 5 minutes per side. Remove chops from pan; keep warm. Carefully add vinegar to skillet, scraping up any brown bits. Stir in marmalade. Return chops to skillet, turning once to coat. Serve immediately.

Exchanges/Choices

1/2 Carbohydrate
2 Lean Meat

Basic Nutritional Values

Calories	95
Calories from Fat	20
Total Fat	2.0 g
Saturated Fat	0.3 g
Trans Fat	0.0 g
Cholesterol	40 mg
Sodium	390 mg
Total Carbohydrate	6 g
Dietary Fiber	0 g
Sugars	3 g
Protein	15 g

Baked Sweet Potato Fries

Serves 4   Serving size: 1/4 recipe

2 medium sweet potatoes	1/4 **tsp** ground turmeric
1 1/2 **Tbsp** Smart Balance Omega oil	1/4 **tsp** cumin seed
1 **tsp** curry powder	1/4 **tsp** ground ginger

Preheat oven to 400°F. Wash and scrub sweet potatoes, leaving the skins on. Cut them into sticks about 1/4–1/2 inch wide and 2–4 inches long; set aside. In a 2-quart mixing bowl, mix together the oil and spices. Add potato sticks to bowl; stir to coat. Arrange sticks on a baking sheet; bake for 30–40 minutes or until fries are tender on the inside and slightly golden on the outside. Halfway through baking, stir with spatula to prevent fries from sticking.

Exchanges/Choices

1 Starch
1 Fat

Basic Nutritional Values

Calories	115
Calories from Fat	45
Total Fat	5.0 g
Saturated Fat	0.4 g
Trans Fat	0.0 g
Cholesterol	0 mg
Sodium	25 mg
Total Carbohydrate	16 g
Dietary Fiber	3 g
Sugars	5 g
Protein	2 g

Green Bean Sesame Salad

Serves 4   Serving size: 1/4 recipe

2 **tsp** Smart Balance Light margarine

2 **Tbsp** sesame seeds

2 **cups** cut green beans

2 **Tbsp** lemon juice

Pepper, to taste

Melt margarine in a skillet and add sesame seeds; cook for about 3 minutes. Bring a pot of water to a boil. Add the green beans and cook until tender, about 5 minutes; drain and rinse under cold water. Place in a bowl and toss with the sesame seeds, lemon juice, and margarine. Season to taste with pepper.

Exchanges/Choices

2 Vegetable
1/2 Fat

Basic Nutritional Values

Calories	70
Calories from Fat	30
Total Fat	3.5 g
Saturated Fat	0.6 g
Trans Fat	0.0 g
Cholesterol	0 mg
Sodium	20 mg
Total Carbohydrate	9 g
Dietary Fiber	4 g
Sugars	2 g
Protein	3 g

Splendid Blueberry Crisp

Serves 9   Serving size: 1/9 recipe

Nonstick cooking spray

4 **Tbsp** Splenda

1 1/2 **Tbsp** whole-wheat flour

1 1/2 **tsp** ground cinnamon

1 **tsp** pure vanilla extract

6 **cups** fresh or frozen (partially thawed) blueberries

1 **cup** old-fashioned oats, uncooked

1/3 **cup** coarsely chopped almonds

1/3 **cup** chopped walnuts

4 **Tbsp** melted Smart Balance Light margarine

1. Lightly coat an 8-inch baking dish with nonstick cooking spray.

2. Combine 2 Tbsp Splenda, flour, 1 tsp cinnamon, and vanilla. Mix well. Fold in blueberries until fruit is evenly coated. Spoon into baking dish.

3. Combine all remaining ingredients; mix well. Sprinkle evenly over fruit. Preheat oven to 350°F. Bake for 35–40 minutes or until topping is golden and filling is bubbly. Serve warm.

Exchanges/Choices

1 1/2 Carbohydrate
1 1/2 Fat

Basic Nutritional Values

Calories	170
Calories from Fat	70
Total Fat	8.0 g
Saturated Fat	1.2 g
Trans Fat	0.0 g
Cholesterol	0 mg
Sodium	40 mg
Total Carbohydrate	23 g
Dietary Fiber	4 g
Sugars	11 g
Protein	4 g

Baked Apples

Serves 4   Serving size: 1/4 recipe

4 medium tart baking apples (Jonathan, York, or Rome Beauty), peeled and cored

1/4 cup Splenda

2 1/2 Tbsp Smart Balance margarine

3 Tbsp sugar-free preserves (any kind)

1 tsp pumpkin pie spice

3 Tbsp raisins

3/4 cup water

1. Preheat oven to 350°F.

2. With the tip of a knife, make six 1/4-inch deep cuts in each apple, from top to halfway down. Place the apples in an 8 × 8 × 2-inch baking dish.

3. In a small bowl, combine the Splenda, margarine, fruit preserves, and spice. Stir in raisins.

4. Stuff each apple with one-fourth of the mixture. Pour water into the bottom of the baking dish; cover with foil and seal tightly. Bake for 50–60 minutes or until fork-tender. Remove foil and gently transfer apples to four small dessert bowls. Spoon a little of the juice from the bottom of the pan over each apple.

Exchanges/Choices

2 Fruit
1 Fat

Basic Nutritional Values

Calories 150
 Calories from Fat 55
Total Fat. . . . . .6.0 g
 Saturated Fat . . . . 1.6 g
 Trans Fat. . . . . 0.0 g
Cholesterol. . . . . 0 mg
Sodium. . . . . 60 mg
Total Carbohydrate. . . 28 g
 Dietary Fiber. . . . . 3 g
 Sugars . . . . 23 g
Protein. . . . . 0 g

Carrot-Raisin Salad

Serves 6   Serving size: 1/6 recipe

1 **lb** carrots, coarsely grated

1 **cup** raisins

1 **cup** crushed pineapple

1 **cup** canola mayonnaise

2 **Tbsp** frozen orange juice concentrate

6 iceberg lettuce leaves

In a large bowl, mix carrots, raisins, and crushed pineapple. In another bowl, combine mayonnaise and orange juice concentrate. Gently fold mayonnaise mixture in with the pineapple mixture. Chill, covered, for 2 hours. Evenly divide salad among lettuce leaves.

Exchanges/Choices

2 Fruit
1 Vegetable
2 1/2 Fat

Basic Nutritional Values

Calories	245
Calories from Fat	110
Total Fat	12.0 g
Saturated Fat	0.0 g
Trans Fat	0.0 g
Cholesterol	0 mg
Sodium	290 mg
Total Carbohydrate	33 g
Dietary Fiber	3 g
Sugars	26 g
Protein	2 g

Banana Baked Chicken

Serves 4   Serving size: 1/4 recipe

1 onion, chopped

1 **Tbsp** Smart Balance Omega oil

1/4 **cup** whole-wheat flour

1 **tsp** sodium-free chicken bouillon

1 **cup** water

1 **lb** boneless, skinless chicken breasts (trimmed of fat)

4 **Tbsp** raisins

4 small bananas, sliced

2 small apples, peeled and grated

1 **Tbsp** grated lemon rind

1 **Tbsp** Splenda

1/2 **Tbsp** curry powder

1 bay leaf

4 peppercorns

1 **cup** fat-free half and half

Fry onions in oil until lightly browned. Add whole-wheat flour and mix well. In a small bowl, combine the bouillon and water to make a broth. Slowly add broth while stirring. Add all remaining ingredients, except half and half. Cover and simmer for 20 minutes. Remove bay leaf. Mix in half and half just before serving.

Exchanges/Choices

1/2 Starch
2 1/2 Fruit
1/2 Fat-Free Milk
3 Lean Meat

Basic Nutritional Values

Calories	385
Calories from Fat	70
Total Fat	8.0 g
Saturated Fat	1.7 g
Trans Fat	0.0 g
Cholesterol	70 mg
Sodium	125 mg
Total Carbohydrate	53 g
Dietary Fiber	6 g
Sugars	29 g
Protein	29 g

Italian Zucchini

Serves 4   Serving size: 1/4 recipe

1   **tsp** Smart Balance Omega oil

4   small zucchini (about 2 cups), sliced into 1/2-inch slices

1/4   **cup** whole-wheat bread crumbs

1/4   **cup** parsley, finely cut

1   **Tbsp** finely crushed almonds

1   **Tbsp** reduced-fat Parmesan cheese

1   **Tbsp** chopped oregano

1   medium clove garlic, minced

Exchanges/Choices
1/2 Carbohydrate
1/2 Fat

Basic Nutritional Values
Calories 65
  Calories from Fat 25
Total Fat . . . . 3.0 g
  Saturated Fat . . . . 0.4 g
  Trans Fat . . . . 0.0 g
Cholesterol . . . . 0 mg
Sodium . . . . 45 mg
Total Carbohydrate . . . 8 g
  Dietary Fiber . . . . 2 g
  Sugars . . . . 1 g
Protein . . . . 2 g

Heat the oil in a large nonstick skillet over medium heat. Cook the zucchini in the skillet for about 10 minutes or until just tender and lightly browned, stirring frequently. While the zucchini is cooking, stir together the remaining ingredients in a bowl. When the zucchini is done, pour the mixture over the zucchini to coat completely. Serve immediately.

Zucchini Carrot Muffins

Serves 8   Serving size: 1 muffin

3/4	**cup** rolled oats
2 1/2	**cups** whole-wheat flour
2/3	**cup** nonfat milk
1/2	**cup** wheat germ, toasted
1	**Tbsp** baking powder
3/4	**cup** Splenda
1	**Tbsp** ground cinnamon

2	**tsp** ground nutmeg
3	**Tbsp** Smart Balance Omega oil
3	egg whites, beaten
1	**cup** carrots, finely shredded
1/2	**cup** zucchini, stemmed and grated

Preheat oven to 350°F. Combine all ingredients and mix well; pour into muffin liners in muffin pans. Bake for about 1 hour. Let cool for about 30 minutes before removing.

Exchanges/Choices

2 1/2 Carbohydrate
1 1/2 Fat

Basic Nutritional Values

Calories 260
Calories from Fat 65
Total Fat . . . . .7.0 g
Saturated Fat . . . . .0.9 g
Trans Fat . . . . .0.0 g
Cholesterol . . . . .0 mg
Sodium . . . . .180 mg
Total Carbohydrate . . .42 g
Dietary Fiber . . . . .7 g
Sugars . . . . .5 g
Protein . . . . .11 g

Chicken, Escarole, and Rice Soup

Serves 4   Serving size: 1/4 recipe

1/2	**Tbsp** Smart Balance Omega oil
1/2	large onion, chopped
1	clove garlic, minced
1/2	head escarole, trimmed and thinly sliced
2	**Tbsp** sodium-free chicken bouillon
2	**cups** water

6	**oz** no-added-salt canned diced tomatoes
3/4	**lb** boneless, skinless chicken breasts (trimmed of fat), cut into 1/2-inch pieces
1/4	**cup** long-grain white rice
	Freshly ground pepper, to taste

Heat oil in a large pot over a medium-high heat. Add onion and garlic; cook, stirring frequently, until softened and just beginning to brown, 2–3 minutes. Add escarole and cook, stirring occasionally, until wilted. Add bouillon, water, tomatoes, and rice; bring to a boil. Reduce heat to low, cover, and simmer until the rice is almost tender, 6–7 minutes. Add chicken and simmer until it is no longer pink in the center and the rice is tender, about 5 minutes. Season with pepper.

Exchanges/Choices

1 Starch
1 Vegetable
2 Lean Meat

Basic Nutritional Values

Calories 200
Calories from Fat 35
Total Fat . . . . .4.0 g
Saturated Fat . . . . .0.8 g
Trans Fat . . . . .0.0 g
Cholesterol . . . . .50 mg
Sodium . . . . .75 mg
Total Carbohydrate . . .20 g
Dietary Fiber . . . . .3 g
Sugars . . . . .4 g
Protein . . . . .20 g

Limed Chicken Breast

Serves 4 　　　Serving size: 1/4 recipe

1/4 **cup** light soy sauce

1/4 **cup** lime juice

1 **Tbsp** Worcestershire sauce

2 medium garlic clove, crushed

1/2 **tsp** dry mustard

1 **lb** boneless, skinless chicken breasts (trimmed of fat)

1/2 **tsp** pepper

Nonstick cooking spray

Mix soy sauce, lime juice, Worcestershire sauce, garlic, and mustard. Place chicken in a bowl and pour sauce over it. Cover and marinate for 30 minutes. Remove chicken from marinade and sprinkle with pepper. Spray a frying pan with nonstick cooking spray and heat over medium heat. Add chicken and cook for about 6 minutes on each side or until done.

Exchanges/Choices

3 Lean Meat

Basic Nutritional Values

Calories 135
　Calories from Fat 25
Total Fat. . . . . 3.0 g
　Saturated Fat . . . . 0.8 g
　Trans Fat. . . . . 0.0 g
Cholesterol. . . . . 65 mg
Sodium. . . . . 265 mg
Total Carbohydrate . . . 1 g
　Dietary Fiber . . . . 0 g
　Sugars . . . . 1 g
Protein. . . . . 25 g

Sautéed Zucchini and Red Peppers

Serves 4 　　　Serving size: 1/4 recipe

2 medium red bell peppers, seeded and cut into 1/2-inch strips

2 medium zucchini, cut into 1/2-inch strips

1 clove garlic, minced

2 **Tbsp** Smart Balance Omega oil

Black pepper, to taste

2 **Tbsp** minced parsley

In a large skillet over medium heat, sauté peppers, zucchini, and garlic in oil until zucchini is golden. Season with pepper and parsley. Serve hot.

Exchanges/Choices

2 Vegetable
1 Fat

Basic Nutritional Values

Calories 95
　Calories from Fat 65
Total Fat. . . . . 7.0 g
　Saturated Fat . . . . 0.6 g
　Trans Fat. . . . . 0.0 g
Cholesterol. . . . . 0 mg
Sodium. . . . . 15 mg
Total Carbohydrate . . . 8 g
　Dietary Fiber . . . . 3 g
　Sugars . . . . 5 g
Protein. . . . . 2 g

Fruit Salad Medley

Serves 4   Serving size: 1/4 recipe

- 1/2 **cup** strawberries, sliced
- 1/4 **cup** Splenda
- 1/2 **cup** blueberries (or canned light)
-   1 banana, sliced
-   1 **Tbsp** lemon juice
-   2 oranges, peeled and sliced crosswise
- 1/2 **cup** blackberries (or canned light)
- 1/2 **cup** pineapple (fresh, frozen, or canned light chunks)
- 1/2 **cup** orange juice
       Sprig mint leaves

In a medium bowl, stir together half of the strawberries and half of the Splenda; set aside. In a 2-quart serving bowl, add blueberries and layer bananas on top; sprinkle with lemon juice. Add a layer of strawberries with remaining Splenda, then oranges and blackberries. Arrange pineapple tidbits around outer edge. Layer remaining strawberry slices around pineapple tidbits. Pour orange juice over all the fruit. Cover and chill for 1 hour. Just before serving, top with mint leaves.

Exchanges/Choices

2 Fruit

Basic Nutritional Values

Calories 120
 Calories from Fat 5
Total Fat . . . . 0.5 g
 Saturated Fat . . . . 0.1 g
 Trans Fat . . . . 0.0 g
Cholesterol . . . . 0 mg
Sodium . . . . 0 mg
Total Carbohydrate . . . 29 g
 Dietary Fiber . . . . 5 g
 Sugars . . . . 21 g
Protein . . . . 2 g

Buttered Parsley Potatoes

Serves 4   Serving size: 1/4 recipe

-   2 **cups** quartered potato
-   2 **Tbsp** Smart Balance Light margarine, melted
- 1/4 **cup** chopped parsley

Peel the potatoes. Cut into quarters and boil in water until tender. Just before serving, toss with margarine and parsley.

Exchanges/Choices

1 Starch
1/2 Fat

Basic Nutritional Values

Calories 85
 Calories from Fat 20
Total Fat . . . . 2.5 g
 Saturated Fat . . . . 0.8 g
 Trans Fat . . . . 0.0 g
Cholesterol . . . . 0 mg
Sodium . . . . 50 mg
Total Carbohydrate . . . 14 g
 Dietary Fiber . . . . 1 g
 Sugars . . . . 1 g
Protein . . . . 1 g

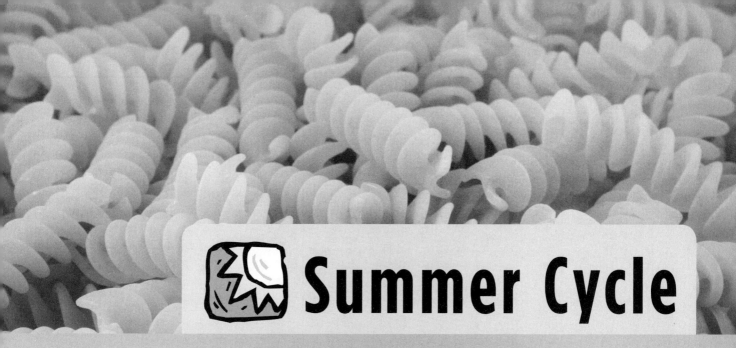

FEATURED RECIPES

Whole-Grain Pancakes or Waffles*

Oven-Fried Chicken

Glazed Carrots

Halibut with Wine Sauce

Sizzlin' Fruit Salad*

Beans and Greens

Roast Pork with Brandied Gravy

Scalloped Jack Potatoes

Whole-Wheat Cornmeal Muffin*

Pizza Muffins*

Tex-Mex Chicken

Carrots in Sherry Wine*

Blueberry Loaf Bread

Baked Haddock

Carrot Slaw*

Beef and Noodles

Pumpkin Spice Muffins*

Tuna Noodle Casserole

Burgundy Citrus Chicken

Seasoned Chilled Vegetables*

Yogurt Muffins

Egg Salad Sandwich

Rigatoni with Tomato-Zucchini Sauce

Marinated Vegetables*

Buttermilk Biscuits

Pasta Primavera with Ham

Key West Shrimp

Chilled Cauliflower Salad*

*Indicates that the recipe has been used previously.

1500 calorie MEAL PLAN SUMMER WEEK 2

	Sunday	Monday	Tuesday	Wednesday	Thursday	Friday	Saturday
Breakfast	**Whole-Grain Pancakes or Waffles*** 1/4 cup sugar-free maple syrup 1/2 cup unsweetened applesauce 1 cup nonfat milk 1/4 tsp margarine	1/2 English muffin 1/2 cup oatmeal 2 Tbsp dried blueberries 1 cup nonfat milk 1 oz Canadian bacon 2 tsp margarine	**Whole-Wheat Cornmeal Muffin*** 1/2 cup shredded wheat 1 small nectarine 1 cup nonfat milk 1 tsp margarine	**Blueberry Loaf Bread** 3/4 cup Multigrain Cheerios 1 medium banana 1 cup nonfat milk 2 tsp peanut butter	**Pumpkin Spice Muffins*** 3/4 cup unsweetened applesauce 1 cup nonfat milk 2 tsp margarine	**Yogurt Muffins** 1/2 Tbsp jam 1 cup cantaloupe cubes 1 cup nonfat milk 1/4 cup egg substitute 1 1/2 tsp margarine	**Buttermilk Biscuits** 1/2 cup bran cereal 3/4 cup pineapple 1 cup nonfat milk 1 oz lean turkey sausage 1 tsp margarine
Lunch	**Oven-Fried Chicken Glazed Carrots** 1 1/2 small dinner rolls 1 small orange	**Beans and Greens** 1 slice oatmeal bread 1 medium banana 1 oz reduced-fat cheese	**Pizza Muffins*** 1/2 cup peas and corn 1/2 cup mango 5 filberts or hazelnuts	**Baked Haddock Carrot Slaw*** 1 whole-wheat sandwich bun 1/2 cup deli-style coleslaw 1 peach	**Tuna Noodle Casserole** 1 small dinner roll 1 1/4 cup strawberries 1 cup salad greens 1 1/2 tsp margarine	**Egg Salad Sandwich** 1/2 cup succotash 1/2 cup mango 1 cup cooked asparagus 1 oz reduced-fat cheese 1/2 tsp margarine	**Pasta Primavera with Ham** 2 small plums 6 almonds
Snack A							
Snack B							
Dinner	**Halibut with Wine Sauce Sizzlin' Fruit Salad** (1/2 serving)* 1/3 cup brown rice 1 cup nonfat milk 1 cup steamed sugar snap peas	**Roast Pork with Brandied Gravy Scalloped Jack Potatoes** 1 slice whole-wheat bread 1 cup mixed melon cubes 1/2 cup nonfat milk 1/2 cup steamed Brussels sprouts 1 tsp margarine	**Tex-Mex Chicken Carrots in Sherry Wine*** 6 oz baked potato 12 sweet cherries 1 cup nonfat milk 1/2 tsp margarine	**Beef and Noodles** 1 slice whole-wheat bread 2 cup mixed salad greens 2 tsp olive oil and vinegar dressing	**Burgundy Citrus Chicken Seasoned Chilled Vegetables*** 2/3 cup brown rice 1/2 cup nonfat milk 1 cup cherry tomatoes 3 cashews	**Rigatoni with Tomato-Zucchini Sauce Marinated Vegetables*** 1/2 cup steamed broccoli 2 oz pork tenderloin 2 tsp margarine	**Key West Shrimp Chilled Cauliflower Salad*** 6 oz baked potato 1 cup nonfat milk 1/2 tsp margarine

*Indicates that the recipe has been used previously.

	Sunday	Monday	Tuesday	Wednesday	Thursday	Friday	Saturday
Breakfast	**Whole-Grain Pancakes or Waffles*** 1/4 cup sugar-free maple syrup 1/2 cup unsweetened applesauce 1 cup nonfat milk 1/4 tsp margarine	1/2 English muffin 1/2 cup oatmeal 2 Tbsp dried blueberries 1 cup nonfat milk 1 oz Canadian bacon 2 tsp margarine	**Whole-Wheat Cornmeal Muffin*** 1/2 cup shredded wheat 1 small nectarine 1 cup nonfat milk 1 oz lean turkey sausage 1 tsp margarine	**Blueberry Loaf Bread** 3/4 cup Multigrain Cheerios 1 medium banana 1 cup nonfat milk 1 Tbsp peanut butter	**Pumpkin Spice Muffins*** 3/4 cup unsweetened applesauce 1 cup nonfat milk 1/4 cup low-fat cottage cheese 2 tsp margarine	**Yogurt Muffins** 1/2 Tbsp jam 1 cup cantaloupe cubes 1 cup nonfat milk 1/4 cup egg substitute 1 1/2 tsp margarine	**Buttermilk Biscuits** 1/2 cup bran cereal 3/4 cup pineapple 1 cup nonfat milk 1 oz lean turkey sausage 1 tsp margarine
Lunch	**Oven-Fried Chicken Glazed Carrots** 1 1/2 small dinner rolls 1 small orange 3/4 tsp margarine	**Beans and Greens** 1 slice oatmeal bread 1 medium banana 1 oz reduced-fat cheese 1 tsp margarine	**Pizza Muffins*** 1/2 cup peas and corn 1/2 cup mango 10 filberts or hazelnuts	**Baked Haddock Carrot Slaw*** 1 whole-wheat sandwich bun 1/2 cup deli-style coleslaw 1 peach 1/2 Tbsp light salad dressing	**Tuna Noodle Casserole** 1 small dinner roll 1 1/4 cup strawberries 1 cup salad greens 1 1/2 tsp margarine	**Egg Salad Sandwich** 1/2 cup succotash 1/2 cup mango 1 cup cooked asparagus 1 oz reduced-fat cheese 1/2 tsp margarine	**Pasta Primavera with Ham** 2 small plums 1 oz reduced-fat cheese 12 almonds
Snack A	6 cashews 1 cup honeydew melon	2 Brazil nuts 2 medium figs	16 pistachios 1/2 cup fruit cocktail in water	3 macadamia nuts 12 cherries	1 1/2 tsp almond butter 1 small apple	16 pistachios 8 dried apricots	5 hazelnuts 3/4 cup blackberries
Snack B	6 oz fat-free yogurt	1 cup nonfat milk	1 cup nonfat milk	1 cup nonfat milk	6 oz fat-free yogurt	1 cup nonfat milk	1 cup nonfat milk
Dinner	**Halibut with Wine Sauce Sizzlin' Fruit Salad** (1/2 serving)* 1/3 cup brown rice 1 cup nonfat milk 1 cup steamed sugar snap peas	**Roast Pork with Brandied Gravy Scalloped Jack Potatoes** 1 slice whole-wheat bread 1 cup mixed melon cubes 1/2 cup nonfat milk 1/2 cup steamed Brussels sprouts 6 medium steamed oysters 1 tsp margarine	**Tex-Mex Chicken Carrots in Sherry Wine*** 6 oz baked potato 12 sweet cherries 1 cup nonfat milk 1/2 tsp margarine	**Beef and Noodles** 2 cup mixed salad greens 2 tsp olive oil and vinegar dressing	**Burgundy Citrus Chicken Seasoned Chilled Vegetables*** 2/3 cup brown rice 1/2 cup nonfat milk 1 cup cherry tomatoes 3 cashews	**Rigatoni with Tomato-Zucchini Sauce Marinated Vegetables*** 1/2 cup steamed broccoli 3 oz pork tenderloin 2 tsp margarine	**Key West Shrimp Chilled Cauliflower Salad*** 6 oz baked potato 1 cup nonfat milk 1/2 tsp margarine

*Indicates that the recipe has been used previously.

2000 calorie MEAL PLAN SUMMER WEEK 2

	Sunday	Monday	Tuesday	Wednesday	Thursday	Friday	Saturday
Breakfast	Whole-Grain Pancakes or Waffles* 1/4 cup sugar-free maple syrup 1/2 cup unsweetened applesauce 1 cup nonfat milk 1/4 tsp margarine	1/2 English muffin 1/2 cup oatmeal 2 Tbsp dried blueberries 1 cup nonfat milk 1 oz Canadian bacon 2 tsp margarine	Whole-Wheat Cornmeal Muffin* 1/2 cup shredded wheat 1 small nectarine 1 cup nonfat milk 1 oz lean turkey sausage 1 tsp margarine	Blueberry Loaf Bread 3/4 cup Multigrain Cheerios 1 medium banana 1 cup nonfat milk 1 Tbsp peanut butter	Pumpkin Spice Muffins* 3/4 cup unsweetened applesauce 1 cup nonfat milk 1/4 cup low-fat cottage cheese 2 tsp margarine	Yogurt Muffins 1/2 Tbsp jam 1 cup cantaloupe cubes 1 cup nonfat milk 1/4 cup egg substitute 1 1/2 tsp margarine	Buttermilk Biscuits 1/2 cup bran cereal 3/4 cup pineapple 1 cup nonfat milk 1 oz lean turkey sausage 1 tsp margarine
Lunch	Oven-Fried Chicken Glazed Carrots 1 1/2 small dinner rolls 1 medium orange 3/4 tsp margarine	Beans and Greens 1 slice oatmeal bread 1 large banana 1/2 cup steamed corn 1 oz reduced-fat cheese 1 tsp margarine	Pizza Muffins* 1/2 cup peas and corn 1 cup mango 10 filberts or hazelnuts	Baked Haddock Carrot Slaw* 1 whole-wheat sandwich bun 1/2 cup deli-style coleslaw 1 peach 1/2 Tbsp light salad dressing	Tuna Noodle Casserole 1 small dinner roll 1 1/4 cup strawberries 1 kiwi fruit 1 cup salad greens 1 1/2 tsp margarine	Egg Salad Sandwich 1/2 cup succotash 1 cup mango 2 cups cooked asparagus 1 oz reduced-fat cheese 1/2 tsp margarine	Pasta Primavera with Ham 2 small plums 1/2 cup unsweetened pears 1 oz reduced-fat cheese 12 almonds
Snack A	1 cup mixed vegetable sticks 1 Tbsp light salad dressing 1 cup honeydew melon	1 cup small tomatoes 2 Brazil nuts 2 medium figs	1 cup mixed raw vegetables 16 pistachios 1/2 cup fruit cocktail in water	3 macadamia nuts 12 cherries	1 cup raw celery sticks 1 1/2 tsp almond butter 1 small apple	1 cup raw vegetable sticks 16 pistachios 8 dried apricots	1 cup carrot sticks 5 hazelnuts 3/4 cup blackberries
Snack B	8 animal crackers 6 cashews 6 oz fat-free yogurt	1 cup oven-baked French fries 1 Tbsp pumpkin seeds 1 cup nonfat milk	1/2 cup tabbouleh 4 pecans 1 cup nonfat milk	1 slice raisin bread 1 tsp margarine 1 cup nonfat milk	5 oz corn on the cob 1 tsp margarine 6 oz fat-free yogurt	1/4 cup low-fat granola 2 Brazil nuts 1 cup nonfat milk	2 oz oven-baked French fries 6 cashews 1 cup nonfat milk
Dinner	Halibut with Wine Sauce Sizzlin' Fruit Salad (1/2 serving)* 1/3 cup brown rice 1 cup nonfat milk 1 cup steamed sugar snap peas	Roast Pork with Brandied Gravy Scalloped Jack Potatoes 1 slice whole-wheat bread 1 cup mixed melon cubes 1/2 cup nonfat milk 1/2 cup steamed Brussels sprouts 6 medium steamed oysters 1 tsp margarine	Tex-Mex Chicken Carrots in Sherry Wine* 6 oz baked potato 12 sweet cherries 1 cup nonfat milk 1/2 tsp margarine	Beef and Noodles 2 cup mixed salad greens 2 tsp olive oil and vinegar dressing	Burgundy Citrus Chicken Seasoned Chilled Vegetables* 2/3 cup brown rice 1/2 cup nonfat milk 1 cup cherry tomatoes 3 cashews	Rigatoni with Tomato-Zucchini Sauce Marinated Vegetables* 1/2 cup steamed broccoli 3 oz pork tenderloin 2 tsp margarine	Key West Shrimp Chilled Cauliflower Salad* 6 oz baked potato 1 cup nonfat milk 1/2 tsp margarine

*Indicates that the recipe has been used previously.

2200 calorie MEAL PLAN

	Sunday	Monday	Tuesday	Wednesday	Thursday	Friday	Saturday
Breakfast	**Whole-Grain Pancakes or Waffles*** 1/4 cup sugar-free maple syrup 1/2 cup unsweetened applesauce 1 cup nonfat milk 1 oz lean ham 1/4 tsp margarine	1/2 English muffin 1/2 cup oatmeal 2 Tbsp dried blueberries 1 cup nonfat milk 2 oz Canadian bacon 2 tsp margarine	**Whole-Wheat Cornmeal Muffin*** 1/2 cup shredded wheat 1 small nectarine 1 cup nonfat milk 2 oz lean turkey sausage 1 tsp margarine	**Blueberry Loaf Bread** 3/4 cup Multigrain Cheerios 1 medium banana 1/4 cup egg substitute, scrambled 1 cup nonfat milk 1 Tbsp peanut butter	**Pumpkin Spice Muffins*** 3/4 cup unsweetened applesauce 1 cup nonfat milk 1/2 low-fat cottage cheese 2 tsp margarine	**Yogurt Muffins** 1/2 Tbsp jam 1 cup cantaloupe cubes 1 cup nonfat milk 1/2 cup egg substitute 1 1/2 tsp margarine	**Buttermilk Biscuits** 1/2 cup bran cereal 3/4 cup pineapple 1 cup nonfat milk 2 oz lean turkey sausage 1 tsp margarine
Lunch	**Oven-Fried Chicken Glazed Carrots** 1 1/2 small dinner rolls 1 medium orange 3/4 tsp margarine	**Beans and Greens** 1 slice oatmeal bread 1 large banana 1/2 cup steamed corn 1 oz reduced-fat cheese 1 tsp margarine	**Pizza Muffins*** 1/2 cup peas and corn 1 cup mango 10 filberts or hazelnuts	**Baked Haddock Carrot Slaw*** 1 whole-wheat sandwich bun 1/2 cup deli-style coleslaw 1 peach 1/2 Tbsp light salad dressing	**Tuna Noodle Casserole** 1 small dinner roll 1 1/4 cup strawberries 1 kiwi fruit 2 cups salad greens 1 1/2 tsp margarine	**Egg Salad Sandwich** 1/2 cup succotash 1 cup mango 2 cups cooked asparagus 1 oz reduced-fat cheese 1/2 tsp margarine	**Pasta Primavera with Ham** 2 small plums 1/2 cup unsweetened pears 1 oz reduced-fat cheese 12 almonds
Snack A	1 cup mixed vegetable sticks 1 Tbsp light salad dressing 1 cup honeydew melon	1 cup small tomatoes 2 Brazil nuts 2 medium figs	1 cup mixed raw vegetables 16 pistachios 1/2 cup fruit cocktail in water	3 macadamia nuts 12 cherries	1 cup raw celery sticks 1 1/2 tsp almond butter 1 small apple	1 cup raw vegetable sticks 16 pistachios 8 dried apricots	1 cup carrot sticks 5 hazelnuts 3/4 cup blackberries
Snack B	8 animal crackers 6 cashews 6 oz fat-free yogurt	1 cup oven-baked French fries 1 Tbsp pumpkin seeds 1 cup nonfat milk	1/2 cup tabbouleh on a lettuce leaf 4 pecans 1 cup nonfat milk	1 slice raisin bread 1 tsp margarine 1 cup nonfat milk	5 oz corn on the cob 1 tsp margarine 6 oz fat-free yogurt	1/4 cup low-fat granola 2 Brazil nuts 1 cup nonfat milk	2 oz oven-baked French fries 6 cashews 1 cup nonfat milk
Dinner	**Halibut with Wine Sauce Sizzlin' Fruit Salad** (1/2 serving)* 2/3 cup brown rice 1 cup nonfat milk 1 cup steamed sugar snap peas	**Roast Pork with Brandied Gravy Scalloped Jack Potatoes** 1 slice whole-wheat bread 1/3 cup baked beans 1 cup mixed melon cubes 1/2 cup nonfat milk 1/2 cup steamed Brussels sprouts 1 tsp margarine	**Tex-Mex Chicken Carrots in Sherry Wine*** 6 oz baked potato 1 small dinner roll 12 sweet cherries 1 cup nonfat milk 1/2 tsp margarine	**Beef and Noodles** 1 slice whole-wheat bread 2 cup mixed salad greens 2 tsp olive oil and vinegar dressing	**Burgundy Citrus Chicken Seasoned Chilled Vegetables*** 2/3 cup brown rice 1/2 cup nonfat milk 1 cup cherry tomatoes 3 cashews	**Rigatoni with Tomato-Zucchini Sauce Marinated Vegetables*** 1/2 cup steamed broccoli 3 oz pork tenderloin 2 tsp margarine	**Key West Shrimp Chilled Cauliflower Salad*** 6 oz baked potato 1/2 cup green peas 1 cup nonfat milk 1/2 tsp margarine

*Indicates that the recipe has been used previously.

SHOPPING LIST SUMMER WEEK 2

VEGETABLES

____ asparagus
____ bell peppers, green
____ bell peppers, yellow
____ broccoli
____ Brussels sprouts
____ carrots
____ carrots, baby
____ cauliflower
____ celery
____ corn
____ cucumber
____ garlic
____ lettuce
____ mushrooms
____ onions, yellow or white
____ onions, green
____ onions, purple or red
____ peas
____ potatoes
____ sugar snap peas
____ tomatoes
____ tomatoes, cherry
____ tomatoes, plum,
       no-added-salt can
____ zucchini

MEATS

____ bacon, Canadian
____ chicken breasts, boneless,
       skinless
____ chicken, fryer
____ fish fillets (haddock, perch,
       or whiting)
____ halibut steaks
____ ham, lean
____ oysters, steamed
____ pork tenderloin, boneless
____ shrimp, peeled
       and deveined
____ stew beef or sirloin cubes
____ tuna, packed in water
____ turkey sausage, lean

FRUITS

____ bananas
____ blueberries
____ blueberries, dried
____ cantaloupe
____ cherries
____ kiwi fruit
____ mango
____ nectarines
____ oranges
____ peaches
____ pears
____ pineapple, crushed
       or cubed
____ plums
____ raisins
____ strawberries

DAIRY

____ buttermilk, fat-free
____ canola mayonnaise
____ egg substitute
____ egg whites
____ milk, nonfat
____ Smart Balance Light
       margarine
____ sour cream, fat-free
____ yogurt, fat-free, vanilla

CHEESE

____ cheese, any kind,
       reduced-fat
____ Colby and Monterey Jack,
       reduced-fat, shredded
____ cottage cheese, low-fat
____ mozzarella, fat-free
____ mozzarella, reduced-fat
____ Parmesan, reduced-fat

BREAD, GRAINS, & PASTA

____ bread, oatmeal
____ bread, whole-wheat,
       whole-grain
____ dinner rolls, small, wheat
____ English muffins, multigrain
____ noodles, whole-wheat,
       wide
____ rice, brown
____ rigatoni pasta
____ sandwich buns,
       whole-wheat

BEANS

____ cannellini,
     no-added-salt can
____ kidney, no-added-salt can

NUTS

____ almonds
____ cashews
____ hazelnuts (or filberts)

CONDIMENTS

____ mustard
____ mustard, Dijon
____ mustard, prepared
____ sweet pickle relish

SPICES & HERBS

____ basil
____ black pepper
____ caraway seeds
____ cayenne pepper
____ chili powder
____ cinnamon
____ cumin seeds
____ dill seeds
____ garlic powder
____ ginger, ground
____ nutmeg
____ onion powder
____ oregano
____ paprika
____ parsley
____ rosemary
____ thyme

OTHER

____ applesauce, unsweetened
____ brandy
____ bread crumbs
____ cereal, bran
____ cereal, Multigrain Cheerios
____ cereal, shredded wheat
____ coleslaw, deli-style
____ honey
____ jam, sugar-free
____ maple syrup, sugar-free
____ olives, black, pitted
____ orange marmalade,
     sugar-free
____ peanut butter
____ pumpkin, canned
____ salad dressing, light, Italian
____ spaghetti sauce, light,
     no-salt-added
____ succotash, frozen or fresh

STAPLES

____ baking powder
____ baking soda
____ bouillon, beef, sodium-free
____ bouillon, chicken,
     sodium-free
____ cornmeal, yellow
____ cornstarch
____ flour, all-purpose
____ flour, whole-wheat
____ juice, lemon
____ juice, lime
____ juice, orange, frozen
     concentrate
____ nonstick cooking spray
____ oats, old-fashioned
____ olive oil
____ sherry, dry cooking
____ Smart Balance Omega oil
____ Splenda
____ Splenda Brown
     Sugar Blend
____ vanilla extract
____ vinegar, white
____ vinegar, white wine
____ wine, dry white
____ wine, red

SUNDAY

Whole-Wheat Pancakes or Waffles

Serves 4   Serving size: 2 pancakes or waffles

1/2 **cup** rolled oats

1/2 **cup** whole-wheat flour, sifted

2 **tsp** baking powder

2 **Tbsp** Splenda

1/2 **cup** egg substitute, beaten well

3/4 **cup** nonfat milk

2 **Tbsp** Smart Balance Omega oil

Nonstick cooking spray

Stir together dry ingredients. Combine egg substitute, milk, and oil; stir into flour mixture. Cook on a griddle lightly coated with nonstick spray until golden brown, then turn. Can also be made in a waffle iron.

Exchanges/Choices

1 1/2 Starch
1 1/2 Fat

Basic Nutritional Values

Calories 185
  Calories from Fat 70
Total Fat. . . . . 8.0 g
  Saturated Fat . . . . 0.7 g
  Trans Fat. . . . . 0.0 g
Cholesterol . . . . 0 mg
Sodium. . . . . 265 mg
Total Carbohydrate . . . 22 g
  Dietary Fiber. . . . . 3 g
  Sugars . . . . 3 g
Protein . . . . 8 g

Oven-Fried Chicken

Serves 4   Serving size: 1/4 recipe

3 **lb** frying chicken, skin removed, trimmed of fat, and cut into parts

1/2 **cup** whole-wheat flour

1 **tsp** paprika

1/8 **tsp** black pepper

Nonstick cooking spray

2 **Tbsp** Smart Balance Omega oil

Wash chicken pieces and pat dry. Combine flour, paprika, and pepper in paper bag. Shake 2–3 pieces at a time in flour mixture. Spray a shallow pan with nonstick cooking spray. Arrange chicken pieces in pan in a single layer. Pour oil over chicken. Bake, uncovered, at 350°F for 60 minutes or until chicken is brown and tender.

Exchanges/Choices

1 Starch
4 Lean Meat
1 1/2 Fat

Basic Nutritional Values

Calories 320
  Calories from Fat 135
Total Fat. . . . . 15.0 g
  Saturated Fat . . . . 2.8 g
  Trans Fat. . . . . 0.0 g
Cholesterol . . . . 95 mg
Sodium. . . . . 95 mg
Total Carbohydrate . . . 11 g
  Dietary Fiber. . . . . 2 g
  Sugars . . . . 0 g
Protein . . . . 34 g

Glazed Carrots

Serves 4   Serving size: 1/4 recipe

- **1 lb** carrots, sliced or diced
- **2 Tbsp** Smart Balance Light Spread
- **1/4 cup** Splenda Brown Sugar Blend

Cook carrots in boiling water until nearly soft. In a large skillet melt margarine and add Splenda Brown Sugar Blend. Stir mixture until smooth, taking care not to burn. Add carrots and simmer over low heat. If it starts to burn, add a little water. Serve hot.

Exchanges/Choices

1 Carbohydrate
2 Vegetable
1/2 Fat

Basic Nutritional Values

Calories	115
Calories from Fat	20
Total Fat	2.5 g
Saturated Fat	0.8 g
Trans Fat	0.0 g
Cholesterol	0 mg
Sodium	115 mg
Total Carbohydrate	22 g
Dietary Fiber	3 g
Sugars	17 g
Protein	1 g

Halibut with Wine Sauce

Serves 4   Serving size: 1/4 recipe

- **1 cup** dry white wine
- **1 lb** halibut steaks
- **1/4 cup** dry bread crumbs
- **1/2 cup** fat-free sour cream
- **1/2 cup** canola mayonnaise
- **1/4 cup** minced green onions
- Paprika, to taste

Pour wine over halibut. Marinate in refrigerator at least 1 hour. Dip both sides of halibut in bread crumbs. Place halibut in a shallow baking dish. Combine sour cream, mayonnaise, and green onions; spread over halibut. Sprinkle with paprika. Bake at 450°F for 10 minutes per inch of thickness (measured at the thickest part of the steaks) or until fish flakes when tested with a fork.

Exchanges/Choices

1/2 Starch
4 Lean Meat
1 Fat

Basic Nutritional Values

Calories	270
Calories from Fat	110
Total Fat	12.0 g
Saturated Fat	0.5 g
Trans Fat	0.0 g
Cholesterol	40 mg
Sodium	310 mg
Total Carbohydrate	7 g
Dietary Fiber	0 g
Sugars	3 g
Protein	27 g

Sizzlin' Fruit Salad

Serves 4   Serving size: 1/4 recipe

1/2 **cup** sliced pears (can use fresh, frozen, or canned light, drained)

1/2 **cup** cherries (or canned light, drained)

1/2 **cup** cubed pineapple (or canned light, drained)

2 medium oranges, peeled and cut into cubes

1 **cup** water

1/2 **cup** Splenda

2 **Tbsp** Smart Balance margarine

1 **Tbsp** cornstarch

1 **Tbsp** lemon juice

1/4 **cup** dry cooking sherry

1/2 **cup** raisins

Exchanges/Choices

3 Fruit
1 Fat

Basic Nutritional Values

Calories 205
 Calories from Fat 45
Total Fat . . . . 5.0 g
 Saturated Fat . . . . 1.3 g
 Trans Fat . . . . 0.0 g
Cholesterol . . . . 0 mg
Sodium . . . . 55 mg
Total Carbohydrate . . . 42 g
 Dietary Fiber . . . . 4 g
 Sugars . . . . 34 g
Protein . . . . 2 g

1. Combine pears, cherries, and pineapple in an ovenproof glass bowl.

2. Combine orange cubes and water in a saucepan. Heat to boiling and simmer 5–10 minutes or until oranges are tender. Strain; add to pears, cherries, and pineapple. Sprinkle the Splenda on top.

3. Melt the margarine and combine with cornstarch in a saucepan. Add lemon juice, sherry, and raisins; cook, stirring consistently, until thickened. Pour over fruit and bake at 350°F for 30–45 minutes. Cool slightly before serving.

Beans and Greens

Serves 4 Serving size: 1/4 recipe

- **2 cups** mixed salad greens
- **8 oz** no-added-salt kidney beans, drained and rinsed
- **8 oz** no-added-salt cannellini beans, drained and rinsed
- **1** medium purple onion, thinly sliced
- **2 Tbsp** Smart Balance Omega oil

Combine ingredients in a large serving bowl. Can be served slightly chilled.

Exchanges/Choices

1 1/2 Starch
1 Vegetable
1 Lean Meat
1 Fat

Basic Nutritional Values

Calories 225
  Calories from Fat 70
Total Fat . . . . 8.0 g
  Saturated Fat . . . . 0.6 g
  Trans Fat . . . . 0.0 g
Cholesterol . . . . 0 mg
Sodium . . . . 5 mg
Total Carbohydrate . . . 30 g
  Dietary Fiber . . . . 9 g
  Sugars . . . . 5 g
Protein . . . . 10 g

Roast Pork with Brandied Gravy

Serves 4   Serving size: 1/4 recipe

1 **Tbsp** Smart Balance Omega oil	1 **Tbsp** brandy
1/2 **tsp** dried thyme	1 **Tbsp** sodium-free chicken bouillon
1/2 **tsp** oregano	1/2 **cup** water
1/2 **tsp** caraway seeds	2 **tsp** Smart Balance margarine
1/4 **cup** minced onion	1 **Tbsp** whole-wheat flour
1 medium clove garlic, minced	1/2 **cup** chopped green onion
3/4 **lb** boneless pork tenderloin (trimmed of fat)	

Exchanges/Choices

1/2 Carbohydrate
2 Lean Meat
1 Fat

Basic Nutritional Values

Calories 160
  Calories from Fat 65
Total Fat . . . . .7.0 g
  Saturated Fat . . . . .1.4 g
  Trans Fat . . . . .0.0 g
Cholesterol . . . . .45 mg
Sodium . . . . .255 mg
Total Carbohydrate . . .5 g
  Dietary Fiber . . . . .1 g
  Sugars . . . . .2 g
Protein . . . . .17 g

1. In a small bowl, combine the oil, thyme, oregano, caraway seeds, onion, and garlic. Rub the mixture on the pork loin and place in a large roasting pan and cover. Chill overnight.

2. Roast the pork in the middle of a preheated 350°F oven for 50 minutes to 1 hour or until a meat thermometer registers 155°F. Remove from oven and transfer to a cutting board. Let the pork stand, covered loosely with foil, for 10 minutes. Drain away any fat.

3. While the pork stands, add brandy, bouillon, and water to the pan juices. Boil the mixture for 1 minute, scraping up the brown bits, and strain it through a sieve into a bowl.

4. In a heavy saucepan, combine the margarine and flour, cook the mixture over medium-low heat for 3 minutes; add the broth mixture. Bring the gravy to a boil, whisking constantly, and add the green onions; simmer for 1 minute. Cut pork into 1/2-inch-thick slices and serve topped with gravy.

Scalloped Jack Potatoes

Serves 4   Serving size: 1/4 recipe

2 large potatoes

1/2 cup nonfat milk

1 Tbsp whole-wheat flour

1 Tbsp sodium-free chicken bouillon

1/2 cup water

Pepper, to taste

1/4 cup chopped onion

2 Tbsp reduced-fat Parmesan cheese

1/4 cup reduced-fat shredded Colby and Monterey Jack cheese

Exchanges/Choices

1 1/2 Starch
1/2 Fat

Basic Nutritional Values

Calories 140
 Calories from Fat 20
Total Fat . . . . .2.0 g
 Saturated Fat . . . . .1.3 g
 Trans Fat . . . . .0.0 g
Cholesterol . . . . .10 mg
Sodium . . . . .140 mg
Total Carbohydrate . . .25 g
 Dietary Fiber . . . . .2 g
 Sugars . . . . .4 g
Protein . . . . .5 g

1. Preheat oven to 350°F. Wash potatoes and peel skins. Slice into 1/8-inch slices and place in an oven-proof dish.

2. In a medium saucepan, whisk together the milk and the flour. Whisk in the bouillon, water, pepper, and onion. Cook over medium-high heat for 5–6 minutes or until thickened, stirring occasionally. Add Parmesan cheese and remove from the heat.

3. Bake covered for about 15 minutes. Gently stir in the remaining cheese and bake 30–40 minutes more, uncovered, until the potatoes are tender and lightly browned.

Whole-Wheat Cornmeal Muffin

Serves 8   Serving size: 1 muffin

2/3 **cup** yellow cornmeal

2/3 **cup** whole-wheat flour

1 **Tbsp** Splenda

2 **tsp** baking powder

2/3 **cup** nonfat milk

1/4 **cup** egg substitute

2 **Tbsp** Smart Balance Omega oil

Preheat oven to 400°F. Place paper liners in muffin trays. Thoroughly mix dry ingredients. Combine milk, egg substitute, and oil; add to dry ingredients. Stir until dry ingredients are just moistened. Batter will be lumpy. Fill muffin tins 2/3 full. Bake until slightly browned, about 20 minutes.

Exchanges/Choices

1 Carbohydrate
1 Fat

Basic Nutritional Values

Calories	120
Calories from Fat	35
Total Fat	4.0 g
Saturated Fat	0.3 g
Trans Fat	0.0 g
Cholesterol	0 mg
Sodium	115 mg
Total Carbohydrate	18 g
Dietary Fiber	2 g
Sugars	1 g
Protein	4 g

Pizza Muffins

Serves 4   Serving size: 1 muffin

4 light multigrain English muffins

1 **cup** no-salt-added spaghetti sauce

4 **oz** fat-free shredded mozzarella cheese

4 **oz** reduced-fat shredded mozzarella cheese

1/4 **cup** sliced mushrooms

1 small onion, sliced into thin rings

4 green bell pepper rings

Exchanges/Choices

2 Starch
2 Vegetable
2 Lean Meat

Basic Nutritional Values

Calories	305
Calories from Fat	65
Total Fat	7.0 g
Saturated Fat	2.4 g
Trans Fat	0.0 g
Cholesterol	15 mg
Sodium	660 mg
Total Carbohydrate	42 g
Dietary Fiber	12 g
Sugars	8 g
Protein	25 g

1. Preheat the oven to 400°F.

2. Split the English muffins in half and put on a baking sheet, cut sides up. Spread spaghetti sauce over muffins. Top with 1 ounce of each of the cheeses. Top with mushrooms, onion rings, and pepper rings. Place pizzas in oven and bake for about 5 minutes or until cheese melts.

This recipe is high in sodium.

Tex-Mex Chicken

Serves 4   Serving size: 1/4 recipe

1/4 **cup** canola mayonnaise

1/4 **cup** lime juice

1 **tsp** chili powder

1/2 **tsp** cumin seed, ground

1/2 **tsp** garlic powder

1 **lb** boneless, skinless chicken breasts (trimmed of fat)

Preheat the broiler. Combine all ingredients, except chicken. Place chicken on the slotted rack of a broiler pan. Brush with half of the mayonnaise mixture. Broil 5–7 inches from heat for 8–10 minutes. Turn and brush with remaining mayonnaise mixture. Continue broiling 8–10 minutes or until tender.

Exchanges/Choices

3 Lean Meat
1 Fat

Basic Nutritional Values

Calories 180
  Calories from Fat 65
Total Fat . . . . 7.0 g
  Saturated Fat . . . . 0.8 g
  Trans Fat . . . . 0.0 g
Cholesterol . . . . 65 mg
Sodium . . . . 155 mg
Total Carbohydrate . . . 2 g
  Dietary Fiber . . . . 0 g
  Sugars . . . . 1 g
Protein . . . . 24 g

Carrots in Sherry Wine

Serves 4   Serving size: 1/4 recipe

2 **cups** baby carrots

2 **Tbsp** Smart Balance Light margarine

1/2 **cup** dry cooking sherry

Combine all ingredients and cook carrots over medium heat until tender.

Exchanges/Choices

2 Vegetable
1/2 Fat

Basic Nutritional Values

Calories 70
  Calories from Fat 20
Total Fat . . . . 2.5 g
  Saturated Fat . . . . 0.8 g
  Trans Fat . . . . 0.0 g
Cholesterol . . . . 0 mg
Sodium . . . . 85 mg
Total Carbohydrate . . . 8 g
  Dietary Fiber . . . . 2 g
  Sugars . . . . 4 g
Protein . . . . 1 g

Blueberry Loaf Bread

Serves 6   Serving size: 1/6 recipe

2/3 **cup** whole-wheat flour
1/2 **tsp** baking powder
1/4 **tsp** baking soda
1/4 **cup** Splenda
1/4 **cup** fat-free yogurt
2 **tsp** Smart Balance Omega oil

1/2 **tsp** vanilla extract
1 egg white, lightly beaten
1/2 **cup** blueberries
Nonstick cooking spray

Exchanges/Choices
1 Carbohydrate

Basic Nutritional Values
Calories 80
Calories from Fat 20
Total Fat . . . . 2.0 g
Saturated Fat . . . . 0.2 g
Trans Fat . . . . 0.0 g
Cholesterol . . . . 0 mg
Sodium . . . . 100 mg
Total Carbohydrate . . . 14 g
Dietary Fiber . . . . 2 g
Sugars . . . . 3 g
Protein . . . . 3 g

Combine flour, baking powder, baking soda, and Splenda in a medium bowl; make a well in center of mixture. Combine yogurt, oil, vanilla, and egg white; add to dry ingredients, stirring just until dry ingredients are moistened. Fold in blueberries. Spoon batter into a 6 × 3 × 2-inch loaf pan coated with nonstick cooking spray. Bake at 350°F for 35–40 minutes or until a wooden pick inserted in the center comes out clean. Remove from pan immediately and let cool on a wire rack.

Baked Haddock

Serves 4   Serving size: 1/4 recipe

1 **lb** fish fillets (such as haddock, perch, or whiting)
2 **Tbsp** lemon juice
1 **tsp** onion powder

1 **Tbsp** Smart Balance margarine, melted
Dash pepper
Dash paprika

Exchanges/Choices
3 Lean Meat

Basic Nutritional Values
Calories 120
Calories from Fat 25
Total Fat . . . . 3.0 g
Saturated Fat . . . . 0.8 g
Trans Fat . . . . 0.0 g
Cholesterol . . . . 65 mg
Sodium . . . . 100 mg
Total Carbohydrate . . . 1 g
Dietary Fiber . . . . 0 g
Sugars . . . . 0 g
Protein . . . . 21 g

Preheat oven to 350°F. Cut fish into serving-size pieces and place in a pan. Mix lemon juice, onion powder, and margarine and spread over fish. Bake uncovered for 20 minutes or until fish flakes with a fork. Season with pepper and paprika to taste.

Carrot Slaw

Serves 4   Serving size: 1/4 recipe

1/2 **cup** crushed pineapple
(or can of no-added-sugar
crushed pineapple)

1 **tsp** honey

1 **tsp** lemon juice

1/4 **tsp** nutmeg

1/2 **cup** fat-free sour cream

2 **cups** carrots, grated

Drain pineapple. In a medium bowl, mix honey, lemon juice, and nutmeg.
Blend in sour cream. Add carrots and pineapple. Serve chilled.

Exchanges/Choices

1/2 Carbohydrate
1 Vegetable

Basic Nutritional Values

Calories 65
 Calories from Fat 0
Total Fat . . . . 0.0 g
 Saturated Fat . . . . 0.1 g
 Trans Fat . . . . 0.0 g
Cholesterol . . . . 5 mg
Sodium . . . . 55 mg
Total Carbohydrate . . . 11 g
 Dietary Fiber . . . . 2 g
 Sugars . . . . 8 g
Protein . . . . 3 g

Beef and Noodles

Serves 4   Serving size: 1/4 recipe

1 **Tbsp** Smart Balance
margarine

2 **oz** mushrooms

1/4 **cup** onion

1 1/2 **lb** stew beef cubes or sirloin
cubes (trimmed of fat)

1 **Tbsp** sodium-free beef
bouillon

1 **cup** water

1 clove garlic, minced

2 **Tbsp** whole-wheat flour

2 **cups** cooked noodles

Melt margarine in a large skillet. Add mushrooms and onions; cook until
onions are tender and then remove from skillet. Add the meat to the skillet
and cook until done. In a bowl, combine the bouillon and water to form
a broth. Reserve 1/3 cup broth. Pour remaining broth over the meat; add
garlic. Cover and simmer 15 minutes. Blend the remaining broth with the
flour and stir into the meat mixture. Add cooked mushrooms and onions.
Heat to boiling, stirring constantly. Serve over hot noodles.

Exchanges/Choices

2 Starch
4 Lean Meat

Basic Nutritional Values

Calories 325
 Calories from Fat 90
Total Fat . . . . 10.0 g
 Saturated Fat . . . . 2.9 g
 Trans Fat . . . . 0.0 g
Cholesterol . . . . 110 mg
Sodium . . . . 85 mg
Total Carbohydrate . . . 26 g
 Dietary Fiber . . . . 1 g
 Sugars . . . . 2 g
Protein . . . . 31 g

Pumpkin Spice Muffins

Serves 8　　　Serving size: 2 muffins

1 **cup** whole-wheat flour	1 **cup** canned pumpkin
3 **tsp** baking powder	1/2 **cup** nonfat milk
2 **tsp** ground cinnamon	1/4 **cup** unsweetened
2 **tsp** ground nutmeg	applesauce
1/4 **cup** egg substitute	1/4 **cup** raisins or chopped nuts
2 **Tbsp** Splenda	

Preheat oven to 400°F. Line sixteen muffin-pan cups with paper liners or spray with nonstick cooking spray. In a large bowl, stir together the flour, baking powder, cinnamon, and nutmeg. In a medium bowl, beat egg substitute with a whisk. Add Splenda, pumpkin, milk, and applesauce; stir until well blended. Stir in raisins. Stir into flour mixture until just blended. Fill muffin-pan cups 2/3 full. Bake 20–25 minutes until a wooden toothpick inserted in the center comes out clean. Remove muffins from muffin pans. Serve warm or at room temperature.

Exchanges/Choices

1 1/2 Carbohydrate

Basic Nutritional Values

Calories 95
  Calories from Fat 5
Total Fat . . . . 0.5 g
  Saturated Fat . . . . 0.2 g
  Trans Fat . . . . 0.0 g
Cholesterol . . . . 0 mg
Sodium . . . . 160 mg
Total Carbohydrate . . . 20 g
  Dietary Fiber . . . . 3 g
  Sugars . . . . 6 g
Protein . . . . 4 g

Tuna Noodle Casserole

Serves 4　　　Serving size: 1/4 recipe

4 **oz** dry whole-wheat noodles, narrow or wide	1 **cup** low-fat cottage cheese
1 **(6-oz)** can tuna packed in water, drained	1/2 **cup** nonfat milk
	1/4 **cup** bread crumbs
4 **oz** mushrooms	1/4 **cup** reduced-fat Parmesan cheese

Cook noodles according to package directions. Drain. Mix the cooked noodles with the tuna, mushrooms, cottage cheese, milk, and any other seasoning you may desire in a large casserole. Sprinkle the bread crumbs and cheese over the top. Bake uncovered at 350°F until hot and bubbly, about 40 minutes. Let stand 5 minutes before serving.

Exchanges/Choices

2 Starch
2 Lean Meat
1/2 Fat

Basic Nutritional Values

Calories 280
  Calories from Fat 65
Total Fat . . . . 7.0 g
  Saturated Fat . . . . 2.2 g
  Trans Fat . . . . 0.0 g
Cholesterol . . . . 20 mg
Sodium . . . . 455 mg
Total Carbohydrate . . . 34 g
  Dietary Fiber . . . . 3 g
  Sugars . . . . 4 g
Protein . . . . 22 g

Burgundy Citrus Chicken

Serves 4   Serving size: 1/4 recipe

1 **Tbsp** Smart Balance margarine

1 **lb** boneless, skinless chicken breasts

1 **tsp** pepper

2 **Tbsp** Splenda

1/3 **cup** sugar-free orange marmalade

1 1/2 **Tbsp** cornstarch

1 **tsp** ginger

1/4 **cup** orange juice concentrate

1 **Tbsp** lemon juice

1/4 **cup** red wine

2/3 medium orange

Exchanges/Choices

1 1/2 Fruit
3 Lean Meat

Basic Nutritional Values

Calories 225
  Calories from Fat 45
Total Fat. . . . . .5.0 g
  Saturated Fat . . . . .1.4 g
  Trans Fat. . . . . .0.0 g
Cholesterol. . . . . .65 mg
Sodium. . . . . .80 mg
Total Carbohydrate . . .21 g
  Dietary Fiber. . . . . .1 g
  Sugars . . . . .13 g
Protein . . . . .25 g

In large skillet, melt margarine and then brown the chicken. Sprinkle with pepper. In a small bowl, combine remaining ingredients, except wine and orange. Pour over chicken. Cover and simmer 25–35 minutes or until tender, stirring occasionally. Slice orange and add to the skillet; add wine. Continue simmering 10 minutes.

Seasoned Chilled Vegetables

Serves 4   Serving size: 1/4 recipe

1/2 **cup** carrots, thinly sliced

1/2 **cup** cauliflower florets

1/2 **cup** zucchini, quartered and thickly sliced

1 **Tbsp** sodium-free chicken bouillon

1/2 **cup** water

1/4 **cup** sliced celery

1/4 **cup** white vinegar

2 **Tbsp** red onions, coarsely chopped

2 **Tbsp** Smart Balance Omega oil

1 **tsp** Splenda

1 **tsp** prepared mustard

1/2 **tsp** dill seeds

1/2 **tsp** dried rosemary, crushed

1/2 **tsp** dried thyme, crushed

1/2 **tsp** black pepper

Exchanges/Choices

1 Vegetable
1 1/2 Fat

Basic Nutritional Values

Calories 85
  Calories from Fat 65
Total Fat. . . . . .7.0 g
  Saturated Fat . . . . .0.5 g
  Trans Fat. . . . . .0.0 g
Cholesterol. . . . . .0 mg
Sodium. . . . . .40 mg
Total Carbohydrate . . .6 g
  Dietary Fiber. . . . . .1 g
  Sugars . . . . .3 g
Protein . . . . .1 g

Place all ingredients in a 3-quart saucepan. Bring to a boil; reduce heat to low, cover, and simmer for 10 minutes or until vegetables are crisp-tender. Pour into a bowl and chill for 2 hours or until cold. Serve.

Yogurt Muffins

Serves 4   Serving size: 1 muffin

2/3 **cup** all-purpose flour
1/2 **tsp** baking powder
1/4 **tsp** baking soda
2 **Tbsp** Splenda
6 **Tbsp** vanilla fat-free yogurt

2 **Tbsp** Smart Balance Omega oil
1/2 **tsp** vanilla extract
2 egg whites
Nonstick cooking spray

Combine the flour, baking powder, baking soda, and Splenda in a medium bowl; make a well in center of mixture. Combine yogurt, oil, vanilla, and egg whites; add to dry ingredients, stirring just until dry ingredients are moistened. Spoon batter evenly into 4 muffin pan cups coated with cooking spray. Bake at 400°F for 30–36 minutes or until golden. Remove from pan immediately.

Exchanges/Choices

1 1/2 Starch
1 Fat

Basic Nutritional Values

Calories 165
 Calories from Fat 65
Total Fat . . . . 7.0 g
 Saturated Fat . . . . 0.5 g
 Trans Fat . . . . 0.0 g
Cholesterol . . . . 0 mg
Sodium . . . . 165 mg
Total Carbohydrate . . . 20 g
 Dietary Fiber . . . . 1 g
 Sugars . . . . 3 g
Protein . . . . 5 g

Egg Salad Sandwich

Serves 4   Serving size: 1 sandwich

1 **cup** egg substitute
1/4 **cup** canola mayonnaise
1/8 **cup** green onion, minced
1 **Tbsp** mustard

1 **Tbsp** vinegar
1/4 **tsp** pepper
1/2 **cups** shredded carrots
8 slices whole-grain bread

Cook egg substitute according to package directions. In a medium bowl, combine all ingredients except bread and mix until well blended. Refrigerate 2 hours and then serve between slices of bread.

Exchanges/Choices

2 Starch
1 Lean Meat
1/2 Fat

Basic Nutritional Values

Calories 220
 Calories from Fat 65
Total Fat . . . . 7.0 g
 Saturated Fat . . . . 0.4 g
 Trans Fat . . . . 0.0 g
Cholesterol . . . . 0 mg
Sodium . . . . 520 mg
Total Carbohydrate . . . 27 g
 Dietary Fiber . . . . 4 g
 Sugars . . . . 5 g
Protein . . . . 14 g

Rigatoni with Tomato-Zucchini Sauce

Serves 4   Serving size: 1/4 recipe

- 2 **Tbsp** sodium-free chicken bouillon
- 2 **cups** water
- 1/2 **cup** finely chopped onion
- 3 cloves garlic, minced
- 1 zucchini, halved lengthwise and cut into 1/4-inch slices

- 2 **lb** canned no-added-salt plum tomatoes, juice reserved
- 1/8 **tsp** cayenne pepper
- 1/2 **tsp** dried basil
- 1/4 **tsp** ground black pepper
- 8 **oz** rigatoni, cooked

Heat bouillon and 1/4 cup water in a large skillet over medium heat. Add onion, garlic, and zucchini. Sauté until onion is lightly golden, about 6 minutes. Remove zucchini, leaving onion-garlic mixture in skillet. Add remaining water and heat in skillet. Add tomatoes and cayenne pepper. Cook over medium heat for 20 minutes. Stir in zucchini, basil, and black pepper and cook for 5 more minutes. Toss cooked pasta with sauce.

Exchanges/Choices

3 Starch
2 Vegetable

Basic Nutritional Values

Calories	290
Calories from Fat	15
Total Fat	1.5 g
Saturated Fat	0.2 g
Trans Fat	0.0 g
Cholesterol	0 mg
Sodium	100 mg
Total Carbohydrate	61 g
Dietary Fiber	7 g
Sugars	12 g
Protein	10 g

Marinated Vegetables

Serves 4   Serving size: 1/4 recipe

- 1/2 **cup** carrots, sliced
- 1/2 medium yellow bell pepper
- 1/2 **cup** light Italian dressing
- 1 **Tbsp** Dijon mustard

- 1/2 **cup** broccoli
- 1/2 cucumber, sliced
- 10 small cherry tomatoes
- 1 **Tbsp** parsley

Diagonally slice the carrots. Cut yellow pepper into strips. Combine dressing and mustard. Combine all other ingredients in a bowl, and pour the dressing and mustard mixture over all remaining ingredients; cover. Refrigerate 2 hours to marinate. Serve immediately.

Exchanges/Choices

2 Vegetable

Basic Nutritional Values

Calories	65
Calories from Fat	20
Total Fat	2.5 g
Saturated Fat	0.3 g
Trans Fat	0.0 g
Cholesterol	0 mg
Sodium	460 mg
Total Carbohydrate	11 g
Dietary Fiber	2 g
Sugars	7 g
Protein	2 g

Buttermilk Biscuits
Serves 6   Serving size: 1 biscuit

1 **cup** all-purpose flour	3 1/3 **Tbsp** Smart Balance margarine
1 **Tbsp** Splenda	1/2 **cup** fat-free buttermilk
1 1/2 **tsp** baking powder	
1/4 **tsp** baking soda	

Preheat oven to 450°F. In a medium bowl combine flour, Splenda, baking powder, and baking soda. With a pastry blender, cut in margarine until mixture resembles coarse crumbs. Stir in buttermilk. Place on a lightly floured surface; knead 3–4 times and roll or pat to a 1/2- to 3/4-inch thickness. Cut with a 2 1/2-inch biscuit cutter dipped in flour. Bake on an ungreased baking sheet for 12–15 minutes or until golden brown.

Exchanges/Choices
1 Starch
1 Fat

Basic Nutritional Values
Calories 135
  Calories from Fat 45
Total Fat. . . . . 5.0 g
  Saturated Fat . . . . 1.4 g
  Trans Fat. . . . . 0.0 g
Cholesterol. . . . . 0 mg
Sodium. . . . . 215 mg
Total Carbohydrate . . . 19 g
  Dietary Fiber. . . . . 1 g
  Sugars . . . . 3 g
Protein . . . . 3 g

Pasta Primavera with Ham
Serves 4   Serving size: 1/4 recipe

8 **oz** whole-wheat noodles, wide	2 medium zucchini, diced
16 **oz** light spaghetti sauce	1/2 **cup** sliced mushrooms
2 large carrots, diced	1/2 **lb** lean ham, trimmed of fat and diced

Cook noodles according to package directions; drain. In a separate pan, bring spaghetti sauce to a boil. Add carrots, zucchini, and mushrooms to sauce. Slowly cook for 30 minutes and then mix with the noodles. Add diced ham and serve.

This recipe is high in sodium.

Exchanges/Choices
3 Starch
2 Vegetable
1 Lean Meat

Basic Nutritional Values
Calories 330
  Calories from Fat 20
Total Fat. . . . . 2.5 g
  Saturated Fat . . . . 0.8 g
  Trans Fat. . . . . 0.0 g
Cholesterol. . . . . 25 mg
Sodium. . . . . 835 mg
Total Carbohydrate . . . 61 g
  Dietary Fiber. . . . . 10 g
  Sugars . . . . 15 g
Protein . . . . 21 g

Key West Shrimp

Serves 4   Serving size: 1/4 recipe

1 **Tbsp** Smart Balance Omega oil

2 medium cloves garlic, crushed

1/4 **tsp** pepper

1 **lb** large cooked shrimp, peeled and deveined

1 bunch green onions, whole

Juice of 1 lime

Exchanges/Choices

3 Lean Meat

Basic Nutritional Values

Calories 125
 Calories from Fat 40
Total Fat . . . . 4.5 g
 Saturated Fat . . . . 0.5 g
 Trans Fat . . . . 0.0 g
Cholesterol . . . . 160 mg
Sodium . . . . 190 mg
Total Carbohydrate . . . 3 g
 Dietary Fiber . . . . 1 g
 Sugars . . . . 1 g
Protein . . . . 18 g

Start fire in a grill, placing rack 6 inches above coals. In small bowl, stir together oil, garlic, and pepper; set aside. Arrange an equal amount of shrimp on four 12-inch skewers. When coals are white-hot, place shrimp skewers on grill rack. Brush with oil mixture and cook 1 1/2–2 minutes. Turn shrimp; add green onions to grill rack; brush both with oil mixture. Cook shrimp 1 1/2–2 minutes more, until just pink and cooked through. Cook green onions 2–3 minutes without turning, until slightly charred and tender. Chop green onions and sprinkle on top of grilled shrimp. Drizzle lime juice over shrimp and serve.

Chilled Cauliflower Salad

Serves 4   Serving size: 1/4 recipe

1 medium cauliflower head, broken into florets

2 medium tomatoes, cut into wedges

2 **Tbsp** Smart Balance Omega oil

3 **Tbsp** white wine vinegar

3 **Tbsp** black pitted olives, sliced

3 **Tbsp** sweet pickle relish

1/2 **tsp** Splenda

1 **tsp** paprika

1/2 **tsp** black pepper

4 lettuce leaves

Exchanges/Choices

3 Vegetable
1 Fat

Basic Nutritional Values

Calories 125
 Calories from Fat 65
Total Fat . . . . 7.0 g
 Saturated Fat . . . . 0.5 g
 Trans Fat . . . . 0.0 g
Cholesterol . . . . 0 mg
Sodium . . . . 160 mg
Total Carbohydrate . . . 16 g
 Dietary Fiber . . . . 5 g
 Sugars . . . . 9 g
Protein . . . . 4 g

1. In a covered saucepan, cook cauliflower in small amount of boiling water, 9–10 minutes or until crisp-tender. Drain. In large bowl, combine the cooked cauliflower and tomato wedges.

2. Combine the oil, vinegar, olives, relish, Splenda, paprika, and pepper. Mix well. Pour dressing over cauliflower and tomatoes. Cover and refrigerate 24 hours, stirring occasionally. To serve, lift vegetables from dressing with slotted spoon; place in a lettuce-lined bowl.

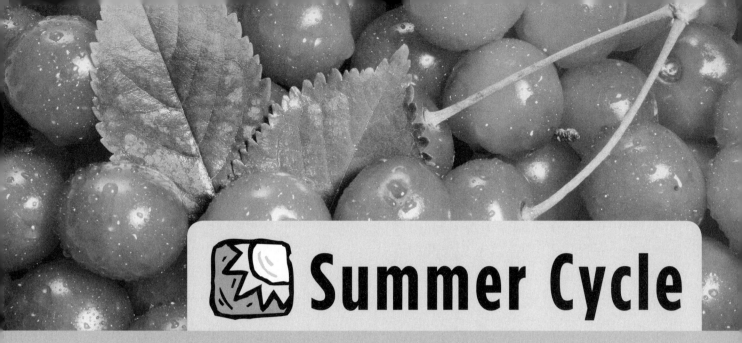

Summer Cycle

FEATURED RECIPES

All-Natural High-Fiber Peach Squares*
Honey-Mustard Lamb Chops
Low-Fat, Low-Sugar Carrot Cake*
Stuffed Cantaloupe Chicken
Stir-Fry Vegetables
Bran Muffins*
Open-Faced Chicken and Almond Sandwich*
Baked Lemon Flounder
Green Beans and Red Peppers*
Chocolate Dream Cake
Whole-Wheat Pancakes or Waffles*
Macaroni and Cheese
Chicken Cacciatore
Blueberry Loaf Bread*
Tuna-Stuffed Tomatoes
Kidney Bean Salad

Veal Scaloppini
Mexican Coleslaw*
Banana Bran Muffin*
Healthy Club Sandwich
Chicken Tetrazzini
Southwest Tomato Salad*
Fried Bananas*
Chicken Salad
Dilled Cucumber Salad*
Greek Halibut Fillet
Italian-Style Zucchini with Whole-Wheat Pasta*
Cherry Crisp Dessert*
Whole-Wheat Blueberry Muffins*
Sliced Steak Hoagie
Tex-Mex Turkey Burgers
Gram's Gingerbread*

*Indicates that the recipe has been used previously.

1500 calorie MEAL PLAN SUMMER WEEK 3

	Sunday	Monday	Tuesday	Wednesday	Thursday	Friday	Saturday
Breakfast	All-Natural High-Fiber Peach Squares (2 servings)* 17 small grapes 1 cup nonfat milk 1 oz lean turkey ham	Bran Muffins* 1/2 cup oatmeal 12 cherries 1 cup nonfat milk 1/4 egg substitute 1 Tbsp cashew butter	Whole-Wheat Pancakes or Waffles* 1/4 cup sugar-free maple syrup 1 1/4 cup strawberries 1 cup nonfat milk 1 oz lean beef sausage 1/2 tsp margarine	Blueberry Loaf Bread (2 servings)* 1 cup cantaloupe 1 cup nonfat milk	Banana Bran Muffin* 1/2 cup shredded wheat 1 cup nonfat milk 1/2 oz reduced-fat cheese 12 almonds	Fried Bananas* 1 slice whole-wheat bread 1 cup nonfat milk 1/4 cup low-fat cottage cheese 1/2 tsp margarine	Whole-Wheat Blueberry Muffins (2 muffins)* 1/2 cup oatmeal 2 small plums 1 cup nonfat milk 1 1/2 tsp margarine
Lunch	Honey-Mustard Lamb Chops Low-Fat, Low-Sugar Carrot Cake* 1 slice whole-wheat bread 1/2 cup mango 1/2 cup steamed Brussels sprouts 1 tsp margarine	Open-Faced Chicken and Almond Sandwich* 1 cup tomato soup 3/4 oz pretzels 3/4 cup blueberries 1 cup grape tomatoes 1/2 tsp light salad dressing	Macaroni and Cheese 1 slice whole-grain bread 1 kiwi fruit 1 cup steamed cabbage	Tuna-Stuffed Tomatoes Kidney Bean Salad 1 slice whole-wheat bread 1/2 cup fruit cocktail in water 1/4 cup low-fat cottage cheese	Healthy Club Sandwich 1 large corn on the cob 1 small apple	Chicken Salad Dilled Cucumber Salad* 1/2 whole-grain bagel 17 grapes 1 cup cherry tomatoes 1/2 Tbsp pumpkin seeds	Sliced Steak Hoagie 1/2 cup peas and corn 1 cup honeydew melon
Snack A							
Snack B							
Dinner	Stuffed Cantaloupe Chicken (1/2 serving) Stir-Fry Vegetables 1 slice multigrain bread 1/3 cup cooked brown rice 1 cup nonfat milk 1 tsp margarine	Baked Lemon Flounder Green Beans and Red Peppers* Chocolate Dream Cake 1 slice whole-grain bread 4 Brazil nuts	Chicken Cacciatore 1/3 cup pasta 1/2 large pear 1 cup nonfat milk 1 cup steamed peas and carrots 1/2 tsp margarine	Veal Scaloppini Mexican Coleslaw* 1/2 cup whole-wheat pasta 1/2 cup fruit cocktail in water 1 cup nonfat milk 1/2 cup steamed green beans	Chicken Tetrazzini (1/2 serving) Southwest Tomato Salad* 1 slice oatmeal bread 3/4 cup blueberries 1 cup nonfat milk 1 1/2 tsp margarine	Greek Halibut Fillet Italian-Style Zucchini with Whole-Wheat Pasta* Cherry Crisp Dessert* 5 peanuts	Tex-Mex Turkey Burgers Gram's Gingerbread* 1/2 cup nonfat milk 1 cup steamed broccoli 2 tsp margarine

*Indicates that the recipe has been used previously.

	Sunday	Monday	Tuesday	Wednesday	Thursday	Friday	Saturday
Breakfast	All-Natural High-Fiber Peach Squares (2 servings)* 17 small grapes 1 cup nonfat milk	Bran Muffins* 1/2 cup oatmeal 12 cherries 1 cup nonfat milk 1 Tbsp cashew butter	Whole-Wheat Pancakes or Waffles* 1/4 cup sugar-free maple syrup 1 1/4 cup strawberries 1 cup nonfat milk 1/2 tsp margarine	Blueberry Loaf Bread (2 servings)* 1 cup cantaloupe 1 cup nonfat milk 1 oz Canadian bacon 1 tsp margarine	Banana Bran Muffin* 1/2 cup shredded wheat 1 cup nonfat milk 1 1/2 oz reduced-fat cheese 12 almonds	Fried Bananas* 1 slice whole-wheat bread 1 cup nonfat milk 1/4 cup low-fat cottage cheese 1/2 tsp margarine	Whole-Wheat Blueberry Muffins (2 muffins)* 1/2 cup oatmeal 2 small plums 1 cup nonfat milk 1 1/2 tsp margarine
Lunch	Honey-Mustard Lamb Chops Low-Fat, Low-Sugar Carrot Cake* 1 slice whole-wheat bread 1/2 cup mango 1/2 cup steamed Brussels sprouts 2 tsp margarine	Open-Faced Chicken and Almond Sandwich* 1 cup tomato soup 3/4 oz pretzels 3/4 cup blueberries 1 cup grape tomatoes 1 1/2 tsp light salad dressing	Macaroni and Cheese 1 slice whole-grain bread 1 kiwi fruit 1 cup steamed cabbage 1 tsp margarine	Tuna-Stuffed Tomatoes Kidney Bean Salad 1 slice whole-wheat bread 1/2 cup fruit cocktail in water 1/4 cup low-fat cottage cheese	Healthy Club Sandwich 1 large corn on the cob 1 small apple 1 tsp margarine	Chicken Salad Dilled Cucumber Salad* 1/2 whole-grain bagel 17 grapes 1 cup cherry tomatoes 1 1/2 Tbsp pumpkin seeds	Sliced Steak Hoagie 1/2 cup peas and corn 1 cup honeydew melon 1 tsp margarine
Snack A	10 peanuts 1 medium banana	3 macadamia nuts 1 kiwi fruit	4 walnut halves 3 dates	3 macadamia nuts 4 dried apple rings	4 pecans 1 1/4 cup watermelon	16 pistachios 2 Tbsp raisins	5 hazelnuts 1 cup papaya
Snack B	6 oz fat-free yogurt	1 cup nonfat milk	1 cup nonfat milk	1 cup nonfat milk	1 cup nonfat milk	1 cup nonfat milk	1 cup nonfat milk
Dinner	Stuffed Cantaloupe Chicken Stir-Fry Vegetables 1 slice multigrain bread 1/3 cup cooked brown rice 1 cup nonfat milk 1/2 tsp margarine	Baked Lemon Flounder Green Beans and Red Peppers* Chocolate Dream Cake 1 slice whole-grain bread 4 Brazil nuts	Chicken Cacciatore 1/2 large pear 1 cup nonfat milk 1 cup steamed peas and carrots 2 tsp margarine	Veal Scaloppini Mexican Coleslaw* 1/2 cup whole-wheat pasta 1/2 cup fruit cocktail in water 1 cup nonfat milk 1/2 cup steamed green beans	Chicken Tetrazzini (1/2 serving) Southwest Tomato Salad* 1 slice oatmeal bread 3/4 cup blueberries 1 cup nonfat milk 1 1/2 tsp margarine	Greek Halibut Fillet Italian-Style Zucchini with Whole-Wheat Pasta* Cherry Crisp Dessert* 5 peanuts	Tex-Mex Turkey Burgers Gram's Gingerbread* 1/2 cup nonfat milk 1 cup steamed broccoli 2 tsp margarine

*Indicates that the recipe has been used previously.

2000 calorie MEAL PLAN SUMMER WEEK 3

	Sunday	Monday	Tuesday	Wednesday	Thursday	Friday	Saturday
Breakfast	All-Natural High-Fiber Peach Squares (2 servings)* 17 small grapes 1 cup nonfat milk	Bran Muffins* 1/2 cup oatmeal 12 cherries 1 cup nonfat milk 1 Tbsp cashew butter	Whole-Wheat Pancakes or Waffles* 1/4 cup sugar-free maple syrup 1 1/4 cup strawberries 1 cup nonfat milk 1/2 tsp margarine	Blueberry Loaf Bread (2 servings)* 1 cup cantaloupe 1 cup nonfat milk 1 oz Canadian bacon 1 tsp margarine	Banana Bran Muffin* 1/2 cup shredded wheat 1 cup nonfat milk 1 1/2 oz reduced-fat cheese 12 almonds	Fried Bananas* 1 slice whole-wheat bread 1 cup nonfat milk 1/4 cup low-fat cottage cheese 1/2 tsp margarine	Whole-Wheat Blueberry Muffins (2 muffins)* 1/2 cup oatmeal 2 small plums 1 cup nonfat milk 1 1/2 tsp margarine
Lunch	Honey-Mustard Lamb Chops Low-Fat, Low-Sugar Carrot Cake* 1 slice whole-wheat bread 1 cup mango 1 cup steamed Brussels sprouts 2 tsp margarine	Open-Faced Chicken and Almond Sandwich* 1 cup tomato soup 3/4 oz pretzels 3/4 cup blueberries 1 cup honeydew melon 2 cups grape tomatoes 1 1/2 tsp light salad dressing	Macaroni and Cheese 1 slice whole-grain bread 2 kiwi fruit 2 cups steamed cabbage 1 tsp margarine	Tuna-Stuffed Tomatoes Kidney Bean Salad 1 slice whole-wheat bread 1 cup fruit cocktail in water 1/4 cup low-fat cottage cheese	Healthy Club Sandwich 1 large corn on the cob 1 medium apple 1/2 cup artichoke hearts 1 tsp margarine	Chicken Salad Dilled Cucumber Salad* 1/2 whole-grain bagel 17 grapes 3/4 cup blackberries 1 cup cherry tomatoes 1 1/2 Tbsp pumpkin seeds	Sliced Steak Hoagie 1/2 cup peas and corn 1 cup honeydew melon 1 tsp margarine
Snack A	1 cup mixed vegetable sticks 10 peanuts 1 medium banana	1 cup raw carrots 3 macadamia nuts 1 kiwi fruit	1 cup raw vegetable sticks 4 walnut halves 3 dates	8 oz grape tomatoes 3 macadamia nuts 4 dried apple rings	1 cup cauliflower 4 pecans 1 1/4 cup watermelon	1 cup celery sticks 16 pistachios 2 Tbsp raisins	1 cup cucumber slices 5 hazelnuts 1 cup papaya
Snack B	3 ginger snaps 1 1/2 tsp cashew butter 6 oz fat-free yogurt	3/4 oz baked tortilla chips 2 Tbsp avocado 1 cup nonfat milk	3 cups popcorn 10 peanuts 1 cup nonfat milk	3/4 oz baked pita chips 2 Tbsp avocado 1 cup nonfat milk	1 slice raisin bread 1 tsp margarine 1 cup nonfat milk	1 4-inch waffle 1 1/2 tsp peanut butter 1 cup nonfat milk	3 ginger snaps 1 1/2 tsp cashew butter 1 cup nonfat milk
Dinner	Stuffed Cantaloupe Chicken Stir-Fry Vegetables 1 slice multigrain bread 1/3 cup cooked brown rice 1 cup nonfat milk 1/2 tsp margarine	Baked Lemon Flounder Green Beans and Red Peppers* Chocolate Dream Cake 1 slice whole-grain bread 4 Brazil nuts	Chicken Cacciatore 1/2 large pear 1 cup nonfat milk 1 cup steamed peas and carrots 2 tsp margarine	Veal Scaloppini Mexican Coleslaw* 1/2 cup whole-wheat pasta 1/2 cup fruit cocktail in water 1 cup nonfat milk 1/2 cup steamed green beans	Chicken Tetrazzini (1/2 serving) Southwest Tomato Salad* 1 slice oatmeal bread 3/4 cup blueberries 1 cup nonfat milk 1 1/2 tsp margarine	Greek Halibut Fillet Italian-Style Zucchini with Whole-Wheat Pasta* Cherry Crisp Dessert* 5 peanuts	Tex-Mex Turkey Burgers Gram's Gingerbread* 1/2 cup nonfat milk 1 cup steamed broccoli 2 tsp margarine

*Indicates that the recipe has been used previously.

	Sunday	Monday	Tuesday	Wednesday	Thursday	Friday	Saturday
Breakfast	All-Natural High-Fiber Peach Squares (2 servings)* 17 small grapes 1 cup nonfat milk 1 oz lean turkey ham	Bran Muffins* 1/2 cup oatmeal 12 cherries 1 cup nonfat milk 1 Tbsp cashew butter	Whole-Wheat Pancakes or Waffles* 1/4 cup sugar-free maple syrup 1 1/4 cup strawberries 1 cup nonfat milk 1 oz lean beef sausage 1/2 tsp margarine	Blueberry Loaf Bread (2 servings)* 1 cup cantaloupe 1 cup nonfat milk 2 oz Canadian bacon 1 tsp margarine	Banana Bran Muffin* 1/2 cup shredded wheat 1 cup nonfat milk 2 1/2 oz reduced-fat cheese 12 almonds	Fried Bananas* 1 slice whole-wheat bread 1 cup nonfat milk 1/2 cup low-fat cottage cheese 1/2 tsp margarine	Whole-Wheat Blueberry Muffins (2 muffins)* 1/2 cup oatmeal 2 small plums 1 cup nonfat milk 1 oz lean turkey sausage 1 1/2 tsp margarine
Lunch	Honey-Mustard Lamb Chops Low-Fat, Low-Sugar Carrot Cake* 1 slice whole-wheat bread 1 cup mango 1 cup steamed Brussels sprouts 2 tsp margarine	Open-Faced Chicken and Almond Sandwich* 1 cup tomato soup 3/4 oz pretzels 3/4 cup blueberries 1 cup honeydew melon 2 cups grape tomatoes 1 1/2 tsp light salad dressing	Macaroni and Cheese 1 slice whole-grain bread 2 kiwi fruit 2 cups steamed cabbage 1 tsp margarine	Tuna-Stuffed Tomatoes Kidney Bean Salad 1 slice whole-wheat bread 1 cup fruit cocktail in water 1/4 cup low-fat cottage cheese	Healthy Club Sandwich 1 large corn on the cob 1 medium apple 1/2 cup artichoke hearts 1 tsp margarine	Chicken Salad Dilled Cucumber Salad* 1/2 whole-grain bagel 17 grapes 3/4 cup blackberries 1 cup cherry tomatoes 1 1/2 Tbsp pumpkin seeds	Sliced Steak Hoagie 1/2 cup peas and corn 1 cup honeydew melon 1 tsp margarine
Snack A	1 cup mixed vegetable sticks 10 peanuts 1 medium banana	1 cup raw carrots 3 macadamia nuts 1 kiwi fruit	1 cup raw vegetable sticks 4 walnut halves 3 dates	8 oz grape tomatoes 3 macadamia nuts 4 dried apple rings	1 cup cauliflower 4 pecans 1 1/4 cup watermelon	1 cup celery sticks 16 pistachios 2 Tbsp raisins	1 cup cucumber slices 5 hazelnuts 1 cup papaya
Snack B	3 ginger snaps 1 1/2 tsp cashew butter 6 oz fat-free yogurt	3/4 oz baked tortilla chips 2 Tbsp avocado 1 cup nonfat milk	3 cups popcorn 10 peanuts 1 cup nonfat milk	3/4 oz baked pita chips 2 Tbsp avocado 1 cup nonfat milk	1 slice raisin bread 1 tsp margarine 1 cup nonfat milk	1 4-inch waffle 1 1/2 tsp peanut butter 1 cup nonfat milk	3 ginger snaps 1 1/2 tsp cashew butter 1 cup nonfat milk
Dinner	Stuffed Cantaloupe Chicken (1/2 serving) Stir-Fry Vegetables 1 slice multigrain bread 2/3 cup cooked brown rice 1 cup nonfat milk 1/2 tsp margarine	Baked Lemon Flounder Green Beans and Red Peppers* Chocolate Dream Cake 2 slices whole-grain bread 4 Brazil nuts	Chicken Cacciatore 1/3 cup pasta 1/2 large pear 1 cup nonfat milk 1 cup steamed peas and carrots 2 tsp margarine	Veal Scaloppini Mexican Coleslaw* 1/2 cup whole-wheat pasta 1 whole-wheat dinner roll 1/2 cup fruit cocktail in water 1 cup nonfat milk 1/2 cup steamed green beans	Chicken Tetrazzini (1/2 serving) Southwest Tomato Salad* 2 slices oatmeal bread 3/4 cup blueberries 1 cup nonfat milk 1 1/2 tsp margarine	Greek Halibut Fillet Italian-Style Zucchini with Whole-Wheat Pasta* Cherry Crisp Dessert* 1 cup nonfat milk 5 peanuts	Tex-Mex Turkey Burgers Gram's Gingerbread* 3/4 cup pineapple 1/2 cup nonfat milk 1 cup steamed broccoli 2 tsp margarine

*Indicates that the recipe has been used previously.

SHOParchShopping LIST SUMMER WEEK 3

VEGETABLES
_____ artichoke hearts
_____ bell peppers, green
_____ bell peppers, red
_____ broccoli
_____ Brussels sprouts
_____ cabbage
_____ carrots
_____ celery
_____ corn on the cob
_____ cucumbers
_____ mushrooms
_____ garlic
_____ green beans, frozen
_____ lettuce, romaine
_____ onion, red
_____ onions, yellow or white
_____ onions, green
_____ peas
_____ pepper, jalapeño
_____ spinach
_____ tomatoes
_____ tomatoes, cherry
_____ tomatoes, grape
_____ water chestnuts
_____ zucchini

MEATS
_____ bacon, Canadian
_____ bacon, turkey
_____ chicken breasts, skinless, boneless
_____ flounder
_____ halibut steaks
_____ lamb chops, about 5 oz each
_____ steak, top sirloin
_____ tuna, packed in water, 6-oz can
_____ turkey breast, light, deli-style
_____ turkey, lean, ground
_____ veal cutlets

FRUITS
_____ apples
_____ bananas
_____ blackberries
_____ blueberries
_____ cantaloupe
_____ cherries
_____ grapes, seedless
_____ honeydew melon
_____ kiwi fruit
_____ mango
_____ peaches
_____ pears
_____ pineapple, crushed
_____ plums
_____ prunes, pitted
_____ strawberries

DAIRY
_____ egg substitute
_____ egg white substitute
_____ milk, nonfat
_____ Smart Balance margarine
_____ sour cream, fat-free
_____ whipped topping, fat-free
_____ yogurt, fat-free, plain
_____ yogurt, fat-free, vanilla

CHEESE
_____ American, fat-free, shredded
_____ cheddar, sharp, fat-free
_____ cottage cheese, low-fat
_____ Monterey Jack, reduced-fat, shredded
_____ mozzarella, fat-free, shredded
_____ Parmesan, reduced-fat

BREAD, GRAINS, & PASTA
_____ bagel, whole-grain
_____ bread, oatmeal
_____ bread, whole-grain, whole-wheat
_____ English muffins, whole-wheat
_____ hoagie rolls, whole-grain
_____ pasta, linguini, whole-wheat
_____ pasta, macaroni or elbows, whole-wheat
_____ pasta, spaghetti, whole-wheat
_____ pocket pita breads, whole-grain, 6-inch
_____ rice, brown

BEANS
_____ red kidney, 16-oz can

NUTS
_____ almonds
_____ Brazil nuts
_____ peanuts

CONDIMENTS
_____ canola mayonnaise
_____ hot pepper sauce
_____ mustard, Dijon
_____ soy sauce, light
_____ sweet pickle relish

SPICES & HERBS
_____ basil
_____ black pepper
_____ chili powder
_____ cilantro
_____ cinnamon, ground
_____ coriander
_____ dill weed
_____ fennel seeds
_____ garlic powder
_____ ginger, ground
_____ mint
_____ nutmeg, ground
_____ onion powder
_____ oregano
_____ parsley
_____ poultry seasoning
_____ red pepper flakes
_____ rosemary

OTHER
_____ almond extract
_____ applesauce, unsweetened
_____ cashew butter
_____ cereal, bran
_____ cereal, shredded wheat
_____ club soda
_____ cocoa powder, unsweetened
_____ fruit cocktail in water
_____ honey
_____ limeade concentrate, frozen
_____ maple syrup, sugar-free
_____ marinara sauce, no-added-salt, 8-oz can
_____ molasses
_____ pie filling, cherry, light, 20-oz can
_____ pimiento
_____ pretzels
_____ pumpkin seeds
_____ raspberry preserves, sugar-free
_____ salad dressing, Italian, light
_____ seasoned croutons
_____ soup, tomato
_____ sweet pickles
_____ tomatoes, Italian-style stewed, 16-oz can
_____ tortillas, flour, whole-wheat, 6-inch
_____ wine, marsala

STAPLES
_____ baking powder
_____ baking soda
_____ bouillon, beef, sodium-free
_____ bouillon, chicken, sodium-free
_____ cornstarch
_____ flour, whole-wheat
_____ juice, lemon
_____ juice, lime
_____ nonstick cooking spray
_____ oats, old-fashioned
_____ Smart Balance Omega oil
_____ Splenda
_____ vanilla extract
_____ vinegar, rice

All-Natural High-Fiber Peach Squares

Serves 9   Serving Size: 1 square

3/4 **cup** fresh or frozen peaches, diced

1 **cup** Splenda

3/4 **cup** + 3/4 **Tbsp** whole-wheat flour

3/4 **cup** warm water

1 **cup** old-fashioned oats

1/4 **cup** Smart Balance margarine

1 **tsp** baking soda

1 **tsp** pure vanilla extract

1. Prepare the filling: bring the peaches, 1/2 cup Splenda, 3/4 Tbsp flour, and 3/4 cup water to a boil in a double boiler. Stir continuously until thickened.

2. Prepare the crumb base and topping: combine oats, margarine, 1/2 cup Splenda, 3/4 cup flour, baking soda, and vanilla; halve the mixture. Place half in the bottom of a 9-inch square baking dish. Layer the thickened filling on top. Add the remaining crumb base to the top.

3. Bake at 350°F for 30 minutes.

Exchanges/Choices

1 Starch
1 Fat

Basic Nutritional Values

Calories	125
Calories from Fat	45
Total Fat	5.0 g
Saturated Fat	1.2 g
Trans Fat	0.0 g
Cholesterol	0 mg
Sodium	180 mg
Total Carbohydrate	18 g
Dietary Fiber	2 g
Sugars	4 g
Protein	3 g

Honey-Mustard Lamb Chops

Serves 4   Serving size: 1 lamb chop

2 **Tbsp** honey

2 **Tbsp** lemon juice

2 **Tbsp** minced rosemary

1 **tsp** Dijon mustard

1 clove garlic, crushed

1 **tsp** onion powder

4 **(5-oz)** lamb chops, about 1 lb (trimmed of fat)

4 mint sprigs

In a small bowl, combine all ingredients except mint and lamb. Microwave on high power for 1 minute. Brush the mixture on both sides of the chops and either grill or broil for about 15 minutes. Garnish with mint sprigs.

Exchanges/Choices

1/2 Carbohydrate
3 Lean Meat

Basic Nutritional Values

Calories	170
Calories from Fat	55
Total Fat	6.0 g
Saturated Fat	2.1 g
Trans Fat	0.0 g
Cholesterol	55 mg
Sodium	85 mg
Total Carbohydrate	10 g
Dietary Fiber	0 g
Sugars	9 g
Protein	18 g

Low-Fat, Low-Sugar Carrot Cake
Serves 12   Serving size: 1 slice

1 **cup** pitted prunes

3 **Tbsp** water

4 **cups** carrots, coarsely shredded

2 **cups** Splenda

1 **tsp** pure vanilla extract

1 **cup** egg white substitute

1 **cup** crushed pineapple (fresh, frozen, or canned light, drained)

2 **cups** whole-wheat flour

2 **tsp** baking powder

2 **tsp** ground cinnamon

1/2 **tsp** baking soda

Exchanges/Choices

2 Carbohydrate

Basic Nutritional Values

Calories	150
Calories from Fat	5
Total Fat	0.5 g
Saturated Fat	0.1 g
Trans Fat	0.0 g
Cholesterol	0 mg
Sodium	175 mg
Total Carbohydrate	33 g
Dietary Fiber	5 g
Sugars	14 g
Protein	6 g

Place prunes and water in a blender or food processor and process until smooth. Combine the prunes, carrots, Splenda, vanilla, egg white substitute, and pineapple; mix well. Sift together the whole-wheat flour, baking powder, cinnamon, and baking soda. Stir into carrot mixture. Spoon batter into a 9 × 13-inch baking dish. Bake at 375°F for 45 minutes.

Stuffed Cantaloupe Chicken
Serves 4   Serving size: 1/4 recipe

1 **lb** boneless, skinless chicken breasts (trimmed of fat)

1 **cup** seedless grapes

2 celery stalks, fine dice

4 green onions, finely chopped

2 **Tbsp** chopped almonds

1/4 **tsp** poultry seasoning

1/4 **cup** canola mayonnaise

Black ground pepper, to taste

2 whole cantaloupes, halved and seeded

4 strawberries, sliced

Exchanges/Choices

2 Fruit
4 Lean Meat
1 Fat

Basic Nutritional Values

Calories	335
Calories from Fat	100
Total Fat	11.0 g
Saturated Fat	1.2 g
Trans Fat	0.0 g
Cholesterol	65 mg
Sodium	195 mg
Total Carbohydrate	34 g
Dietary Fiber	4 g
Sugars	29 g
Protein	28 g

Cook chicken in a skillet until done; allow to cool and then cut into cubes. In a large bowl, combine the grapes, celery, green onions, almonds, poultry seasoning, mayonnaise, and pepper. Fold in cubed meat. Scoop the filling mixture into the centers of the cantaloupes. Garnish with strawberries.

Stir-Fry Vegetables

Serves 4   Serving size: 1/4 recipe

1 Tbsp Smart Balance Omega oil

1 small onion, peeled, quartered, and thinly sliced

2 cloves garlic, minced

3/4 cup carrots, pared and thinly sliced

3/4 cup zucchini, thinly sliced

3/4 cup celery, thinly sliced

3/4 cup broccoli florets

1 Tbsp sodium-free chicken bouillon

1/4 cup water

2 tsp ground ginger

1/3 cup sliced water chestnuts

3 green onions, sliced

2 tsp light soy sauce

Heat oil in a large heavy skillet; sauté onion and garlic for 2 minutes. Add carrots, zucchini, celery, and broccoli; mix well. In a small bowl, combine bouillon and water to form a broth. Add broth and ginger to skillet; cover and cook 3 minutes. Add water chestnuts, green onions, and soy sauce. Stir until chestnuts and onions are heated through and vegetables are crisp-tender.

Exchanges/Choices

2 Vegetable
1/2 Fat

Basic Nutritional Values

Calories 85
  Calories from Fat 35
Total Fat . . . . 4.0 g
  Saturated Fat . . . . 0.3 g
  Trans Fat . . . . 0.0 g
Cholesterol . . . . 0 mg
Sodium . . . . 140 mg
Total Carbohydrate . . . 12 g
  Dietary Fiber . . . . 3 g
  Sugars . . . . 5 g
Protein . . . . 2 g

Bran Muffins

Serves 4   Serving size: 3 muffins

Nonstick cooking spray

3/4 **cup** whole-wheat flour

2 **tsp** baking powder

1 1/2 **Tbsp** Splenda

2/3 **cup** all-bran cereal

2/3 **cup** nonfat milk

1/4 **cup** egg substitute

1/4 **cup** unsweetened applesauce

Spray twelve 2-inch muffin-pan cups with nonstick cooking spray; set aside. Stir together flour, baking powder, and Splenda; set aside. Add cereal and milk to a large mixing bowl. Stir to combine and then allow it to stand until cereal is softened, 1–2 minutes. Add egg substitute and applesauce; beat well. Add flour mixture and stir only enough to combine. Divide batter evenly among prepared muffin cups. Bake at 400°F for 25 minutes or until lightly browned.

Exchanges/Choices

1/2 Starch

Basic Nutritional Values

Calories 45
 Calories from Fat 0
Total Fat . . . . .0.0 g
 Saturated Fat . . . . .0.1 g
 Trans Fat . . . . .0.0 g
Cholesterol . . . . .0 mg
Sodium . . . . .85 mg
Total Carbohydrate . . . 10 g
 Dietary Fiber . . . . .2 g
 Sugars . . . . .2 g
Protein . . . . .2 g

Open-Faced Chicken and Almond Sandwich

Serves 4   Serving size: 1 sandwich

1 **lb** boneless, skinless chicken breasts (trimmed of fat)

1/3 **cup** canola mayonnaise

1/4 **cup** toasted slivered almonds

1 celery stalk, thinly sliced

1 green onion (with top), thinly sliced

1 medium tomato, sliced

2 whole-wheat English muffins, split and toasted

Boil chicken in water until thoroughly cooked; then transfer to refrigerator to chill. When chicken has cooled, dice and mix with mayonnaise, almonds, celery, and onion. Arrange tomato slices on muffin halves. Spoon chicken onto tomato and serve.

Exchanges/Choices

1 Starch
4 Lean Meat
1 Fat

Basic Nutritional Values

Calories 310
 Calories from Fat 125
Total Fat . . . . .14.0 g
 Saturated Fat . . . . .1.2 g
 Trans Fat . . . . .0.0 g
Cholesterol . . . . .65 mg
Sodium . . . . .345 mg
Total Carbohydrate . . . 17 g
 Dietary Fiber . . . . .4 g
 Sugars . . . . .5 g
Protein . . . . .29 g

Baked Lemon Flounder

Serves 4   Serving size: 1/4 recipe

- 3 medium tomatoes, diced
- 3 medium cloves garlic, minced
- 3 **Tbsp** lemon juice
- 1/4 **cup** whole-wheat flour
- 1 **lb** flounder
- 1 **Tbsp** Smart Balance Omega oil
- 1 **cup** spinach
- 3/4 **cup** fat-free sour cream
- 3 **Tbsp** grated reduced-fat Parmesan cheese

In a 9 × 13-inch baking dish, arrange tomatoes and garlic evenly on bottom. Sprinkle 1 Tbsp lemon juice on tomatoes. Lightly dust fish fillets with flour. In a separate frying pan, brown fillets in oil and drain. Place fillets on top of tomatoes. Combine spinach, sour cream, Parmesan cheese, and remaining 2 Tbsp lemon juice; top fillets with mixture. Bake uncovered at 375°F until bubbly (about 20 minutes).

Exchanges/Choices

1 Carbohydrate
4 Lean Meat

Basic Nutritional Values

Calories 240
 Calories from Fat 55
Total Fat. . . . . 6.0 g
 Saturated Fat . . . . 1.2 g
 Trans Fat. . . . . 0.0 g
Cholesterol . . . . 70 mg
Sodium. . . . . 220 mg
Total Carbohydrate . . . 15 g
 Dietary Fiber. . . . . 2 g
 Sugars . . . . 4 g
Protein . . . . 28 g

Green Beans and Red Peppers

Serves 4   Serving size: 1/4 recipe

- 1/2 medium red bell pepper
- 1/2 **cup** water
- 1 **Tbsp** sodium-free chicken bouillon
- 16 **oz** frozen green beans
- 1/2 **Tbsp** Smart Balance Light margarine
- 1/4 **tsp** garlic powder

Cut bell pepper into strips. In a medium saucepan, combine water and bouillon to make a broth; bring to a boil. Add green beans. Cover and cook over medium heat for 8–12 minutes or until beans are crisp-tender. Drain. Meanwhile, melt margarine in a small skillet. Add pepper strips and cook until just tender. In a serving bowl, combine green beans, pepper strips, and garlic powder; toss gently.

Exchanges/Choices

2 Vegetable

Basic Nutritional Values

Calories 45
 Calories from Fat 10
Total Fat. . . . . 1.0 g
 Saturated Fat . . . . 0.2 g
 Trans Fat. . . . . 0.0 g
Cholesterol . . . . 0 mg
Sodium. . . . . 20 mg
Total Carbohydrate . . . 9 g
 Dietary Fiber. . . . . 3 g
 Sugars . . . . 4 g
Protein . . . . 2 g

Chocolate Dream Cake

Serves 6   Serving size: 1 slice

Nonstick cooking spray

1 **cup** whole-wheat flour

1 **cup** Splenda

3 **Tbsp** unsweetened cocoa powder

1 **tsp** cinnamon

1 **tsp** baking powder

1/2 **cup** egg substitute

8 **oz** fat-free vanilla yogurt

2 **Tbsp** unsweetened applesauce

1 **tsp** pure vanilla extract

4 **Tbsp** sugar-free raspberry preserves

6 **Tbsp** fat-free whipped topping

Exchanges/Choices

2 Carbohydrate

Basic Nutritional Values

Calories 130
 Calories from Fat 10
Total Fat . . . . 1.0 g
 Saturated Fat . . . . 0.4 g
 Trans Fat . . . . 0.0 g
Cholesterol . . . . 0 mg
Sodium . . . . 120 mg
Total Carbohydrate . . . 27 g
 Dietary Fiber . . . . 4 g
 Sugars . . . . 8 g
Protein . . . . 6 g

Preheat oven 350°F. Spray an 8-inch round cake pan with nonstick cooking spray. In a medium bowl, combine flour, Splenda, cocoa powder, cinnamon, and baking powder. Beat egg substitute in a medium bowl. In another bowl, combine yogurt, applesauce, and vanilla. Stir flour mixture into yogurt mixture until just blended. Fold egg substitute into the flour and yogurt batter. Pour into prepared cake pan. Bake 35 minutes or until a toothpick inserted in the center comes out clean. Cool for 5 minutes. Remove from pan and allow to cool completely before topping with raspberry preserves and whipped topping.

Whole-Wheat Pancakes or Waffles

Serves 4   Serving size: 2 pancakes or waffles

1/2 **cup** rolled oats

1/2 **cup** whole-wheat flour, sifted

2 **tsp** baking powder

2 **Tbsp** Splenda

1/2 **cup** egg substitute, beaten well

3/4 **cup** nonfat milk

2 **Tbsp** Smart Balance Omega oil

Nonstick cooking spray

Stir together dry ingredients. Combine egg substitute, milk, and oil; stir into flour mixture. Cook on a griddle lightly coated with nonstick spray until golden brown, then turn. Can also be made in a waffle iron.

Exchanges/Choices

1 1/2 Starch
1 1/2 Fat

Basic Nutritional Values

Calories 185
  Calories from Fat 70
Total Fat . . . . 8.0 g
  Saturated Fat . . . . 0.7 g
  Trans Fat . . . . 0.0 g
Cholesterol . . . . 0 mg
Sodium . . . . 265 mg
Total Carbohydrate . . . 22 g
  Dietary Fiber . . . . 3 g
  Sugars . . . . 3 g
Protein . . . . 8 g

Macaroni and Cheese

Serves 4   Serving size: 1/4 recipe

4 **oz** macaroni, elbows or shells

6 **Tbsp** Smart Balance Light margarine

1 small onion, diced

Pepper, to taste

1/4 **cup** whole-wheat flour

1 **cup** nonfat milk

2 **oz** fat-free shredded American cheese

2 **oz** fat-free sharp cheddar cheese

Cook macaroni according to package directions. Drain. In a large skillet, cook margarine, onion, and pepper over medium heat until onion is tender. Stir in flour and milk; cook over low heat until mixture is smooth and bubbly. Stir in cheese until melted. Add cooked macaroni; stir to mix thoroughly. Transfer mixture to a baking dish and bake at 375°F for 30 minutes.

Exchanges/Choices

2 Starch
2 Lean Meat
1 Fat

Basic Nutritional Values

Calories 280
  Calories from Fat 70
Total Fat . . . . 8.0 g
  Saturated Fat . . . . 2.4 g
  Trans Fat . . . . 0.0 g
Cholesterol . . . . 5 mg
Sodium . . . . 490 mg
Total Carbohydrate . . . 35 g
  Dietary Fiber . . . . 3 g
  Sugars . . . . 5 g
Protein . . . . 15 g

Chicken Cacciatore

Serves 4   Serving size: 1/4 recipe

Nonstick cooking spray

2 **Tbsp** reduced-fat Parmesan cheese

2 **Tbsp** nonfat milk

1/4 **cup** egg substitute

1 **Tbsp** Smart Balance margarine

4 **oz** linguini, cooked and drained

1 **lb** boneless, skinless chicken breasts (trimmed of fat)

2 **Tbsp** Smart Balance Omega oil

1/4 **cup** chopped onions

2 **oz** mushrooms, sliced (about 1 cup)

8 **oz** no-added-salt marinara sauce

1 **Tbsp** sodium-free chicken bouillon

1 **cup** water

1/2 **tsp** basil

1/8 **tsp** oregano

Exchanges/Choices

2 Starch
4 Lean Meat
1 Fat

Basic Nutritional Values

Calories 375
  Calories from Fat 115
Total Fat . . . . .13.0 g
  Saturated Fat . . . . .2.4 g
  Trans Fat . . . . .0.0 g
Cholesterol . . . . .70 mg
Sodium . . . . .185 mg
Total Carbohydrate . . .31 g
  Dietary Fiber . . . . .2 g
  Sugars . . . . .6 g
Protein . . . . .32 g

1. Lightly spray a large casserole dish with nonstick cooking spray. In a large bowl, beat together the Parmesan cheese, nonfat milk, egg substitute, and margarine until blended. Add cooked linguini and toss until evenly coated. Spread in casserole dish; set aside.

2. Cut chicken into 1-inch pieces. In a 10-inch skillet over medium-high heat, sauté the chicken in oil until chicken is no longer pink on the inside. Remove chicken and set aside.

3. Lower heat to medium. In same skillet, sauté onion for 1–2 minutes or until just beginning to brown. Add mushrooms and sauté for 1 minute. Add marinara sauce, bouillon, water, basil, and oregano. Stirring frequently over low heat, cook for 10 minutes. Stir in chicken and spoon spaghetti mixture over chicken.

4. Transfer chicken mixture to casserole dish, layering on top of linguini. Cover with foil and bake at 350°F for 30–40 minutes or until hot and bubbly around edges.

Blueberry Loaf Bread
Serves 6   Serving size: 1/6 recipe

2/3 **cup** whole-wheat flour

1/2 **tsp** baking powder

1/4 **tsp** baking soda

1/4 **cup** Splenda

1/4 **cup** fat-free yogurt

2 **tsp** Smart Balance Omega oil

1/2 **tsp** vanilla extract

1 egg white, lightly beaten

1/2 **cup** blueberries

Nonstick cooking spray

Combine flour, baking powder, baking soda, and Splenda in a medium bowl; make a well in center of mixture. Combine yogurt, oil, vanilla, and egg white; add to dry ingredients, stirring just until dry ingredients are moistened. Fold in blueberries. Spoon batter into a 6 × 3 × 2-inch loaf pan coated with nonstick cooking spray. Bake at 350°F for 35–40 minutes or until a wooden pick inserted in the center comes out clean. Remove from pan immediately and let cool on a wire rack.

Exchanges/Choices
1 Carbohydrate

Basic Nutritional Values
Calories 80
  Calories from Fat 20
Total Fat . . . . 2.0 g
  Saturated Fat . . . . 0.2 g
  Trans Fat . . . . 0.0 g
Cholesterol . . . . 0 mg
Sodium . . . . 100 mg
Total Carbohydrate . . . 14 g
  Dietary Fiber . . . . 2 g
  Sugars . . . . 3 g
Protein . . . . 3 g

Tuna-Stuffed Tomatoes
Serves 4   Serving size: 1/4 recipe

6 medium ripe tomatoes, washed

2 celery stalks, washed

1 (6-oz) can tuna packed in water, drained

3 **Tbsp** sweet pickle relish

1 **tsp** lemon juice

2/3 **cup** canola mayonnaise

1/4 **tsp** freshly ground pepper

1/2 **cup** parsley, snipped into tiny bits

4 lettuce leaves

Cut the top 1/2 inch off four tomatoes. Cut around the inside of the tomatoes; scoop out seeds and pulp and discard. Drain tomato cups upside down for 20 minutes. Dice the remaining tomatoes and celery. In a medium bowl, mix diced vegetables with tuna, relish, lemon juice, mayonnaise, and pepper. Fill each tomato cup with tuna mixture. Sprinkle with parsley for garnish. Place each stuffed tomatoes on a lettuce leaf and serve.

Exchanges/Choices
1/2 Carbohydrate
1 Vegetable
1 Lean Meat
2 Fat

Basic Nutritional Values
Calories 195
  Calories from Fat 115
Total Fat . . . . 13.0 g
  Saturated Fat . . . . 0.1 g
  Trans Fat . . . . 0.0 g
Cholesterol . . . . 10 mg
Sodium . . . . 385 mg
Total Carbohydrate . . . 12 g
  Dietary Fiber . . . . 2 g
  Sugars . . . . 9 g
Protein . . . . 8 g

Kidney Bean Salad

Serves 4   Serving size: 1/4 recipe

- 1 **(16-oz)** can red kidney beans, drained
- 1/2 **cup** sliced celery
- 1/4 **cup** chopped sweet pickles
- 3 **Tbsp** chopped pimiento
- 1/4 **cup** thinly sliced green onions
- 1/4 **cup** coarsely chopped green bell pepper
- 1/3 **cup** canola mayonnaise
- 4 romaine lettuce leaves
  Freshly ground pepper, to taste

Gently toss together beans, celery, pickles, pimiento, green onions, and green pepper. Season to taste. Blend in mayonnaise and chill. Serve on lettuce leaves and sprinkle with pepper to taste.

Exchanges/Choices

1 Starch
1 Vegetable
1 Fat

Basic Nutritional Values

Calories	180
Calories from Fat	55
Total Fat	6.0 g
Saturated Fat	0.0 g
Trans Fat	0.0 g
Cholesterol	0 mg
Sodium	360 mg
Total Carbohydrate	24 g
Dietary Fiber	6 g
Sugars	3 g
Protein	7 g

Veal Scaloppini

Serves 4   Serving size: 1/4 recipe

- 4 **oz** mushrooms, sliced
- 2 **Tbsp** lemon juice
- 1 **Tbsp** Smart Balance Omega oil
- 1 **Tbsp** cornstarch
- 1/8 **tsp** pepper
- 1 **lb** veal cutlets (trimmed of fat)
- 2 **tsp** sodium-free beef bouillon
- 1/4 **cup** water
- 1/4 **cup** marsala wine
- 1 clove garlic, minced

Sauté mushrooms in lemon juice and oil. Remove from pan. Combine cornstarch and pepper. Cut veal into 1-inch thick strips; coat evenly with cornstarch mixture. Brown the veal in the remaining oil in the skillet. Remove from pan when done. Combine beef bouillon and water; add to pan. Add wine and garlic. Cook, stirring, for 1 minute. Add cooked mushrooms and veal; heat until hot.

Exchanges/Choices

1/2 Carbohydrate
3 Lean Meat
1/2 Fat

Basic Nutritional Values

Calories	195
Calories from Fat	65
Total Fat	7.0 g
Saturated Fat	1.4 g
Trans Fat	0.0 g
Cholesterol	90 mg
Sodium	50 mg
Total Carbohydrate	5 g
Dietary Fiber	0 g
Sugars	2 g
Protein	25 g

Mexican Coleslaw

Serves 4   Serving size: 1/4 recipe

4 **cups** thinly sliced green cabbage

1 **cup** grated carrots

1 **Tbsp** cilantro

1/4 **cup** rice vinegar

2 **Tbsp** Smart Balance Omega oil

Place cabbage and carrots in a colander; rinse with cold water. Allow to drain for 5 minutes. Meanwhile, whisk together cilantro, vinegar, and oil in a large bowl. Add cabbage; toss well to coat. Toss again just before serving.

Exchanges/Choices

1 Vegetable
1 1/2 Fat

Basic Nutritional Values

Calories 90
 Calories from Fat 65
Total Fat . . . . 7.0 g
 Saturated Fat . . . . 0.5 g
 Trans Fat . . . . 0.0 g
Cholesterol . . . . 0 mg
Sodium . . . . 35 mg
Total Carbohydrate . . . 7 g
 Dietary Fiber . . . . 2 g
 Sugars . . . . 4 g
Protein . . . . 1 g

Banana Bran Muffin

Serves 8   Serving size: 1 muffin

2/3 **cup** bran cereal

2/3 **cup** plain fat-free yogurt

5/8 **cup** whole-wheat flour

5 **Tbsp** Splenda

1 **tsp** ground cinnamon

1/2 **tsp** baking soda

3/16 **tsp** ground nutmeg

2 **cups** bananas, mashed

1/4 **cup** unsweetened applesauce

1/2 **cup** egg substitute, beaten

1. Preheat oven to 375°F. Place paper liners in muffin pan cups.

2. In a medium bowl, mix cereal and yogurt. Let stand for 5 minutes or until cereal is softened and breaks up.

3. Meanwhile, in a small bowl, combine the flour, Splenda, cinnamon, baking soda, and nutmeg; set aside.

4. Stir banana, applesauce, and egg substitute into cereal mixture. Stir in flour mixture until moistened. Fill muffin cups to about 2/3 full. Bake for 20–25 minutes or until muffins are lightly browned on top. Remove from pan and let cool on a wire rack before serving.

Exchanges/Choices

1 Starch
1 Fruit

Basic Nutritional Values

Calories 120
  Calories from Fat 5
Total Fat . . . . .0.5 g
  Saturated Fat . . . . .0.2 g
  Trans Fat . . . . .0.0 g
Cholesterol . . . . .0 mg
Sodium . . . . .135 mg
Total Carbohydrate . . .27 g
  Dietary Fiber . . . . .5 g
  Sugars . . . . .11 g
Protein . . . . .5 g

Healthy Club Sandwich

Serves 4   Serving size: 1 pita sandwich

2 (**6-inch**) whole-grain pocket pita breads

1/2 lb deli-style light turkey breast

1 medium tomato, sliced

1 cup romaine lettuce, finely shredded

4 oz turkey bacon, cooked

4 Tbsp canola mayonnaise

Cut each pita in half and place turkey in pita, followed with tomato and lettuce. Crumble bacon and sprinkle on each pita. Top with 1 Tbsp mayonnaise.

This recipe is high in sodium.

Exchanges/Choices

1 Starch
1 Vegetable
2 Lean Meat
1 Fat

Basic Nutritional Values

Calories 230
 Calories from Fat 80
Total Fat . . . . 9.0 g
 Saturated Fat . . . . 1.2 g
 Trans Fat . . . . 0.0 g
Cholesterol . . . . 35 mg
Sodium . . . . 1225 mg
Total Carbohydrate . . . 23 g
 Dietary Fiber . . . . 4 g
 Sugars . . . . 4 g
Protein . . . . 16 g

Chicken Tetrazzini

Serves 4   Serving size: 1/4 recipe

Nonstick cooking spray

4 **oz** spaghetti

4 **oz** mushrooms, sliced

1 **Tbsp** Smart Balance margarine

1/4 **cup** whole-wheat flour

1 **cup** water

1 **cup** nonfat milk

2 **tsp** sodium-free chicken bouillon

1/4 **tsp** ground nutmeg

2 **oz** fat-free shredded mozzarella cheese

2 **oz** reduced-fat shredded Monterey Jack cheese

1 **lb** boneless, skinless chicken breasts, cooked and cut into bite-size pieces (trimmed of fat)

Exchanges/Choices

2 Starch
5 Lean Meat

Basic Nutritional Values

Calories 380
  Calories from Fat 70
Total Fat. . . . . 8.0 g
  Saturated Fat . . . . 3.3 g
  Trans Fat. . . . . 0.0 g
Cholesterol . . . . 75 mg
Sodium. . . . . 400 mg
Total Carbohydrate . . . 34 g
  Dietary Fiber . . . . 3 g
  Sugars . . . . 5 g
Protein . . . . 39 g

Preheat oven to 350°F. Lightly spray a shallow 1 1/2-quart baking dish with nonstick cooking spray. Break spaghetti in half and cook according to package directions. Drain, cover, and keep warm. Meanwhile, in a 3-quart saucepan over medium heat, sauté mushrooms in margarine for 3 minutes or until soft; add flour. Cook and stir 1–2 minutes. Add water, nonfat milk, bouillon, and nutmeg. While stirring, bring to a boil until thickened. Reduce heat to low. Add cheeses. Stir until cheese just melts. Remove from heat. Stir in spaghetti and chicken until well coated. Spoon into baking dish. Bake 40 minutes or until very bubbly and heated through.

Southwest Tomato Salad

Serves 4   Serving size: 1/4 recipe

2 **cups** diced tomatoes (about 4 medium tomatoes)

1/2 **cup** diced green bell pepper

1/2 **cup** chopped, peeled cucumber

1/2 **cup** finely chopped red onion

1 **Tbsp** minced jalapeño

1/2 **cup** seasoned croutons

1/4 **cup** light Italian salad dressing

In a large bowl, combine tomatoes, green bell pepper, cucumber, onion, and jalapeño. Add croutons and dressing; toss thoroughly to combine.

Exchanges/Choices

2 Vegetable
1/2 Fat

Basic Nutritional Values

Calories 70
 Calories from Fat 20
Total Fat. . . . . 2.0 g
 Saturated Fat . . . . 0.4 g
 Trans Fat. . . . . 0.0 g
Cholesterol . . . . 0 mg
Sodium. . . . . 245 mg
Total Carbohydrate . . . 12 g
 Dietary Fiber. . . . . 2 g
 Sugars . . . . 6 g
Protein . . . . 2 g

Fried Bananas

Serves 4   Serving size: 1 banana

4 small bananas (or plantains)	**1/4 cup** whole-wheat flour
1/4 cup nonfat milk	**1/4 cup** Smart Balance
1/4 cup egg substitute	Omega oil (for frying)
1 Tbsp Splenda	

Peel the bananas and cut diagonally into half-inch-thick slices. Mix milk, egg substitute, Splenda, and flour until smooth. Heat oil in large skillet over medium heat. Dip each banana slice into batter and then drop into oil. Fry until browned, about 2 minutes on each side. Drain on paper towels. Serve warm or at room temperature.

Exchanges/Choices

1/2 Starch
1 1/2 Fruit
1 1/2 Fat

Basic Nutritional Values

Calories 190	
Calories from Fat 65	
Total Fat . . . . 7.0 g	
Saturated Fat . . . . 0.6 g	
Trans Fat . . . . 0.0 g	
Cholesterol . . . . 0 mg	
Sodium . . . . 40 mg	
Total Carbohydrate . . . 30 g	
Dietary Fiber . . . . 4 g	
Sugars . . . . 14 g	
Protein . . . . 4 g	

Chicken Salad

Serves 4   Serving size: 1/4 recipe

1/2 lb boneless, skinless chicken breasts (trimmed of fat)	**1/2 cup** crushed pineapple (or canned light, drained)
1 Tbsp lemon juice	Pepper, to taste
1/2 cup diced celery	**1/4 cup** canola mayonnaise
1/2 cup diced onion	**1/2 cup** plain fat-free yogurt

Place chicken breasts in boiling water and thoroughly cook; then put chicken in refrigerator to cool. Combine all other ingredients in large bowl and mix well. When chicken is cool to the touch, cut into small chunks. Add to large bowl and mix thoroughly. Refrigerate for 2 hours before serving.

Exchanges/Choices

1/2 Carbohydrate
2 Lean Meat
1/2 Fat

Basic Nutritional Values

Calories 145	
Calories from Fat 55	
Total Fat . . . . 6.0 g	
Saturated Fat . . . . 0.4 g	
Trans Fat . . . . 0.0 g	
Cholesterol . . . . 35 mg	
Sodium . . . . 155 mg	
Total Carbohydrate . . . 8 g	
Dietary Fiber . . . . 1 g	
Sugars . . . . 7 g	
Protein . . . . 14 g	

Dilled Cucumber Salad

Serves 4   Serving size: 1/4 recipe

1/4	**cup** fat-free sour cream		1 1/2	**Tbsp** dill weed
1	**Tbsp** canola mayonnaise			Black pepper, to taste
1/4	**cup** plain fat-free yogurt		1 1/2	medium cucumber
1 1/2	**Tbsp** lime juice			

In a bowl, whisk together sour cream, mayonnaise, yogurt, lime juice, dill, and pepper. Peel the cucumbers and cut crosswise into 1/8-inch-thick slices. Stir them into the dressing. Serve chilled.

Exchanges/Choices

1 Vegetable

Basic Nutritional Values

Calories	40
Calories from Fat	15
Total Fat	1.5 g
Saturated Fat	0.0 g
Trans Fat	0.0 g
Cholesterol	5 mg
Sodium	45 mg
Total Carbohydrate	4 g
Dietary Fiber	1 g
Sugars	3 g
Protein	2 g

Greek Halibut Fillet

Serves 4   Serving size: 1/4 recipe

6	**oz** frozen limeade concentrate, thawed		2	**tsp** oregano
1/4	**cup** Smart Balance Omega oil		1	**tsp** coriander
2	**Tbsp** minced garlic		1	**lb** halibut steaks

Combine limeade, oil, garlic, oregano, and coriander in a shallow baking dish. Place fish in dish and turn over several times to coat; refrigerate for 30–45 minutes. Remove fish; discard leftover marinade. Cook fish on a grill over medium-high heat, turning once during cooking, about 6–12 minutes per inch of thickness. Grill until fish flakes with a fork. Do not overcook.

Exchanges/Choices

1/2 Carbohydrate
3 Lean Meat

Basic Nutritional Values

Calories	175
Calories from Fat	55
Total Fat	6.0 g
Saturated Fat	0.6 g
Trans Fat	0.0 g
Cholesterol	35 mg
Sodium	60 mg
Total Carbohydrate	6 g
Dietary Fiber	0 g
Sugars	5 g
Protein	24 g

Italian-Style Zucchini with Whole-Wheat Pasta

Serves 6   Serving size: 1/6 recipe

6 **oz** whole-wheat pasta, macaroni or elbows

1 large onion, chopped

1 clove garlic, minced

1 medium carrot, thinly chopped

2 **Tbsp** Smart Balance Omega oil

1 **(16-oz)** can Italian-style stewed tomatoes

1 zucchini, halved lengthwise and sliced in 1/4-inch pieces

1/2 **tsp** fennel seeds, crushed

1/4 **tsp** red pepper flakes

Exchanges/Choices

1 1/2 Starch
2 Vegetable
1/2 Fat

Basic Nutritional Values

Calories 185
 Calories from Fat 45
Total Fat . . . . 5.0 g
 Saturated Fat . . . . 0.5 g
 Trans Fat . . . . 0.0 g
Cholesterol . . . . 0 mg
Sodium . . . . 255 mg
Total Carbohydrate . . . 33 g
 Dietary Fiber . . . . 5 g
 Sugars . . . . 8 g
Protein . . . . 6 g

Cook the pasta according to package directions; drain and set aside. In a large skillet, cook the onion, garlic, and carrot in hot oil for 5 minutes or until tender. Add tomatoes, zucchini, fennel seeds, and red pepper flakes. Bring to a boil and reduce heat. Simmer uncovered for about 3 minutes. Stir in pasta and heat through.

Cherry Crisp Dessert

Serves 8   Serving size: 1/8 recipe

1 **(20-oz)** can light cherry pie filling

3/8 **tsp** almond extract

3 1/2 **Tbsp** Smart Balance margarine, melted

2 **cups** rolled oats, dry

1/4 **cup** Splenda

Exchanges/Choices

2 Carbohydrate
1 Fat

Basic Nutritional Values

Calories 165
 Calories from Fat 45
Total Fat . . . . 5 g
 Saturated Fat . . . . 1.3 g
 Trans Fat . . . . 0 g
Cholesterol . . . . 0 mg
Sodium . . . . 55 mg
Total Carbohydrate . . . 27 g
 Dietary Fiber . . . . 3 g
 Sugars . . . . 13 g
Protein . . . . 4 g

Place pie filling and almond extract in a baking dish that has sides about 2 inches high. Stir until blended; set aside. Place melted margarine in a small bowl; add oats and Splenda. Stir until well mixed. Spoon mixture evenly over pie filling. Bake at 350°F for about 30 minutes. Serve warm.

Whole-Wheat Blueberry Muffins

Serves 12   Serving size: 1 muffin

1 cup whole-wheat flour	**3 Tbsp** Smart Balance margarine
5 1/2 Tbsp Splenda	**1/2 cup** egg substitute
1 tsp baking powder	**1/2 cup** blueberries
6 Tbsp nonfat milk	

Preheat oven to 400°F. In a medium bowl, combine flour, Splenda, and baking powder. In a small bowl, beat milk, margarine, and egg substitute; stir into dry ingredients until just moist. Fold in blueberries and spoon batter into 12 paper-lined muffin cups. Bake for 20–25 minutes or until golden brown. Serve immediately.

Exchanges/Choices

1/2 Starch
1/2 Fat

Basic Nutritional Values

Calories 70
  Calories from Fat 20
Total Fat . . . . .2.5 g
  Saturated Fat . . . . .0.7 g
  Trans Fat . . . . .0.0 g
Cholesterol . . . . .0 mg
Sodium . . . . .75 mg
Total Carbohydrate . . .9 g
  Dietary Fiber . . . . .1 g
  Sugars . . . . .2 g
Protein . . . . .3 g

Sliced Steak Hoagie

Serves 4   Serving size: 1 hoagie

1 Tbsp Smart Balance Omega oil	**1 cup** fat-free shredded mozzarella cheese
2 medium onions, sliced	**4** whole-grain hoagie rolls
3/4 lb top sirloin steak (trimmed of fat)	

Heat the oil in a skillet; add onions and steak and cook until meat is browned. Reduce heat; cover to cook to desired doneness. Remove from heat, slice steak very thinly, and place in the buns. Top with cooked onions and cheese. Bake hoagies at 400°F for about 5 minutes to melt the cheese. Serve hot.

This recipe is high in sodium.

Exchanges/Choices

2 Starch
2 Vegetable
3 Lean Meat
1 Fat

Basic Nutritional Values

Calories 380
  Calories from Fat 90
Total Fat . . . . .10.0 g
  Saturated Fat . . . . .2.0 g
  Trans Fat . . . . .0.1 g
Cholesterol . . . . .35 mg
Sodium . . . . .690 mg
Total Carbohydrate . . .43 g
  Dietary Fiber . . . . .6 g
  Sugars . . . . .9 g
Protein . . . . .31 g

Tex-Mex Turkey Burgers
Serves 4   Serving size: 1 burger

1 **tsp** Smart Balance Omega oil

2/3 **cup** chopped onion

2 medium cloves garlic, crushed

2 **tsp** chili powder

2 slices whole-wheat bread

3 **Tbsp** club soda

1 **lb** lean ground turkey

1/4 **tsp** pepper

1/4 **tsp** hot pepper sauce

4 **(6-inch)** whole-wheat flour tortillas

Preheat a grill or broiler (this recipe can be prepared in either). In a small skillet over medium heat, heat oil; add onion, garlic, and chili powder; cook 4 minutes, stirring frequently, until onion is softened. Remove from heat; let cool slightly. Tear bread into crumbs; about 1 1/4 cup. In a medium bowl, toss bread crumbs with club soda to moisten; add turkey, onion mixture, pepper, and hot pepper sauce; mix well. Shape mixture into four 3/4-inch-thick patties. Cook patties 4–6 minutes on each side until browned and cooked through. While burgers are cooking, warm the tortillas. Fold each warm tortilla into quarters; insert burgers and serve hot.

Exchanges/Choices
1 1/2 Starch
3 Lean Meat

Basic Nutritional Values
Calories 235
 Calories from Fat 35
Total Fat. . . . . .4.0 g
 Saturated Fat . . . . .0.5 g
 Trans Fat. . . . . .0.0 g
Cholesterol. . . . . .55 mg
Sodium. . . . . .315 mg
Total Carbohydrate . . .24 g
 Dietary Fiber. . . . . .4 g
 Sugars . . . . .3 g
Protein . . . . .24 g

Gram's Gingerbread
Serves 8   Serving size: 1 square

1/2 **cup** Splenda

1/2 **cup** molasses

1/4 **cup** unsweetened applesauce

1/2 **cup** egg substitute or egg whites, beaten

1 1/2 **cup** whole-wheat flour

1 **tsp** ginger, ground

1 **tsp** baking soda

1/2 **cup** boiling water

Mix together all ingredients (except water); then add water. Mix thoroughly. Bake at 350°F until a toothpick inserted into the center comes out clean.

Exchanges/Choices
2 Carbohydrate

Basic Nutritional Values
Calories 155
 Calories from Fat 0
Total Fat. . . . . .0.0 g
 Saturated Fat . . . . .0.1 g
 Trans Fat. . . . . .0.0 g
Cholesterol. . . . . .0 mg
Sodium. . . . . .195 mg
Total Carbohydrate . . .35 g
 Dietary Fiber. . . . . .3 g
 Sugars . . . . .14 g
Protein . . . . .5 g

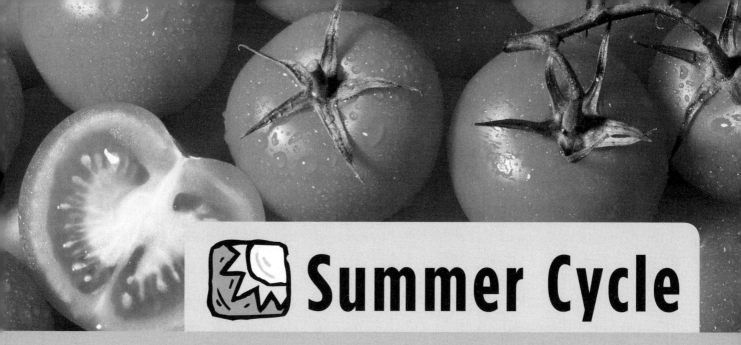

Summer Cycle

WEEK 4

FEATURED RECIPES

Lemon Baked Chicken

Oven-Baked Potatoes*

Cinnamon Apple Yogurt*†

Red Snapper with Cinnamon

Multigrain Rice Pilaf*

Colorful Coleslaw*

Zucchini Carrot Muffins*

Broccoli Floret Salad*

Frozen Pumpkin Dessert*

Sesame Yogurt Chicken

Cold Spinach with Yogurt

Oatmeal and Apple Muffins*

Bacon, Lettuce, and Tomato Sandwich

Ambrosia Salad*

Southwestern Fajitas with Pico de Gallo

Baked Tomatoes and Squash*

Bread Pudding

Deli Turkey and Swiss on Rye

Parmesan Pork Cutlet

Three Bean Salad*

French Toast*

Spicy Whole-Grain Rice with Peanuts*

Sweet and Sour Red Cabbage*

Cashew Chicken

Fiesta Pasta Salad*

Peach and Apple Crisp*

Turkey Reuben Sandwich

Perfection Salad*

Tuna Noodle Casserole*

Chicken and White Bean Soup

German Potato Salad*

Baked Ziti

*Indicates that the recipe has been used previously.

†This recipe is used as a snack, but its ingredients are in the shopping list.

	Sunday	Monday	Tuesday	Wednesday	Thursday	Friday	Saturday
Breakfast	1 English muffin 1/2 cup unsweetened peaches 1 cup nonfat milk 1/2 tsp margarine	Zucchini Carrot Muffins* 1 cup raspberries 1/2 cup nonfat milk 1/2 tsp margarine	Oatmeal and Apple Muffins* 1 cup nonfat milk 1 1/2 tsp margarine	Bread Pudding 1 slice raisin bread 1 medium banana 1/2 cup nonfat milk 1 tsp margarine	French Toast* 1/4 cup sugar-free maple syrup 1 1/4 cup strawberries 1/2 cup nonfat milk 1/2 tsp margarine	Peach and Apple Crisp* 1/2 bagel 1 cup nonfat milk 1 1/2 tsp margarine	1 whole-grain English muffin 3/4 cup berries and melon cubes 1 cup nonfat milk 2 tsp margarine
Lunch	Lemon Baked Chicken Oven-Baked Potatoes* 1 slice whole-wheat bread 3/4 cup blackberries 1/2 cup steamed spinach 1/2 tsp margarine	Broccoli Floret Salad* Frozen Pumpkin Dessert* 1 slice whole-wheat bread 3/4 cup blueberries 2 oz grilled buffalo burger/patty 1 1/2 tsp margarine	Bacon, Lettuce, and Tomato Sandwich Ambrosia Salad* 3 macadamia nuts	Deli Turkey and Swiss on Rye 8 animal crackers 3/4 cup pineapple 1 cup cauliflower florets 1/2 tsp margarine	Spicy Whole-Grain Rice with Peanuts* Sweet and Sour Red Cabbage* 1/2 cup cantaloupe 1 cup pepper slices 1 oz reduced-fat cheese	Turkey Reuben Sandwich Perfection Salad* 3/4 oz baked pita chips 1 medium banana 2 Brazil nuts	Chicken and White Bean Soup German Potato Salad* 1 1/4 cup watermelon 4 walnut halves
Snack A							
Snack B							
Dinner	Red Snapper with Cinnamon Multigrain Rice Pilaf* Colorful Coleslaw* 1 cup nonfat milk	Sesame Yogurt Chicken Cold Spinach with Yogurt 3/4 cup unsweetened mandarin oranges 1/2 cup carrots 1 tsp margarine 2 Brazil nuts	Southwestern Fajitas with Pico de Gallo Baked Tomatoes and Squash* 1/2 large pear 1 cup nonfat milk	Parmesan Pork Cutlet Three Bean Salad* 1 medium ear corn on the cob 1 small nectarine 1 cup nonfat milk 1/2 cup cooked okra 1/2 tsp margarine	Cashew Chicken Fiesta Pasta Salad* 1/2 cup nonfat milk	Tuna Noodle Casserole* 2 tangerines 1 cup nonfat milk 2 cups tomato and cucumber slices 9 cashews	Baked Ziti (1/2 serving) 1 small dinner roll 1/2 cup unsweetened applesauce 1 cup nonfat milk 1/2 cup vegetable sticks 1 1/2 tsp margarine

*Indicates that the recipe has been used previously.

	Sunday	Monday	Tuesday	Wednesday	Thursday	Friday	Saturday
Breakfast	1 English muffin 1/2 cup unsweetened peaches 1 cup nonfat milk 1/4 cup egg substitute 1/2 tsp margarine	Zucchini Carrot Muffins* 1 cup raspberries 1/2 cup nonfat milk 1 oz lean turkey sausage 1/2 tsp margarine	Oatmeal and Apple Muffins* 1 cup nonfat milk 1 oz Canadian bacon 1 1/2 tsp margarine	Bread Pudding 1 slice raisin bread 1 medium banana 1/2 cup nonfat milk 1 tsp margarine	French Toast* 1/4 cup sugar-free maple syrup 1 1/4 cup strawberries 1/2 cup nonfat milk 1 1/2 tsp margarine	Peach and Apple Crisp* 1/2 bagel 1 cup nonfat milk 1 1/2 tsp margarine	1 whole-grain English muffin 3/4 cup berries and melon cubes 1 cup nonfat milk 2 tsp margarine
Lunch	Lemon Baked Chicken Oven-Baked Potatoes* 1 slice whole-wheat bread 3/4 cup blackberries 1/2 cup steamed spinach 1 1/2 tsp margarine	Broccoli Floret Salad* Frozen Pumpkin Dessert* 1 slice whole-wheat bread 3/4 cup blueberries 2 oz grilled buffalo burger/patty 1 1/2 tsp margarine	Bacon, Lettuce, and Tomato Sandwich Ambrosia Salad* 6 macadamia nuts	Deli Turkey and Swiss on Rye 8 animal crackers 3/4 cup pineapple 1 cup cauliflower florets 1 1/2 tsp margarine	Spicy Whole-Grain Rice with Peanuts* Sweet and Sour Red Cabbage* 1/2 cup cantaloupe 1 cup pepper slices 2 oz reduced-fat cheese	Turkey Reuben Sandwich Perfection Salad* 3/4 oz baked pita chips 1 medium banana 4 Brazil nuts	Chicken and White Bean Soup German Potato Salad* 1 1/4 cup watermelon 8 walnut halves
Snack A	4 pecans 1/2 cup mango	6 almonds 1/2 cup unsweetened pears	5 hazelnuts 12 cherries	4 walnut halves 1 medium peach	1 Tbsp pumpkin seeds 1/2 cup unsweetened apricots	10 peanuts 17 grapes	6 cashews 3 dates
Snack B	Cinnamon Apple Yogurt*	1 cup nonfat milk	1 cup nonfat milk	1 cup nonfat milk	1 cup nonfat milk	1 cup nonfat milk	6 oz fat-free yogurt
Dinner	Red Snapper with Cinnamon Multigrain Rice Pilaf* Colorful Coleslaw* 1 cup nonfat milk	Sesame Yogurt Chicken Cold Spinach with Yogurt 3/4 cup unsweetened mandarin oranges 1/2 cup carrots 1 tsp margarine 2 Brazil nuts	Southwestern Fajitas with Pico de Gallo Baked Tomatoes and Squash* 1/2 large pear 1 cup nonfat milk	Parmesan Pork Cutlet Three Bean Salad* 1 medium ear corn on the cob 1 small nectarine 1 cup nonfat milk 1/2 cup cooked okra 1/2 tsp margarine	Cashew Chicken Fiesta Pasta Salad* 1/2 cup nonfat milk	Tuna Noodle Casserole* 2 tangerines 1 cup nonfat milk 2 cups tomato and cucumber slices 1 oz reduced-fat cheese 9 cashews	Baked Ziti (1/2 serving) 1 small dinner roll 1/2 cup unsweetened applesauce 1 cup nonfat milk 1 1/2 cup vegetable sticks 1 oz reduced-fat cheese 1 1/2 tsp margarine

*Indicates that the recipe has been used previously.

2000 calorie MEAL PLAN

	Sunday	Monday	Tuesday	Wednesday	Thursday	Friday	Saturday
Breakfast	1 English muffin 1/2 cup unsweetened peaches 1 cup nonfat milk 1/4 cup egg substitute 1/2 tsp margarine	**Zucchini Carrot Muffins*** 1 cup raspberries 1/2 cup nonfat milk 1 oz lean turkey sausage 1/2 tsp margarine	**Oatmeal and Apple Muffins*** 1 cup nonfat milk 1 oz Canadian bacon 1 1/2 tsp margarine	**Bread Pudding** 1 slice raisin bread 1 medium banana 1/2 cup nonfat milk 1 tsp margarine	**French Toast*** 1/4 cup sugar-free maple syrup 1 1/4 cup strawberries 1/2 cup nonfat milk 1 1/2 tsp margarine	**Peach and Apple Crisp*** 1/2 bagel 1 cup nonfat milk 1 1/2 tsp margarine	1 whole-grain English muffin 3/4 cup berries and melon cubes 1 cup nonfat milk 2 tsp margarine
Lunch	**Lemon Baked Chicken** **Oven-Baked Potatoes*** 1 slice whole-wheat bread 1 1/2 cup blackberries 1 cup steamed spinach 1 1/2 tsp margarine	**Broccoli Floret Salad*** **Frozen Pumpkin Dessert*** 1 slice whole-wheat bread 1 1/2 cup blueberries 1 cup grape tomatoes 2 oz grilled buffalo burger/patty 1 1/2 tsp margarine	**Bacon, Lettuce, and Tomato Sandwich** **Ambrosia Salad*** 3/4 oz pretzels 1 cup mixed vegetable sticks 6 macadamia nuts	**Deli Turkey and Swiss on Rye** 8 animal crackers 1 1/2 cup pineapple 2 cups cauliflower florets 1 1/2 tsp margarine	**Spicy Whole-Grain Rice with Peanuts*** **Sweet and Sour Red Cabbage*** 1/2 cup cantaloupe 2 cups pepper and tomato slices 2 oz reduced-fat cheese	**Turkey Reuben Sandwich** **Perfection Salad*** 3/4 oz baked pita chips 1 large banana 4 Brazil nuts	**Chicken and White Bean Soup** **German Potato Salad*** 1 1/4 cup watermelon 1/2 cup steamed green beans 8 walnut halves
Snack A	1 cup carrot sticks 4 pecans 1/2 cup mango	1 cup celery sticks 6 almonds 1/2 cup unsweetened pears	1 cup grape tomatoes 5 hazelnuts 12 cherries	1 cup mixed vegetable sticks 4 walnut halves 1 medium peach	1 cup cucumber sticks 1 Tbsp pumpkin seeds 1/2 cup unsweetened apricots	1 cup zucchini slices 10 peanuts 17 grapes	1 cup cucumber slices 6 cashews 3 dates
Snack B	1 4-inch waffle 1 tsp margarine **Cinnamon Apple Yogurt***	1 cup oven-baked French fries 1 cup nonfat milk	20 oyster crackers 10 peanuts 1 cup nonfat milk	1/4 cup low-fat granola 1 Tbsp sunflower seeds 1 cup nonfat milk	3 cups popcorn 1 tsp margarine 1 cup nonfat milk	2 small sandwich cookies 1 cup nonfat milk	5 vanilla wafers 6 oz fat-free yogurt
Dinner	**Red Snapper with Cinnamon** **Multigrain Rice Pilaf*** **Colorful Coleslaw*** 1 cup nonfat milk	**Sesame Yogurt Chicken** **Cold Spinach with Yogurt** 3/4 cup unsweetened mandarin oranges 1/2 cup carrots 1 tsp margarine 2 Brazil nuts	**Southwestern Fajitas with Pico de Gallo** **Baked Tomatoes and Squash*** 1/2 large pear 1 cup nonfat milk	**Parmesan Pork Cutlet** **Three Bean Salad*** 1 medium ear corn on the cob 1 small nectarine 1 cup nonfat milk 1/2 cup cooked okra 1/2 tsp margarine	**Cashew Chicken** **Fiesta Pasta Salad*** 1/2 cup nonfat milk	**Tuna Noodle Casserole*** 2 tangerines 1 cup nonfat milk 2 cups tomato and cucumber slices 1 oz reduced-fat cheese 9 cashews	**Baked Ziti** (1/2 serving) 1 small dinner roll 1/2 cup unsweetened applesauce 1 cup nonfat milk 1 1/2 cup vegetable sticks 1 oz reduced-fat cheese 1 1/2 tsp margarine

*Indicates that the recipe has been used previously.

	Sunday	Monday	Tuesday	Wednesday	Thursday	Friday	Saturday
Breakfast	1 English muffin 1/2 cup unsweetened peaches 1 cup nonfat milk 1/2 cup egg substitute 1/2 tsp margarine	**Zucchini Carrot Muffins*** 1 cup raspberries 1/2 cup nonfat milk 2 oz lean turkey sausage 1/2 tsp margarine	**Oatmeal and Apple Muffins*** 1 cup nonfat milk 2 oz Canadian bacon 1 1/2 tsp margarine	**Bread Pudding** 1 slice raisin bread 1 medium banana 1/2 cup nonfat milk 1 oz reduced-fat cheese 1 tsp margarine	**French Toast*** 1/4 cup sugar-free maple syrup 1 1/4 cup strawberries 1/2 cup nonfat milk 1/4 cup egg substitute 1 1/2 tsp margarine	**Peach and Apple Crisp*** 1/2 bagel 1 cup nonfat milk 1/4 cup egg substitute 1 1/2 tsp margarine	1 whole-grain English muffin 3/4 cup berries and melon cubes 1 cup nonfat milk 1 oz lean beef sausage 2 tsp margarine
Lunch	**Lemon Baked Chicken Oven-Baked Potatoes*** 1 slice whole-wheat bread 1 1/2 cup blackberries 1 cup steamed spinach 1 1/2 tsp margarine	**Broccoli Floret Salad* Frozen Pumpkin Dessert*** 1 slice whole-wheat bread 1 1/2 cup blueberries 1 cup grape tomatoes 2 oz grilled buffalo burger/patty 1 1/2 tsp margarine	**Bacon, Lettuce, and Tomato Sandwich Ambrosia Salad*** 3/4 oz pretzels 1 cup mixed vegetable sticks 6 macadamia nuts	**Deli Turkey and Swiss on Rye** 8 animal crackers 1 1/2 cup pineapple 2 cups cauliflower florets 1 1/2 tsp margarine	**Spicy Whole-Grain Rice with Peanuts* Sweet and Sour Red Cabbage*** 1/2 cup cantaloupe 2 cups pepper and tomato slices 2 oz reduced-fat cheese	**Turkey Reuben Sandwich Perfection Salad*** 3/4 oz baked pita chips 1 large banana 4 Brazil nuts	**Chicken and White Bean Soup German Potato Salad*** 1 1/4 cup watermelon 1/2 cup steamed green beans 8 walnut halves
Snack A	1 cup carrot sticks 4 pecans 1/2 cup mango	1 cup celery sticks 6 almonds 1/2 cup unsweetened pears	1 cup grape tomatoes 5 hazelnuts 12 cherries	1 cup mixed vegetable sticks 4 walnut halves 1 medium peach	1 cup cucumber sticks 1 Tbsp pumpkin seeds 1/2 cup unsweetened apricots	1 cup zucchini slices 10 peanuts 17 grapes	1 cup cucumber slices 6 cashews 3 dates
Snack B	1 4-inch waffle 1 tsp margarine **Cinnamon Apple Yogurt***	1 cup oven-baked French fries 1 cup nonfat milk	20 oyster crackers 10 peanuts 1 cup nonfat milk	1/4 cup low-fat granola 1 Tbsp sunflower seeds 1 cup nonfat milk	3 cups popcorn 1 tsp margarine 1 cup nonfat milk	2 small sandwich cookies 1 cup nonfat milk	5 vanilla wafers 6 oz fat-free yogurt
Dinner	**Red Snapper with Cinnamon Multigrain Rice Pilaf* Colorful Coleslaw*** 1 small orange 1 cup nonfat milk	**Sesame Yogurt Chicken Cold Spinach with Yogurt** 1 slice whole-wheat bread 3/4 cup unsweetened mandarin oranges 1/2 cup nonfat milk 1/2 cup carrots 1 tsp margarine 2 Brazil nuts	**Southwestern Fajitas with Pico de Gallo Baked Tomatoes and Squash*** 3/4 oz baked tortilla chips 1/2 large pear 1 cup nonfat milk	**Parmesan Pork Cutlet Three Bean Salad*** 1 large ear corn on the cob 1 small nectarine 1 cup nonfat milk 1/2 cup cooked okra 1/2 tsp margarine	**Cashew Chicken Fiesta Pasta Salad*** 3/4 cup blackberries 1/2 cup nonfat milk	**Tuna Noodle Casserole*** 2 tangerines 1 cup nonfat milk 2 cups tomato and cucumber slices 1 oz reduced-fat cheese 9 cashews	**Baked Ziti** (1/2 serving) 2 small dinner rolls 1/2 cup unsweetened applesauce 1 cup nonfat milk 1 1/2 cup vegetable sticks 1 oz reduced-fat cheese 1 1/2 tsp margarine

*Indicates that the recipe has been used previously.

SHOPPING LIST SUMMER WEEK 4

VEGETABLES
____ bell peppers, green
____ bell peppers, red
____ bell peppers, yellow
____ broccoli
____ cabbage, green
____ cabbage, purple
____ cabbage, red
____ carrots
____ cauliflower
____ celery
____ corn on the cob
____ corn, frozen
____ cucumber
____ garlic
____ green beans
____ leeks
____ lettuce, romaine
____ mushrooms
____ okra
____ onion, purple
____ onions, yellow or white
____ onions, green
____ onions, red
____ potatoes
____ spinach
____ squash, summer
____ tomatoes
____ tomatoes, grape
____ zucchini

MEATS
____ bacon, Canadian
____ bacon, turkey
____ beef steak, top round
    or top sirloin
____ beef, ground, 96% lean
____ buffalo burger
____ chicken breasts, boneless,
    skinless
____ pork chops, boneless,
    sirloin
____ red snapper fillets
____ sausage, turkey, lean
____ turkey breast, deli-style,
    light

FRUITS
____ apples
____ bananas
____ blackberries
____ blueberries
____ cantaloupe
____ grapes, green, seedless
____ lemons
____ limes
____ nectarines
____ oranges
____ oranges, mandarin,
    unsweetened
____ peaches, unsweetened
____ pears
____ pineapple
____ raisins
____ raspberries
____ strawberries
____ tangerines
____ watermelon

DAIRY
____ egg substitute
____ egg whites
____ ice cream, vanilla, fat-free
____ milk, nonfat
____ Smart Balance Light
    margarine
____ Smart Balance Light
    Spread
____ whipped topping, fat-free
____ yogurt, fat-free, plain
____ yogurt, fat-free, vanilla

CHEESE
____ cheese, any kind,
    reduced-fat
____ cottage cheese, low-fat
____ feta, reduced-fat
____ mozzarella, fat-free,
    shredded
____ Parmesan, reduced-fat
____ Swiss, reduced-fat

BREAD, GRAINS, & PASTA
____ bagels, whole-grain
____ bread, raisin
____ bread, whole-grain,
    whole-wheat
____ dinner rolls, whole-wheat
____ English muffins,
    whole-grain
____ pasta, any noodles,
    whole-grain
____ pasta, ziti, whole-grain
____ pearl barley
____ rice, brown/whole-grain
____ rice, wild

BEANS

____ cannellini (white kidney), no-added-salt, 15 1/2-oz can
____ garbanzo beans
____ kidney beans

NUTS

____ Brazil nuts
____ cashews
____ macadamia nuts
____ peanuts, dry roasted
____ walnuts

CONDIMENTS

____ canola mayonnaise

SPICES & HERBS

____ basil
____ bay leaf
____ black pepper
____ cayenne pepper
____ chili powder
____ cilantro
____ cinnamon, ground
____ cloves, ground
____ cloves, whole
____ cumin seeds
____ dill weed
____ fines herbes
____ garlic powder
____ ginger, ground
____ Italian seasoning
____ nutmeg, ground
____ paprika
____ parsley
____ pumpkin pie spice
____ red pepper flakes
____ sage
____ sesame seeds
____ thyme, ground

OTHER

____ animal crackers
____ applesauce, unsweetened
____ cereal, cornflakes
____ gelatin, raspberry, sugar-free, 0.3-oz box
____ graham crackers
____ honey
____ maple syrup, sugar-free
____ oats, old-fashioned
____ pita chips, baked
____ pretzels
____ pumpkin, canned
____ salad dressing, Italian, light
____ salad dressing, thousand island, light
____ salsa, mild or hot
____ sauerkraut
____ tomato paste, no-added-salt
____ tortillas, flour, whole-wheat, small
____ tuna, packed in water, 6-oz can
____ vanilla extract
____ wheat germ

STAPLES

____ baking powder
____ bouillon, chicken, sodium-free
____ cornstarch
____ flour, whole-wheat
____ juice, lemon
____ juice, lime
____ juice, orange
____ nonstick cooking spray
____ Smart Balance Omega oil
____ Splenda
____ Splenda Brown Sugar Blend
____ vinegar, cider
____ vinegar, white

Lemon Baked Chicken

Serves 4   Serving size: 1/4 recipe

1   **lb** boneless, skinless chicken breasts (trimmed of fat)

1   **Tbsp** grated lemon peels

1/3 **cup** lemon juice (about 2 large lemons)

2   **Tbsp** water

1   **Tbsp** minced parsley

1   **tsp** fines herbes, crushed (a blend of parsley, chives, tarragon, and chervil)

1/2 **tsp** black pepper

Exchanges/Choices

3 Lean Meat

Basic Nutritional Values

Calories 135
  Calories from Fat 25
Total Fat . . . . 3.0 g
  Saturated Fat . . . . 0.8 g
  Trans Fat . . . . 0.0 g
Cholesterol . . . . 65 mg
Sodium . . . . 65 mg
Total Carbohydrate . . . 2 g
  Dietary Fiber . . . . 0 g
  Sugars . . . . 0 g
Protein . . . . 24 g

Preheat oven to 375°F. Place the chicken in a small roasting pan. In a small bowl, combine lemon peels, lemon juice, water, parsley, and fines herbes. Pour over chicken. Bake, basting every 20 minutes with juices, for 1 hour or until tender. Spoon juices and herbs over chicken just before serving.

Oven-Baked Potatoes

Serves 4   Serving size: 1/4 recipe

4   medium potatoes

1/4 **cup** Smart Balance Light margarine

1/8 **tsp** black pepper

Exchanges/Choices

2 1/2 Starch
1/2 Fat

Basic Nutritional Values

Calories 205
  Calories from Fat 45
Total Fat . . . . 5.0 g
  Saturated Fat . . . . 1.6 g
  Trans Fat . . . . 0.0 g
Cholesterol . . . . 0 mg
Sodium . . . . 100 mg
Total Carbohydrate . . . 37 g
  Dietary Fiber . . . . 4 g
  Sugars . . . . 2 g
Protein . . . . 4 g

Wash potatoes and cut into small cubes, leaving the skins on. Place margarine on top of potatoes and bake at 350°F for about 1 hour. Check frequently and spoon the melted margarine over the potatoes. Season with pepper.

Cinnamon Apple Yogurt

Serves 4   Serving size: 1/4 serving

2 **cups** vanilla fat-free yogurt

1/2 **cup** unsweetened applesauce

4 **tsp** Splenda

2 **tsp** ground cinnamon

Spoon 1/2 cup yogurt into each of four dessert dishes. Top each with 2 Tbsp applesauce, 1 tsp Splenda, and 1/2 tsp cinnamon.

Exchanges/Choices

1 Carbohydrate

Basic Nutritional Values

Calories	90
Calories from Fat	0
Total Fat	0.0 g
Saturated Fat	0.0 g
Trans Fat	0.0 g
Cholesterol	0 mg
Sodium	65 mg
Total Carbohydrate	18 g
Dietary Fiber	0 g
Sugars	14 g
Protein	4 g

Red Snapper with Cinnamon

Serves 4   Serving size: 1/4 recipe

1 **lb** red snapper fillets

4 **tsp** Smart Balance Omega oil

1 **cup** sliced onion

2 medium cloves garlic, minced

1/2 **tsp** cinnamon

1 medium tomato, diced

1/3 **cup** orange juice

1 medium orange, peeled

In a skillet, cook fish in 3 tsp oil over medium-high heat for 3 minutes per side or until fish flakes easily with fork. Remove when done and keep warm. In the same skillet, cook the onion, garlic, and cinnamon in 1 tsp oil until soft. Stir in tomato and orange juice. Cook, uncovered, over medium-high heat for 10 minutes or until thickened, stirring occasionally. Spoon sauce over fish. Peel and cut oranges into pieces. Top fish with oranges.

Exchanges/Choices

1/2 Fruit
1 Vegetable
3 Lean Meat

Basic Nutritional Values

Calories	205
Calories from Fat	55
Total Fat	6.0 g
Saturated Fat	0.7 g
Trans Fat	0.0 g
Cholesterol	40 mg
Sodium	55 mg
Total Carbohydrate	13 g
Dietary Fiber	2 g
Sugars	8 g
Protein	25 g

Multigrain Rice Pilaf

Serves 6   Serving size: 1/6 recipe

1/2 **cup** pearl barley

1/2 **cup** parsley

1/2 **cup** wild rice, uncooked

1/2 **cup** brown rice, uncooked

2 **Tbsp** Smart Balance Light margarine

1/2 **cup** diced onion

1/4 **cup** diced celery

1 **Tbsp** sodium-free chicken bouillon

1 **cup** water

1/2 **tsp** ground thyme

1/2 **tsp** pepper

Rinse the pearl barley. Chop the parsley. Bring a large pot of water to a full boil and add the wild rice first. Let it cook for about 10 minutes and then add the barley and the brown rice (wild rice takes longer to cook). Reduce heat; simmer until tender. Drain and rinse under cold water. Melt margarine in a large skillet over medium heat. Add onions and celery; cook until tender, about 4 minutes. In a small bowl, combine the bouillon and water to create a broth. Add cooked rice mixture, broth, thyme, and pepper to the skillet; cook, stirring occasionally, until heated through, about 5 minutes. Add parsley just before serving.

Exchanges/Choices

2 1/2 Starch

Basic Nutritional Values

Calories 190
  Calories from Fat 20
Total Fat. . . . . 2.5 g
  Saturated Fat . . . . 0.7 g
  Trans Fat. . . . . 0.0 g
Cholesterol . . . . 0 mg
Sodium. . . . . 40 mg
Total Carbohydrate . . . 38 g
  Dietary Fiber. . . . . 4 g
  Sugars . . . . 2 g
Protein . . . . 4 g

Colorful Coleslaw

Serves 4   Serving size: 1/4 recipe

1 **cup** green cabbage, finely chopped

1 **cup** purple cabbage, finely chopped

1/2 **cup** diced red pepper

1/2 **cup** shredded carrots

1/2 **cup** diced onions

1/2 **cup** diced celery

1/4 **cup** cider vinegar

2 **Tbsp** water

3 **Tbsp** Splenda

1/4 **cup** Smart Balance Omega oil

Combine the vegetables in a large bowl. In a separate bowl, mix the vinegar, water, Splenda, and oil. Then toss together and chill before serving.

Exchanges/Choices

2 Vegetable
2 1/2 Fat

Basic Nutritional Values

Calories 160
  Calories from Fat 125
Total Fat. . . . . 14.0 g
  Saturated Fat . . . . 1.0 g
  Trans Fat. . . . . 0.0 g
Cholesterol . . . . 0 mg
Sodium. . . . . 30 mg
Total Carbohydrate . . . 8 g
  Dietary Fiber. . . . . 2 g
  Sugars . . . . 5 g
Protein . . . . 1 g

Zucchini Carrot Muffins

Serves 8   Serving size: 1 muffin

- **3/4 cup** rolled oats
- **2 1/2 cups** whole-wheat flour
- **2/3 cup** nonfat milk
- **1/2 cup** wheat germ, toasted
- **3 tsp** baking powder
- **3/4 cup** Splenda
- **1 Tbsp** ground cinnamon

- **2 tsp** ground nutmeg
- **3 Tbsp** Smart Balance Omega oil
- **3** egg whites, beaten
- **1 cup** carrots, finely shredded
- **1/2 cup** zucchini, stemmed and grated

Preheat oven to 350°F. Combine all ingredients and mix well; pour into muffin liners in muffin pans. Bake for about 1 hour. Let cool for about 30 minutes before removing.

Exchanges/Choices

2 1/2 Carbohydrate
1 1/2 Fat

Basic Nutritional Values

Calories	260
Calories from Fat	65
Total Fat	7.0 g
Saturated Fat	0.9 g
Trans Fat	0.0 g
Cholesterol	0 mg
Sodium	180 mg
Total Carbohydrate	42 g
Dietary Fiber	7 g
Sugars	5 g
Protein	11 g

Broccoli Floret Salad

Serves 4   Serving size: 1/4 recipe

- **2 cups** fresh or frozen broccoli florets, cut small
- **2 Tbsp** chopped parsley
- **1 Tbsp** basil
- **1** medium red pepper, thinly sliced

- Black pepper, to taste
- **1** small purple onion, diced
- **2/3 cup** light Italian salad dressing

Combine all ingredients (except dressing) in a large bowl. Add dressing. Stir well and chill for 2 hours before serving.

Exchanges/Choices

1/2 Carbohydrate
1 Vegetable
1/2 Fat

Basic Nutritional Values

Calories	80
Calories from Fat	25
Total Fat	3.0 g
Saturated Fat	0.3 g
Trans Fat	0.0 g
Cholesterol	0 mg
Sodium	480 mg
Total Carbohydrate	12 g
Dietary Fiber	2 g
Sugars	9 g
Protein	2 g

Frozen Pumpkin Dessert

Serves 4   Serving size: 1/4 recipe

Nonstick cooking spray

1/4 **cup** graham cracker crumbs

1 **tsp** Smart Balance Light Spread, melted

1/2 **cup** canned pumpkin

1/4 **cup** Splenda

1 **tsp** pumpkin pie spice

2 **cups** fat-free vanilla ice cream, softened

Lightly coat an 8-inch square baking dish with nonstick cooking spray. Mix the crumbs with the margarine. Evenly pat the crumbs into the bottom of the dish. In a medium bowl, stir together the pumpkin, Splenda, and pumpkin pie spice until well blended. In a large bowl, stir ice cream until smooth but not melted. Add the pumpkin mixture to the ice cream and mix until just well blended. Carefully pour into the baking dish. Cover dish with foil or plastic wrap. Freeze for at least 4 hours. To serve, cut into squares using a sharp knife.

Exchanges/Choices
2 Carbohydrate

Basic Nutritional Values
Calories 135
  Calories from Fat 10
Total Fat . . . . 1.0 g
  Saturated Fat . . . . 0.3 g
  Trans Fat . . . . 0.0 g
Cholesterol . . . . 0 mg
Sodium . . . . 95 mg
Total Carbohydrate . . . 30 g
  Dietary Fiber . . . . 5 g
  Sugars . . . . 17 g
Protein . . . . 4 g

Sesame Yogurt Chicken

Serves 4   Serving size: 1/4 recipe

1 **lb** boneless, skinless chicken breasts (trimmed of fat)

1 **cup** fat-free plain yogurt

3 **Tbsp** honey

1 **cup** cornflakes, crumbled

2 **Tbsp** sesame seeds

1/4 **tsp** ginger

1 **tsp** paprika

1/2 **tsp** cayenne pepper

Nonstick cooking spray

3 **Tbsp** Smart Balance Light Spread

Cut chicken into pieces. Combine honey and yogurt in a small bowl. In another bowl, combine cornflakes, sesame seeds, ginger, paprika, and cayenne pepper. Dip chicken pieces in yogurt mixture and then roll in crumb mixture until well coated. Place in a single layer on a baking sheet sprayed with nonstick cooking spray. Melt light spread and drizzle on chicken. Bake at 350°F for 1 hour or until chicken is tender. Do not cover or turn chicken during baking.

Exchanges/Choices
2 1/2 Carbohydrate
3 Lean Meat

Basic Nutritional Values
Calories 320
  Calories from Fat 65
Total Fat . . . . 7.0 g
  Saturated Fat . . . . 2.0 g
  Trans Fat . . . . 0.0 g
Cholesterol . . . . 70 mg
Sodium . . . . 320 mg
Total Carbohydrate . . . 36 g
  Dietary Fiber . . . . 1 g
  Sugars . . . . 19 g
Protein . . . . 29 g

Cold Spinach with Yogurt

Serves 4   Serving size: 1/4 recipe

16 oz spinach

1 cup fat-free plain yogurt

1 clove garlic, minced

Simmer spinach, uncovered, for 5 minutes, stirring constantly, and then allow to cool. Add yogurt and garlic. Mix thoroughly. Chill 2 hours before serving.

Exchanges/Choices

1/2 Fat-Free Milk
1 Vegetable

Basic Nutritional Values

Calories 55
  Calories from Fat 0
Total Fat . . . . 0.0 g
  Saturated Fat . . . . 0.1 g
  Trans Fat . . . . 0.0 g
Cholesterol . . . . 5 mg
Sodium . . . . 115 mg
Total Carbohydrate . . . 9 g
  Dietary Fiber . . . . 3 g
  Sugars . . . . 4 g
Protein . . . . 6 g

Oatmeal and Apple Muffins

Serves 8   Serving size: 1 muffin

1/4 **cup** egg substitute

2/3 **cup** whole-wheat flour

2 **tsp** baking powder

2 **tsp** cinnamon

1 **tsp** nutmeg

1/2 **cup** nonfat milk

1 **cup** raisins

1 apple, peeled, cored, and chopped

1/4 **cup** unsweetened applesauce

2/3 **cup** rolled oats

4 **Tbsp** Splenda Brown Sugar Blend

Exchanges/Choices

3 Carbohydrate

Basic Nutritional Values

Calories 190
  Calories from Fat 10
Total Fat . . . . 1.0 g
  Saturated Fat . . . . 0.2 g
  Trans Fat . . . . 0.0 g
Cholesterol . . . . 0 mg
Sodium . . . . 120 mg
Total Carbohydrate . . . 44 g
  Dietary Fiber . . . . 3 g
  Sugars . . . . 28 g
Protein . . . . 4 g

Preheat oven to 400°F. Beat egg substitute. Sift together flour, baking powder, cinnamon, and nutmeg. Combine all ingredients, mixing just to moisten. Spoon batter into muffin cups until 3/4 full. Bake for 15–20 minutes.

Bacon, Lettuce, and Tomato Sandwich

Serves 4   Serving size: 1 sandwich

8 **oz** turkey bacon

2 medium tomatoes, sliced

8 romaine lettuce leaves

4 **Tbsp** canola mayonnaise

8 slices light-style soft wheat bread

Exchanges/Choices

1 Starch
1 Vegetable
1 High-Fat Meat

Basic Nutritional Values

Calories 200
  Calories from Fat 80
Total Fat . . . . 9.0 g
  Saturated Fat . . . . 1.3 g
  Trans Fat . . . . 0.0 g
Cholesterol . . . . 20 mg
Sodium . . . . 555 mg
Total Carbohydrate . . . 22 g
  Dietary Fiber . . . . 4 g
  Sugars . . . . 5 g
Protein . . . . 10 g

Cook bacon according to the package directions, drain away excess fat, and pat dry with paper towels to remove any remaining fat. Layer the bacon, tomato slices, and lettuce on a slice of bread. Lightly spread mayonnaise on the other slice of bread and combine to create sandwiches.

Ambrosia Salad

Serves 4   Serving size: 1/4 recipe

1 **cup** diced oranges

2 bananas, sliced

1 **cup** seedless green grapes

1/2 **cup** raisins

2 **Tbsp** lemon juice

1/4 **cup** canola mayonnaise

2/3 **cup** fat-free whipped topping

6 **Tbsp** nonfat milk

4 small lettuce leaves

Combine the oranges, bananas, grapes, and raisins; sprinkle with lemon juice and chill. Stir in mayonnaise and mix with remaining ingredients. Serve on lettuce.

Exchanges/Choices

3 Fruit
1 Fat

Basic Nutritional Values

Calories 235
  Calories from Fat 45
Total Fat . . . . 5.0 g
  Saturated Fat . . . . 0.2 g
  Trans Fat . . . . 0.0 g
Cholesterol . . . . 0 mg
Sodium . . . . 115 mg
Total Carbohydrate . . . 47 g
  Dietary Fiber . . . . 4 g
  Sugars . . . . 33 g
Protein . . . . 3 g

Southwestern Fajitas with Pico de Gallo

Serves 4   Serving size: 1/4 recipe

1 **lb** beef top round or sirloin steak (trimmed of fat), cut into 3/4-inch thick strips

3 **Tbsp** lime juice

2 **Tbsp** Smart Balance Omega oil

2 large cloves garlic, crushed

1 **cup** tomatoes, chopped

1/2 **cup** zucchini, diced

1/4 **cup** cilantro, chopped

1/4 **cup** salsa

8 small whole-wheat flour tortillas

Lime wedges (optional)

Cilantro sprig (optional)

Exchanges/Choices

2 Starch
3 Lean Meat
1 1/2 Fat

Basic Nutritional Values

Calories 360
  Calories from Fat 110
Total Fat . . . . 12.0 g
  Saturated Fat . . . . 1.8 g
  Trans Fat . . . . 0.0 g
Cholesterol . . . . 60 mg
Sodium . . . . 525 mg
Total Carbohydrate . . . 32 g
  Dietary Fiber . . . . 5 g
  Sugars . . . . 4 g
Protein . . . . 29 g

1. Place beef strips in a resealable plastic bag; add 2 Tbsp lime juice, oil, and garlic, turning to coat. Securely close bag and marinate in refrigerator for 2 hours or longer, turning once.

2. In a medium bowl, prepare the pico de gallo: combine tomatoes, zucchini, cilantro, salsa, and 1 Tbsp lime juice, mixing well.

3. Remove steak from marinade, discard marinade. Place steak on a grill over medium ash-covered coals. Grill top round steak, uncovered, for 8–9 minutes (10–12 for top sirloin steak) for medium-rare to medium doneness, turning occasionally.

4. Wrap tortillas in heavy-duty aluminum foil. During the last 5 minutes of cooking, place wrapped tortillas on outer edge of grill, turning occasionally. Serve beef in tortillas with pico de gallo and optional lime wedges and cilantro sprigs.

Baked Tomatoes and Squash

Serves 4   Serving size: 1/4 recipe

2 medium summer squash (about 1/2 lb each)

1 (10-oz) pkg frozen spinach, cooked and drained

3 oz reduced-fat feta cheese, crumbled

1/4 cup dry whole-wheat bread crumbs

1/4 cup green onions, finely chopped

2 Tbsp minced parsley

1/2 tsp dill weed

2 medium tomatoes

4 tsp reduced-fat grated Parmesan cheese

Paprika, to taste

Exchanges/Choices

2 Vegetable
1 Lean Meat
1 Fat

Basic Nutritional Values

Calories 135
  Calories from Fat 40
Total Fat . . . . 4.5 g
  Saturated Fat . . . . 2.6 g
  Trans Fat . . . . 0.0 g
Cholesterol . . . . 10 mg
Sodium . . . . 415 mg
Total Carbohydrate . . . 16 g
  Dietary Fiber . . . . 5 g
  Sugars . . . . 5 g
Protein . . . . 11 g

1. Preheat oven to 375°F.

2. Cut squash in half lengthwise. Scoop out centers (leaving a 1/2-inch shell) and reserve pulp and seeds. In a large skillet over medium heat, bring 1 inch of water to a boil. Add squash shells, cover, and cook for 10 minutes or until fork-tender. Remove shells and drain well; then transfer to a baking dish.

3. In a medium bowl, combine squash pulp with spinach, feta cheese, bread crumbs, green onions, parsley, and dill weed. Mound 1/4 of the mixture into each squash shell, packing lightly. Bake for 10 minutes.

4. Remove stems from tomatoes and cut in half crosswise. Sprinkle top of each half with 1 tsp Parmesan cheese. Place tomatoes beside squash in baking dish. Bake 15–20 minutes longer or until spinach mixture is set and vegetables are heated through. Sprinkle spinach with paprika and serve.

Bread Pudding

Serves 10   Serving size: 1/10 recipe

Nonstick cooking spray

2 **cups** stale whole-wheat bread, cut into 1/2-inch cubes

3/4 **cup** raisins

1/4 **cup** chopped walnuts

4 **cups** nonfat milk

3/4 **cup** Splenda

3/4 **cup** egg substitute

2 **tsp** ground cinnamon

2 **tsp** pure vanilla extract

1/4 **cup** Smart Balance margarine

Preheat oven to 325°F. Spray a shallow 1 1/2-quart casserole with nonstick cooking spray. Place bread cubes, raisins, and nuts in casserole. In a large bowl, combine milk, Splenda, egg substitute, cinnamon, and vanilla. Pour over bread mixture; mix well. Dot with margarine. Place casserole in a large baking pan; fill pan with hot water to a depth of 1 inch. Bake for 45–55 minutes or until a knife inserted halfway between center and edge of casserole comes out clean. Serve warm or cold.

Exchanges/Choices

1/2 Fat-Free Milk
1 Carbohydrate
1 Fat

Basic Nutritional Values

Calories 165
  Calories from Fat 55
Total Fat . . . . 6.0 g
  Saturated Fat . . . . 1.3 g
  Trans Fat . . . . 0.0 g
Cholesterol . . . . 0 mg
Sodium . . . . 175 mg
Total Carbohydrate . . . 21 g
  Dietary Fiber . . . . 2 g
  Sugars . . . . 14 g
Protein . . . . 8 g

Deli Turkey and Swiss on Rye

Serves 4   Serving size: 1 sandwich

8 **oz** deli-style light turkey

4 slices reduced-fat Swiss cheese

4 **Tbsp** canola mayonnaise

4 leaves romaine lettuce

2 medium tomatoes, sliced

8 slices whole-grain bread

Place equal amounts of turkey, cheese, mayonnaise, lettuce, and tomatoes between slices of bread.

This recipe is high in sodium.

Exchanges/Choices

2 Starch
3 Lean Meat
1/2 Fat

Basic Nutritional Values

Calories 300
  Calories from Fat 90
Total Fat . . . . 10.0 g
  Saturated Fat . . . . 2.0 g
  Trans Fat . . . . 0.0 g
Cholesterol . . . . 35 mg
Sodium . . . . 1235 mg
Total Carbohydrate . . 30 g
  Dietary Fiber . . . . 6 g
  Sugars . . . . 8 g
Protein . . . . 24 g

Parmesan Pork Cutlet

Serves 4   Serving size: 1/4 recipe

- 1/2 **cup** egg substitute
- 2 cloves garlic, minced
- 3 **Tbsp** grated Parmesan cheese
- 1 **Tbsp** chopped parsley
  Dash black pepper
- 2 **tsp** Smart Balance margarine
- 3/4 **lb** boneless sirloin pork chops (trimmed of fat)
- 3 **Tbsp** whole-wheat flour
- 1 **Tbsp** lemon juice

Combine egg substitute, garlic, Parmesan cheese, parsley, and pepper. Heat margarine in a large skillet over medium-high heat. Dip pork cutlets in whole-wheat flour and then into egg batter. Sauté cutlets until golden brown, about 2–3 minutes per side, turning once. Serve sprinkled with lemon juice.

Exchanges/Choices

1/2 Carbohydrate
3 Lean Meat

Basic Nutritional Values

Calories 155
  Calories from Fat 45
Total Fat . . . . 5.0 g
  Saturated Fat . . . . 1.3 g
  Trans Fat . . . . 0.0 g
Cholesterol . . . . 45 mg
Sodium . . . . 370 mg
Total Carbohydrate . . . 8 g
  Dietary Fiber . . . . 1 g
  Sugars . . . . 0 g
Protein . . . . 20 g

Three Bean Salad

Serves 4   Serving size: 1/4 recipe

- 1/2 **cup** green beans, drained (if using canned)
- 1/2 **cup** kidney beans, rinsed and drained
- 1/4 **cup** garbanzo beans, rinsed and drained
- 1/4 **cup** green pepper, diced
- 1/2 **cup** onions, diced
- 2 **Tbsp** Smart Balance Omega oil
- 1/2 **cup** cider vinegar
- 1/4 **cup** Splenda
  Pepper, to taste

In a bowl, gently mix together the beans, pepper, and onions. Pour the liquids and other seasonings over the beans. Mix well and chill before serving.

Exchanges/Choices

1/2 Starch
1 Vegetable
1 1/2 Fat

Basic Nutritional Values

Calories 130
  Calories from Fat 65
Total Fat . . . . 7.0 g
  Saturated Fat . . . . 0.5 g
  Trans Fat . . . . 0.0 g
Cholesterol . . . . 0 mg
Sodium . . . . 55 mg
Total Carbohydrate . . . 13 g
  Dietary Fiber . . . . 3 g
  Sugars . . . . 4 g
Protein . . . . 3 g

French Toast

Serves 4   Serving size: 2 slices

- 1 **Tbsp** Splenda
- 1/2 **tsp** pure vanilla extract
- 2 **cups** nonfat milk
- 1 **cup** egg substitute
- 8 slices whole-grain bread
- 2 **Tbsp** Smart Balance Light Spread

Beat Splenda, vanilla, milk, and egg substitute with a beater until well blended and smooth. Soak bread in batter. Heat margarine in skillet and carefully transfer bread to the skillet. Cook bread over medium heat until browned and then flip to cook the other side.

Exchanges/Choices

1 1/2 Starch
1/2 Fat-Free Milk
1 Lean Meat
1/2 Fat

Basic Nutritional Values

Calories	240
Calories from Fat	40
Total Fat	4.5 g
Saturated Fat	1.2 g
Trans Fat	0.0 g
Cholesterol	0 mg
Sodium	485 mg
Total Carbohydrate	31 g
Dietary Fiber	4 g
Sugars	10 g
Protein	18 g

Spicy Whole-Grain Rice with Peanuts

Serves 4   Serving size: 1/4 recipe

- 2 **Tbsp** Smart Balance Omega oil
- 2 **tsp** cumin seed
- 1 **tsp** whole cloves
- 1 bay leaf
- 1 **tsp** red pepper flakes
- 1/2 **cup** onion, minced
- 1 medium garlic clove, minced
- 2/3 **cup** whole-grain rice, uncooked
- 2 1/2 **cups** water
- 1/4 **cup** dry roasted peanuts

Exchanges/Choices

2 Starch
2 Fat

Basic Nutritional Values

Calories	245
Calories from Fat	115
Total Fat	13.0 g
Saturated Fat	1.3 g
Trans Fat	0.0 g
Cholesterol	0 mg
Sodium	80 mg
Total Carbohydrate	29 g
Dietary Fiber	3 g
Sugars	2 g
Protein	5 g

1. In a large heavy saucepan, heat the oil over moderate heat until it is hot. Add cumin seed, cloves, and bay leaf; cook, stirring constantly, for 5–10 seconds or until the cumin seed is a few shades darker and fragrant. Add the red pepper flakes, onion, and garlic; cook, stirring constantly, until the onion has softened. Add the rice and cook, while stirring, for 2 minutes or until it is well coated with the mixture. Add water; bring to a boil. Simmer covered for 35–40 minutes or until the water is absorbed and the rice is fluffy and tender.

2. Put the peanuts in a blender and grind for a few seconds. Fluff the rice with a fork, remove the pan from the heat, and discard the bay leaf. Let the rice stand, covered, for 10 minutes. Stir in the peanuts and serve.

Sweet and Sour Red Cabbage

Serves 4   Serving size: 1/4 recipe

2 medium tart apples	**1 Tbsp** vinegar
1/2 cup water	**1/4 tsp** ground cloves
6 Tbsp chopped onions	**1/2** medium head red cabbage
2 Tbsp Splenda Brown Sugar Blend	(about 2 lb), wedged, cored, and thinly sliced

Peel and slice apples 1/4 inch thick. In a 5-quart Dutch oven over medium heat, combine apples, water, onions, Splenda, vinegar, and cloves. Stir cabbage into apple mixture. Bring to a boil; reduce heat to low, cover, and simmer for 1 hour or until cabbage is tender. Uncover and boil for about 5 minutes more to reduce liquid, stirring occasionally.

Exchanges/Choices

1 1/2 Carbohydrate

Basic Nutritional Values

Calories 95
  Calories from Fat 0
Total Fat. . . . . .0.0 g
  Saturated Fat . . . . .0.0 g
  Trans Fat . . . . .0.0 g
Cholesterol . . . . .0 mg
Sodium. . . . . .15 mg
Total Carbohydrate . . .23 g
  Dietary Fiber . . . . .3 g
  Sugars . . . . .19 g
Protein . . . . .2 g

Cashew Chicken

Serves 4   Serving size: 1/4 recipe

3/4 cup orange juice	**4** green onions, chopped
1/4 cup honey	**3** large carrots, peeled and sliced
1 Tbsp cornstarch	
1 tsp ground ginger	**2** celery stalks, sliced
1 tsp garlic powder	**1 lb** boneless, skinless chicken breasts, cut into 1-inch strips
1/2 tsp pepper	
2 Tbsp Smart Balance Omega oil	**1/4 cup** cashews

In a medium bowl, combine orange juice, honey, cornstarch, ginger, garlic powder, and pepper. Heat 1 Tbsp oil in a skillet. Stir-fry green onions, carrots, and celery for several minutes, until the onions are soft; set aside. Remove vegetables from skillet; heat 1 Tbsp oil and stir-fry chicken strips until browned and tender. Add cooked vegetables, cashews, and sauce mix. Continue cooking until sauce bubbles and thickens.

Exchanges/Choices

2 Carbohydrate
1 Vegetable
3 Lean Meat
1 1/2 Fat

Basic Nutritional Values

Calories 365
  Calories from Fat 125
Total Fat. . . . . .14.0 g
  Saturated Fat . . . . .2.1 g
  Trans Fat . . . . .0.0 g
Cholesterol . . . . .65 mg
Sodium. . . . . .120 mg
Total Carbohydrate . . .35 g
  Dietary Fiber . . . . .3 g
  Sugars . . . . .26 g
Protein . . . . .27 g

Fiesta Pasta Salad

Serves 4   Serving size: 1/4 recipe

4 oz whole-wheat pasta	**1** medium garlic clove, minced
1/2 cup tomato, peeled and diced	**1/2 cup** carrot, shredded
1/2 medium red pepper	**1 Tbsp** cilantro, chopped
1/2 medium green pepper	**1 Tbsp** Smart Balance Omega oil
1/2 medium yellow pepper	
1/2 medium red onion	**1 tsp** ground cumin seed
1/2 cup corn, frozen	**1/4 tsp** cayenne pepper
1/4 cup salsa, mild or hot	**1/4 tsp** chili powder

Cook pasta according to package directions; rinse and drain. Dice tomatoes, chop peppers and red onion. Thaw corn; cook in microwave for about 2 minutes. Place pasta in a large bowl; add all other ingredients and mix to blend. Chill for 1 hour before serving.

Exchanges/Choices

1 1/2 Starch
2 Vegetable
1/2 Fat

Basic Nutritional Values

Calories	185
Calories from Fat	40
Total Fat	4.5 g
Saturated Fat	0.4 g
Trans Fat	0.0 g
Cholesterol	0 mg
Sodium	115 mg
Total Carbohydrate	34 g
Dietary Fiber	6 g
Sugars	5 g
Protein	5 g

Peach and Apple Crisp

Serves 4   Serving size: 1/4 recipe

2 **cups** sliced peaches (fresh, frozen, or canned light)

1 1/2 **cups** apples, peeled and sliced

3 1/2 **Tbsp** Splenda

2 **Tbsp + 2 tsp** whole-wheat flour

1 **tsp** ground cinnamon

1 **tsp** ground nutmeg

3 **Tbsp** old-fashioned oats

2 **Tbsp** Smart Balance Light margarine, melted

Preheat oven to 400°F. Place peaches and apples in a large bowl. In a small bowl, mix 2 Tbsp Splenda, 2 tsp flour, 1/2 tsp cinnamon, and 1/2 tsp nutmeg. Sprinkle over fruit and toss until fruit is evenly coated; mound mixture in a 1-quart casserole. In a small bowl, mix oats, 2 Tbsp flour, 1 1/2 Tbsp Splenda, 1/2 tsp cinnamon, and 1/2 tsp nutmeg. Stir in margarine until mixture is evenly moistened. Spoon over fruit. Bake in lower third of the oven for 30 minutes or until juices are bubbly and topping is browned. Serve warm.

Exchanges/Choices

1 1/2 Carbohydrate
1/2 Fat

Basic Nutritional Values

Calories	130
Calories from Fat	40
Total Fat	4.5 g
Saturated Fat	1.3 g
Trans Fat	0.0 g
Cholesterol	0 mg
Sodium	40 mg
Total Carbohydrate	22 g
Dietary Fiber	3 g
Sugars	14 g
Protein	2 g

Turkey Reuben Sandwich

Serves 4   Serving size: 1 sandwich

1/4 **cup** light thousand island salad dressing

8 slices whole-grain bread

4 **oz** deli-style light turkey breast

1/2 **cup** sauerkraut, rinsed and well drained

3 **oz** reduced-fat Swiss cheese
Nonstick cooking spray

Spread salad dressing on one side of each slice of bread. Top 4 bread slices with turkey, sauerkraut, and cheese. Top with remaining bread slices, dressing side down. Spray a large skillet with nonstick cooking spray. Cook sandwiches over medium heat for 4–6 minutes or until bread is toasted and cheese melted, turning once.

This recipe is high in sodium.

Exchanges/Choices

2 Starch
3 Lean Meat

Basic Nutritional Values

Calories	275
Calories from Fat	55
Total Fat	6.0 g
Saturated Fat	2.0 g
Trans Fat	0.0 g
Cholesterol	35 mg
Sodium	990 mg
Total Carbohydrate	31 g
Dietary Fiber	4 g
Sugars	4 g
Protein	25 g

Perfection Salad

Serves 4   Serving size: 1/4 recipe

1 (0.3-oz) box sugar-free raspberry gelatin

2 tsp vinegar

1/2 head cabbage, shredded

2 carrots, shredded

Make gelatin according to package directions. Add vinegar, cabbage, and carrots. Refrigerate 2 hours before serving.

Exchanges/Choices

2 Vegetable

Basic Nutritional Values

Calories 50
  Calories from Fat 0
Total Fat. . . . . .0.0 g
  Saturated Fat . . . . .0.0 g
  Trans Fat. . . . . .0.0 g
Cholesterol . . . . .0 mg
Sodium. . . . . .105 mg
Total Carbohydrate . . .10 g
  Dietary Fiber. . . . . .4 g
  Sugars . . . . .6 g
Protein . . . . .3 g

Tuna Noodle Casserole

Serves 4   Serving size: 1/4 recipe

4 oz dry whole-wheat noodles, narrow or wide

1 (6-oz) can tuna packed in water, drained

4 oz mushrooms

1 cup low-fat cottage cheese

1/2 cup nonfat milk

1/4 cup bread crumbs

1/4 cup reduced-fat Parmesan cheese

Cook noodles according to package directions. Drain. Mix the cooked noodles with the tuna, mushrooms, cottage cheese, milk, and any other seasoning you may desire in a large casserole. Sprinkle the bread crumbs and cheese over the top. Bake uncovered at 350°F until hot and bubbly, about 40 minutes. Let stand 5 minutes before serving.

Exchanges/Choices

2 Starch
2 Lean Meat
1/2 Fat

Basic Nutritional Values

Calories 280
  Calories from Fat 65
Total Fat. . . . . .7.0 g
  Saturated Fat . . . . .2.2 g
  Trans Fat. . . . . .0.0 g
Cholesterol . . . . .20 mg
Sodium. . . . . .455 mg
Total Carbohydrate . . .34 g
  Dietary Fiber. . . . . .3 g
  Sugars . . . . .4 g
Protein . . . . .22 g

Chicken and White Bean Soup

Serves 4   Serving size: 1/4 recipe

- **3/4 lb** boneless, skinless chicken breasts
- **2 tsp** Smart Balance Omega oil
- **2** leeks, washed and cut into 1/4-inch rounds
- **1 Tbsp** chopped sage (or 1/4 tsp dried sage)
- **2 Tbsp** sodium-free chicken bouillon
- **2 cups** water
- **1** (**15 1/2-oz**) can no-added-salt cannellini (white kidney) beans, rinsed

Boil the chicken breasts until cooked; set aside until cool. When chicken is cool, shred it. Heat oil in a soup pot or large Dutch oven over medium-high heat. Add leeks and cook, stirring often, until soft, about 3 minutes. Stir in sage and continue cooking until aromatic, about 30 seconds. Stir in bouillon and water, increase heat to high, cover, and bring to a boil. Add beans and chicken; cook, stirring occasionally, until heated through, about 3 minutes. Serve hot.

Exchanges/Choices

1 Starch
1 Vegetable
3 Lean Meat

Basic Nutritional Values

Calories	250
Calories from Fat	45
Total Fat	5.0 g
Saturated Fat	0.8 g
Trans Fat	0.0 g
Cholesterol	50 mg
Sodium	60 mg
Total Carbohydrate	26 g
Dietary Fiber	5 g
Sugars	5 g
Protein	25 g

German Potato Salad

Serves 4   Serving size: 1/4 recipe

- **4 cups** potatoes
- **4** slices turkey bacon
- **1/2 cup** chopped onions
- **2 Tbsp** whole-wheat flour
- **1 cup** water
- **1/2 cup** cider vinegar
- **2 1/2 Tbsp** Splenda
- **1/16 tsp** black pepper

Peel and dice the potatoes; place in boiling water. Cook until just soft. Fry bacon in a large skillet until crisp; remove and drain. Place the onions in the skillet and cook until tender. Slowly stir in flour; blend well. Add water and vinegar; cook, stirring, until bubbly and slightly thick. Stir in Splenda and pepper; simmer for 10 minutes. Crumble bacon. Carefully stir bacon and potatoes into hot mixture. Heat through, stirring gently to coat potato slices. Serve warm.

Exchanges/Choices

2 Starch

Basic Nutritional Values

Calories	160
Calories from Fat	25
Total Fat	3.0 g
Saturated Fat	0.8 g
Trans Fat	0.0 g
Cholesterol	15 mg
Sodium	180 mg
Total Carbohydrate	28 g
Dietary Fiber	3 g
Sugars	4 g
Protein	5 g

Baked Ziti

Serves 4   Serving size: 1/4 recipe

1 lb 96% lean ground beef

1/4 cup chopped onions

1 clove garlic, minced

1 cup water

1/2 cup no-added-salt tomato paste

1 tsp Italian seasoning

1/16 tsp black pepper

4 oz dry ziti

2 oz fat-free shredded mozzarella cheese

Preheat oven to 350°F. In a 10-inch skillet over medium heat, cook the beef, onion, and garlic, breaking up meat as it browns. Drain fat. Stir in water, tomato paste, Italian seasoning, and pepper. Stirring occasionally, simmer for 5 minutes or until thickened. Cook ziti noodles according to package directions; drain. Stir ziti into beef mixture. Spoon into a 1-quart casserole. Sprinkle with cheese. Bake for 20 minutes or until cheese is melted and mixture is hot and bubbly.

Exchanges/Choices

1 1/2 Starch
1 Vegetable
4 Lean Meat
1/2 Fat

Basic Nutritional Values

Calories 340
  Calories from Fat 90
Total Fat . . . . 10.0 g
  Saturated Fat . . . . 3.7 g
  Trans Fat . . . . 0.6 g
Cholesterol . . . . 70 mg
Sodium . . . . 250 mg
Total Carbohydrate . . . 30 g
  Dietary Fiber . . . . 3 g
  Sugars . . . . 3 g
Protein . . . . 31 g

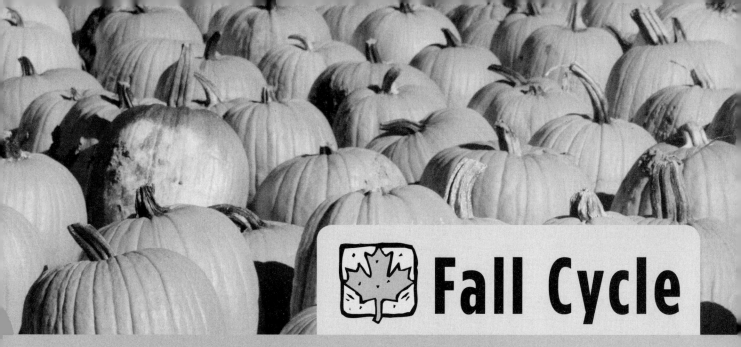

Fall Cycle

WEEK 1

FEATURED RECIPES

Herb Chicken
Ratatouille
Prune Delight Spread*
Stuffed Peppers
Lemon Parsley Carrots*
Whole-Wheat Blueberry Muffins*
Egg Salad
Peas and Cheese Salad*
New Orleans Chilled Rice*
Scallops Provençal
Stir-Fry Vegetables*
Apple Crisp
Sauerkraut Salad*
German Potato Salad*
Baked Sole
Italian-Style Zucchini with Whole-Wheat Pasta*

Low-Fat Corn Bread*
Grilled Vegetable Wrap
Bread Pudding*
Turkey Tetrazzini
Spaghetti with Meat Sauce
Beef Stew
Pumpkin Spice Muffins*
Chicken Pasta Salad
Tangerine Broccoli
Citrus Dijon Pork
Skillet Green Bean Casserole
Whole-Wheat French Toast
Meatloaf
Cauliflower au Gratin
Caribbean Ham Slice

*Indicates that the recipe has been used previously.

1500 calorie MEAL PLAN FALL WEEK 1

	Sunday	Monday	Tuesday	Wednesday	Thursday	Friday	Saturday
Breakfast	1/2 cup grits 1 slice multigrain bread 1 1/4 cup strawberries 1 cup nonfat milk 3 macadamia nuts 1/2 tsp margarine	**Whole-Wheat Blueberry Muffins*** 1 cup Rice Chex cereal 1 medium banana 1 cup nonfat milk 1 oz lean turkey sausage	**Apple Crisp** 1 slice whole-wheat bread 1 Tbsp dried fruit 1 cup nonfat milk 1/2 tsp margarine	**Low-Fat Corn Bread*** 1 kiwi fruit 1 cup nonfat milk 1 Tbsp cashew butter	1 cup Kashi cereal 1 1/4 cup strawberries 1 cup nonfat milk 8 pecans	**Pumpkin Spice Muffins*** 1/2 Tbsp jam 1 cup cantaloupe 1 cup nonfat milk 1 Tbsp peanut butter	**Whole-Wheat French Toast** 2 Tbsp sugar-free maple syrup 3/4 cup pineapple 1 cup nonfat milk
Lunch	**Herb Chicken Ratatouille Prune Delight Spread*** 3/4 cup steamed peas 1/4 cup cranberry sauce	**Egg Salad Peas and Cheese Salad*** **New Orleans Chilled Rice*** 1/2 large pear	**Sauerkraut Salad*** **German Potato Salad*** 4 oz smoked sausage 2 Tbsp raisins 8 large black olives	**Grilled Vegetable Wrap Bread Pudding*** 1 medium peach 1/4 cup low-fat cottage cheese	**Spaghetti with Meat Sauce** 3/4 cup mixed berries 1 Tbsp sunflower seeds	**Chicken Pasta Salad Tangerine Broccoli** (2 servings) 1/2 cup cooked Brussels sprouts 10 peanuts	**Meatloaf** (1/2 serving) **Cauliflower au Gratin** 1/2 cup sweet potatoes 1 dinner roll 1/2 cup unsweetened applesauce 1/2 tsp margarine
Snack A							
Snack B							
Dinner	**Stuffed Peppers Lemon Parsley Carrots*** 4 1/2 oz red potatoes 1/2 cup unsweetened peaches 1 cup nonfat milk	**Scallops Provençal Stir-Fry Vegetables*** 2/3 cup brown rice 1/2 tsp margarine	**Baked Sole Italian-Style Zucchini with Whole-Wheat Pasta*** 1 small nectarine 1 cup nonfat milk 24 pistachios	**Turkey Tetrazzini** 1/2 cup nonfat milk 1 cup steamed carrots	**Beef Stew** 12 cherries 1 cup nonfat milk 1 cup salad greens 1 1/2 Tbsp light salad dressing	**Citrus Dijon Pork Skillet Green Bean Casserole** 2/3 cup brown rice 1/2 cup nonfat milk 10 hazelnuts	**Caribbean Ham Slice** 1/2 cup brown rice 1 cup cooked kale 2 tsp margarine

*Indicates that the recipe has been used previously.

	Sunday	Monday	Tuesday	Wednesday	Thursday	Friday	Saturday
Breakfast	1/2 cup grits 1 slice multigrain bread 1 1/4 cup strawberries 1 cup nonfat milk 3 macadamia nuts 1/2 tsp margarine	**Whole-Wheat Blueberry Muffins*** 1 cup Rice Chex cereal 1 medium banana 1 cup nonfat milk 1 oz lean turkey sausage 3 Brazil nuts	**Apple Crisp** 1 slice whole-wheat bread 1 Tbsp dried fruit 1 cup nonfat milk 1/4 cup egg substitute, scrambled 1/2 tsp margarine	**Low-Fat Corn Bread*** 1 kiwi fruit 1 cup nonfat milk 1 oz Canadian bacon 1 Tbsp cashew butter	1 cup Kashi cereal 1 1/4 cup strawberries 1 cup nonfat milk 1/4 cup egg substitute 8 pecans	**Pumpkin Spice Muffins*** 1/2 Tbsp jam 1 cup cantaloupe 1 cup nonfat milk 1 Tbsp peanut butter	**Whole-Wheat French Toast** 2 Tbsp sugar-free maple syrup 3/4 cup pineapple 1 cup nonfat milk
Lunch	**Herb Chicken Ratatouille Prune Delight Spread*** 3/4 cup steamed peas 1/4 cup cranberry sauce	**Egg Salad Peas and Cheese Salad*** **New Orleans Chilled Rice*** 1/2 large pear	**Sauerkraut Salad*** **German Potato Salad*** 4 oz smoked sausage 2 Tbsp raisins 8 large black olives 5 hazelnuts	**Grilled Vegetable Wrap Bread Pudding*** 1 medium peach 1/4 cup low-fat cottage cheese 4 pecans	**Spaghetti with Meat Sauce** 3/4 cup mixed berries 2 Tbsp sunflower seeds	**Chicken Pasta Salad Tangerine Broccoli** (2 servings) 1/2 cup cooked Brussels sprouts 10 peanuts	**Meatloaf** (1/2 serving) **Cauliflower au Gratin** 1/2 cup sweet potatoes 1 dinner roll 1/2 cup unsweetened applesauce 1/2 tsp margarine
Snack A	10 peanuts 17 grapes	1 1/2 tsp cashew butter 1 small apple	10 peanuts 4 whole apricots	1 Tbsp pine nuts 1 cup papaya	6 almonds 1/2 cup fruit cocktail in light syrup	6 cashews 3 oz frozen juice bar	2 Brazil nuts 3/4 cup blackberries
Snack B	6 oz fat-free yogurt	1 cup nonfat milk	1 cup nonfat milk	1 cup nonfat milk	6 oz fat-free yogurt	1 cup nonfat milk	1 cup nonfat milk
Dinner	**Stuffed Peppers Lemon Parsley Carrots*** 4 1/2 oz red potatoes 1/2 cup unsweetened peaches 1 cup nonfat milk 1 oz reduced-fat cheese	**Scallops Provençal Stir-Fry Vegetables*** 2/3 cup brown rice 1 oz reduced-fat cheese 1/2 tsp margarine	**Baked Sole Italian-Style Zucchini with Whole-Wheat Pasta*** 1 small nectarine 1 cup nonfat milk 24 pistachios	**Turkey Tetrazzini** 1/2 cup nonfat milk 1 cup steamed carrots	**Beef Stew** 12 cherries 1 cup nonfat milk 1 cup salad greens 1 1/2 Tbsp light salad dressing	**Citrus Dijon Pork Skillet Green Bean Casserole** 2/3 cup brown rice 1/2 cup nonfat milk 10 hazelnuts	**Caribbean Ham Slice** 1/2 cup brown rice 1 cup cooked kale 1 oz reduced-fat cheese 2 tsp margarine

*Indicates that the recipe has been used previously.

2000 calorie MEAL PLAN FALL WEEK 1

	Sunday	Monday	Tuesday	Wednesday	Thursday	Friday	Saturday
Breakfast	1/2 cup grits 1 slice multigrain bread 1 1/4 cup strawberries 1 cup nonfat milk 3 macadamia nuts 1/2 tsp margarine	**Whole-Wheat Blueberry Muffins*** 1 cup Rice Chex cereal 1 medium banana 1 cup nonfat milk 1 oz lean turkey sausage 3 Brazil nuts	**Apple Crisp** 1 slice whole-wheat bread 1 Tbsp dried fruit 1 cup nonfat milk 1/4 cup egg substitute, scrambled 1/2 tsp margarine	**Low-Fat Corn Bread*** 1 kiwi fruit 1 cup nonfat milk 1 oz Canadian bacon 1 Tbsp cashew butter	1 cup Kashi cereal 1 1/4 cup strawberries 1 cup nonfat milk 1/4 cup egg substitute 8 pecans	**Pumpkin Spice Muffins*** 1/2 Tbsp jam 1 cup cantaloupe 1 cup nonfat milk 1 Tbsp peanut butter	**Whole-Wheat French Toast** 2 Tbsp sugar-free maple syrup 3/4 cup pineapple 1 cup nonfat milk
Lunch	**Herb Chicken Ratatouille Prune Delight Spread*** 1 cup steamed peas 1/4 cup cranberry sauce 8 grapes	**Egg Salad Peas and Cheese Salad*** **New Orleans Chilled Rice*** 1/2 large pear	**Sauerkraut Salad*** **German Potato Salad*** 4 oz smoked sausage 2 Tbsp raisins 1 small apple 8 large black olives 5 hazelnuts	**Grilled Vegetable Wrap Bread Pudding*** 1 large peach 1/4 cup low-fat cottage cheese 4 pecans	**Spaghetti with Meat Sauce** 1 1/2 cup mixed berries 2 Tbsp sunflower seeds	**Chicken Pasta Salad Tangerine Broccoli** (2 servings) 1 medium banana 1 cup cooked Brussels sprouts 10 peanuts	**Meatloaf** (1/2 serving) **Cauliflower au Gratin** 1/2 cup sweet potatoes 1 dinner roll 1 cup unsweetened applesauce 1/2 tsp margarine
Snack A	1 cup celery sticks 10 peanuts 17 grapes	1 cup carrot sticks 1 1/2 tsp cashew butter 1 small apple	1 cup grape tomatoes 1 Tbsp light salad dressing 4 whole apricots	1 cup broccoli 1 Tbsp pine nuts 1 cup papaya	1 cup raw cauliflower 6 almonds 1/2 cup fruit cocktail in light syrup	1 cup green pepper slices 3 oz frozen juice bar	1 cup cucumber slices 2 Brazil nuts 3/4 cup blackberries
Snack B	3/4 oz whole-wheat crackers 1 1/2 tsp almond butter 6 oz fat-free yogurt	3/4 chewy fruit bar 1 cup nonfat milk	8 animal crackers 10 peanuts 1 cup nonfat milk	1/4 cup granola 1 cup nonfat milk	1 cup oven-baked French fries 6 oz fat-free yogurt	5 vanilla wafers 1 cup nonfat milk	2 small sandwich cookies 1 cup nonfat milk
Dinner	**Stuffed Peppers Lemon Parsley Carrots*** 4 1/2 oz red potatoes 1/2 cup unsweetened peaches 1 cup nonfat milk 1 oz reduced-fat cheese	**Scallops Provençal Stir-Fry Vegetables*** 2/3 cup brown rice 1 oz reduced-fat cheese 1/2 tsp margarine	**Baked Sole Italian-Style Zucchini with Whole-Wheat Pasta*** 1 small nectarine 1 cup nonfat milk 24 pistachios	**Turkey Tetrazzini** 1/2 cup nonfat milk 1 cup steamed carrots	**Beef Stew** 12 cherries 1 cup nonfat milk 1 cup salad greens 1 1/2 Tbsp light salad dressing	**Citrus Dijon Pork Skillet Green Bean Casserole** 2/3 cup brown rice 1/2 cup nonfat milk 10 hazelnuts	**Caribbean Ham Slice** 1/2 cup brown rice 1 cup cooked kale 1 oz reduced-fat cheese 2 tsp margarine

*Indicates that the recipe has been used previously.

	Sunday	Monday	Tuesday	Wednesday	Thursday	Friday	Saturday
Breakfast	1/2 cup grits 1 slice multigrain bread 1 1/4 cup strawberries 1 cup nonfat milk 1/4 cup egg substitute, scrambled 3 macadamia nuts 1/2 tsp margarine	**Whole-Wheat Blueberry Muffins*** 1 cup Rice Chex cereal 1 medium banana 1 cup nonfat milk 2 oz lean turkey sausage 3 Brazil nuts	**Apple Crisp** 1 slice whole-wheat bread 1 Tbsp dried fruit 1 cup nonfat milk 1/2 cup egg substitute, scrambled 1/2 tsp margarine	**Low-Fat Corn Bread*** 1 kiwi fruit 1 cup nonfat milk 2 oz Canadian bacon 1 Tbsp cashew butter	1 cup Kashi cereal 1 1/4 cup strawberries 1 cup nonfat milk 1/2 cup egg substitute 8 pecans	**Pumpkin Spice Muffins*** 1/2 Tbsp jam 1 cup cantaloupe 1 cup nonfat milk 1 oz Canadian bacon 1 Tbsp peanut butter	**Whole-Wheat French Toast** 2 Tbsp sugar-free maple syrup 3/4 cup pineapple 1 cup nonfat milk 1 oz lean turkey sausage
Lunch	**Herb Chicken Ratatouille Prune Delight Spread*** 3/4 cup steamed peas 1/4 cup cranberry sauce 8 small grapes	**Egg Salad Peas and Cheese Salad*** **New Orleans Chilled Rice*** 1/2 large pear	**Sauerkraut Salad*** **German Potato Salad*** 4 oz smoked sausage 2 Tbsp raisins 1 small apple 8 large black olives 5 hazelnuts	**Grilled Vegetable Wrap Bread Pudding*** 1 large peach 1/4 cup low-fat cottage cheese 4 pecans	**Spaghetti with Meat Sauce** 1 1/2 cup mixed berries 2 Tbsp sunflower seeds	**Chicken Pasta Salad Tangerine Broccoli** (2 servings) 1 medium banana 1 cup cooked Brussels sprouts 10 peanuts	**Meatloaf** (1/2 serving) **Cauliflower au Gratin** 1/2 cup sweet potatoes 1 dinner roll 1 cup unsweetened applesauce 1/2 tsp margarine
Snack A	1 cup celery sticks 10 peanuts 17 grapes	1 cup carrot sticks 1 1/2 tsp cashew butter 1 small apple	1 cup grape tomatoes 1 Tbsp light salad dressing 4 whole apricots	1 cup broccoli 1 Tbsp pine nuts 1 cup papaya	1 cup raw cauliflower 6 almonds 1/2 cup fruit cocktail in light syrup	1 cup green pepper slices 3 oz frozen juice bar	1 cup cucumber slices 2 Brazil nuts 3/4 cup blackberries
Snack B	3/4 oz whole-wheat crackers 1 1/2 tsp almond butter 6 oz fat-free yogurt	3/4 chewy fruit bar 1 cup nonfat milk	8 animal crackers 10 peanuts 1 cup nonfat milk	1/4 cup granola 1 cup nonfat milk	1 cup oven-baked French fries 6 oz fat-free yogurt	5 vanilla wafers 1 cup nonfat milk	2 small sandwich cookies 1 cup nonfat milk
Dinner	**Stuffed Peppers Lemon Parsley Carrots*** 4 1/2 oz red potatoes 1 slice pumpernickel bread 1/2 cup unsweetened peaches 1 cup nonfat milk 1 oz reduced-fat cheese	**Scallops Provençal Stir-Fry Vegetables*** 1 cup brown rice 1 oz reduced-fat cheese 1/2 tsp margarine	**Baked Sole Italian-Style Zucchini with Whole-Wheat Pasta*** 1 small dinner roll 1 small nectarine 1 cup nonfat milk 24 pistachios	**Turkey Tetrazzini** 1 slice whole-grain bread 1/2 cup nonfat milk 1 cup steamed carrots	**Beef Stew** 1 small dinner roll 12 cherries 1 cup nonfat milk 1 cup salad greens 1 1/2 Tbsp light salad dressing	**Citrus Dijon Pork Skillet Green Bean Casserole** 1 cup brown rice 1/2 cup nonfat milk 10 hazelnuts	**Caribbean Ham Slice** 1 cup brown rice 1 cup cooked kale 1 oz reduced-fat cheese 2 tsp margarine

*Indicates that the recipe has been used previously.

SHOPPING LIST

VEGETABLES

_____ bell peppers, green
_____ bell peppers, red
_____ broccoli
_____ Brussels sprouts
_____ carrots
_____ cauliflower
_____ celery
_____ eggplant
_____ garlic
_____ green beans
_____ kale
_____ lettuce, romaine
_____ mushrooms
_____ onions, yellow or white
_____ onions, green
_____ onions, red
_____ peas, frozen
_____ potatoes
_____ potatoes, red
_____ potatoes, sweet
_____ shallots
_____ tomatoes
_____ tomatoes, cherry
_____ zucchini

MEATS

_____ bacon, Canadian
_____ bacon, turkey
_____ beef, ground, 96% lean
_____ beef, stew cubes
_____ chicken breasts, boneless, skinless
_____ ham steak
_____ pork chops, sirloin, boneless
_____ sausage, smoked
_____ sausage, turkey, lean
_____ scallops, sea or bay
_____ sole fillets
_____ turkey breast, lean, skinless

FRUITS

_____ apples
_____ bananas
_____ blueberries
_____ cantaloupe
_____ cherries
_____ fruit, dried, mixed
_____ grapes
_____ kiwi fruit
_____ lemons
_____ nectarine
_____ oranges
_____ oranges, mandarin, canned, packed in juice
_____ peaches
_____ pears
_____ pineapple, chunks
_____ prunes, canned in light syrup
_____ raisins
_____ strawberries

DAIRY

_____ egg substitute
_____ egg white substitute
_____ milk, nonfat
_____ Smart Balance Light Spread
_____ Smart Balance margarine
_____ yogurt, fat-free, plain

CHEESE

_____ cheddar, fat-free, shredded
_____ cheddar, fat-free, slices
_____ cheddar, reduced-fat
_____ cheddar, sharp, reduced-fat, shredded
_____ cottage cheese, low-fat
_____ cream cheese, fat-free
_____ mozzarella, fat-free
_____ Parmesan, reduced-fat, grated

BREAD, GRAINS, & PASTA

_____ bread, multigrain
_____ bread, whole-grain, whole-wheat
_____ dinner rolls, whole-wheat
_____ noodles, whole-wheat
_____ pasta, penne, whole-grain
_____ pasta, whole-wheat, macaroni or elbows
_____ rice, brown, whole-grain
_____ rice, long-grain
_____ spaghetti

BEANS

_____ white beans, no-added-salt

NUTS

_____ almonds
_____ Brazil nuts
_____ hazelnuts
_____ macadamia nuts
_____ peanuts
_____ pecans
_____ pistachios
_____ walnuts

CONDIMENTS

_____ canola mayonnaise
_____ mustard, Dijon
_____ mustard, prepared
_____ soy sauce, light

SPICES & HERBS

_____ basil
_____ black pepper
_____ cayenne pepper
_____ chili powder
_____ cinnamon, ground
_____ cloves, ground
_____ cream of tartar
_____ cumin, ground
_____ fennel seeds
_____ ginger, ground
_____ lemon pepper seasoning, no-added-salt
_____ mustard, dry
_____ nutmeg, ground
_____ oregano
_____ parsley
_____ red pepper flakes
_____ tarragon
_____ thyme

OTHER

_____ applesauce, unsweetened
_____ cashew butter
_____ cereal, Kashi
_____ cereal, Rice Chex
_____ crackers, saltine, unsalted
_____ cranberry sauce
_____ dill pickle
_____ gelatin, unflavored
_____ grits
_____ honey
_____ jam
_____ marmalade, orange or tangerine, sugar-free
_____ olives, black
_____ peanut butter
_____ pimento
_____ pumpkin, canned
_____ rum
_____ salad dressing, light
_____ sauerkraut
_____ oats, old-fashioned
_____ sunflower seeds
_____ syrup, maple, sugar-free
_____ tomato paste, no-added-salt
_____ tomato sauce, no-added-salt
_____ tomatoes, diced, no-added-salt
_____ tomatoes, stewed, Italian-style, 16-oz can
_____ tortillas, whole-wheat, low-fat, 6-inch
_____ vanilla extract
_____ water chestnuts
_____ wine, red, dry

STAPLES

_____ baking powder
_____ bouillon, beef, sodium-free
_____ bouillon, chicken, sodium-free
_____ cornmeal
_____ cornstarch
_____ flour, whole-wheat
_____ juice, apple, unsweetened
_____ juice, lemon
_____ juice, orange, frozen concentrate
_____ juice, orange, unsweetened
_____ nonstick cooking spray
_____ Smart Balance Omega oil
_____ Splenda
_____ vinegar, cider
_____ vinegar, white

Herb Chicken

Serves 4   Serving size: 1/4 recipe

- 1 **lb** boneless, skinless chicken breasts (trimmed of fat)
- 1/2 **cup** water
- 1 **Tbsp** sodium-free chicken bouillon
- 1 **lb** mushrooms, sliced
- 1/2 **cup** sliced green onions
- 1/4 **cup** minced garlic
- 2 **tsp** dried tarragon, crushed
- 2 **tsp** dried thyme, crushed

  Black pepper, to taste

Place chicken in a large, cold nonstick skillet. Add water and bouillon. Cover and cook over medium heat for 8–10 minutes or until slightly browned, turning several times. Remove from heat. Reduce heat to low. Add mushrooms, green onions, garlic, tarragon, thyme, and pepper. Cover and simmer for 10 minutes; baste and cook 7 minutes longer or until chicken is tender. Transfer chicken to a serving platter. Spoon liquid over chicken and serve.

Exchanges/Choices

2 Vegetable
3 Lean Meat

Basic Nutritional Values

Calories	180
Calories from Fat	30
Total Fat	3.5 g
Saturated Fat	0.9 g
Trans Fat	0.0 g
Cholesterol	65 mg
Sodium	70 mg
Total Carbohydrate	9 g
Dietary Fiber	2 g
Sugars	3 g
Protein	28 g

Ratatouille

Serves 4   Serving size: 1/4 recipe

- 3/4 medium onion, diced
- 1/4 **cup** Smart Balance Omega oil
- 1 small zucchini, cut into 1/4-inch cubes
- 1 clove garlic, finely chopped
- 1 small green bell pepper, cut into small pieces
- 2 tomatoes, peeled and coarsely chopped
- 3/4 small eggplant, peeled and cubed
- 1/2 **tsp** basil
- 1/2 **tsp** oregano

Sauté onion in oil in a large skillet until transparent. Add all remaining ingredients. Cover and cook over medium heat for about 45 minutes, stirring occasionally. Add a little water if necessary. May be served hot or chilled.

Exchanges/Choices

3 Vegetable
2 1/2 Fat

Basic Nutritional Values

Calories	180
Calories from Fat	125
Total Fat	14.0 g
Saturated Fat	1.1 g
Trans Fat	0.0 g
Cholesterol	0 mg
Sodium	10 mg
Total Carbohydrate	15 g
Dietary Fiber	4 g
Sugars	7 g
Protein	2 g

Prune Delight Spread

Serves 4   Serving size: 1/4 recipe

1 1/2   envelopes unflavored gelatin

2   **cups** canned prunes in light syrup, drained, discard 1/2 juice

3   **Tbsp** Splenda

2/3   **tsp** pure vanilla extract

2   egg whites

1/16   **tsp** cream of tartar

1. In a small saucepan, add gelatin to 1/2 cup water; let stand for 1 minute. Cook and stir over low heat until gelatin is dissolved; set aside. Place drained prunes in a blender. Cover and blend at high speed for 30 seconds or until thickened and well blended.

2. In a large metal bowl, combine 6 Tbsp water, Splenda, vanilla, and gelatin-prune mixture. Place bowl in a larger bowl half filled with ice water. Stir mixture until syrupy. Remove bowl from water bath.

3. In a small mixer bowl at high speed, beat egg whites until foamy. Add cream of tartar and continue beating until stiff but not dry.

4. Return prune mixture to ice water bath and stir until mixture mounds slightly when dropped from a spoon. Fold in egg whites. Spoon into 6 dessert dishes. Chill for 30 minutes or until set.

Exchanges/Choices

1 1/2 Fruit

Basic Nutritional Values

Calories 95
  Calories from Fat 0
Total Fat . . . . 0.0 g
  Saturated Fat . . . . 0.0 g
  Trans Fat . . . . 0.0 g
Cholesterol . . . . 0 mg
Sodium . . . . 60 mg
Total Carbohydrate . . . 19 g
  Dietary Fiber . . . . 1 g
  Sugars . . . . 18 g
Protein . . . . 4 g

Stuffed Peppers

Serves 4   Serving size: 1/4 recipe

2 medium green bell peppers

1/4 **cup** chopped onion

1 **Tbsp** Smart Balance Light Spread

1/2 **lb** 96% lean ground beef

4 **oz** no-added-salt tomato sauce

1/2 **cup** cooked long-grain rice

1 **tsp** chili powder

Preheat oven to 350°F. Cut peppers in half lengthwise and remove membrane and seeds. In a large pot of boiling water, cook the scooped-out peppers for 5 minutes; remove and drain upside-down. In a large skillet over medium-high heat, sauté onion in margarine until tender. Add beef and brown; drain off fat. Stir in tomato sauce, cooked rice, and chili powder; spoon into peppers. Place in a 13 × 9 × 2-inch baking dish; pour water in bottom of dish to a depth of 1/4 inch. Bake for 15 minutes.

Exchanges/Choices

1/2 Starch
1 Vegetable
2 Lean Meat

Basic Nutritional Values

Calories 135
  Calories from Fat 35
Total Fat . . . . 4.0 g
  Saturated Fat . . . . 1.4 g
  Trans Fat . . . . 0.1 g
Cholesterol . . . . 30 mg
Sodium . . . . 80 mg
Total Carbohydrate . . . 12 g
  Dietary Fiber . . . . 2 g
  Sugars . . . . 4 g
Protein . . . . 13 g

Lemon Parsley Carrots

Serves 4   Serving size: 1/4 recipe

2 **cups** carrots, sliced 1/4-inch thick

2 **Tbsp** water

2 **Tbsp** Smart Balance margarine

1 **Tbsp** Splenda

1 **Tbsp** parsley, chopped

1/2 **tsp** lemon peels, grated

1 **Tbsp** lemon juice

Place carrots and water in a 2-quart covered glass casserole. Microwave, covered, at 100% power (700 watts) for 8–9 minutes until crisp-tender, stirring once after 5 minutes. Drain. Stir in margarine, Splenda, parsley, lemon peels, and lemon juice. Microwave again, covered, at 100% power for 1–2 minutes, until heated through.

Exchanges/Choices

1 Vegetable
1 Fat

Basic Nutritional Values

Calories 70
  Calories from Fat 40
Total Fat . . . . 4.5 g
  Saturated Fat . . . . 1.3 g
  Trans Fat . . . . 0.0 g
Cholesterol . . . . 0 mg
Sodium . . . . 90 mg
Total Carbohydrate . . . 7 g
  Dietary Fiber . . . . 2 g
  Sugars . . . . 3 g
Protein . . . . 1 g

Whole-Wheat Blueberry Muffins

Serves 12   Serving size: 1 muffin

1 **cup** whole-wheat flour	3 **Tbsp** Smart Balance margarine
5 1/2 **Tbsp** Splenda	
1 **tsp** baking powder	1/2 **cup** egg substitute
6 **Tbsp** nonfat milk	1/2 **cup** blueberries

Preheat oven to 400°F. In a medium bowl, combine flour, Splenda, and baking powder. In a small bowl, beat milk, margarine, and egg substitute; stir into dry ingredients until just moist. Fold in blueberries and spoon batter into 12 paper-lined muffin cups. Bake for 20–25 minutes or until golden brown. Serve immediately.

Exchanges/Choices

1/2 Starch
1/2 Fat

Basic Nutritional Values

Calories 70
  Calories from Fat 20
Total Fat . . . . .2.5 g
  Saturated Fat . . . . .0.7 g
  Trans Fat . . . . .0.0 g
Cholesterol . . . . .0 mg
Sodium . . . . .75 mg
Total Carbohydrate . . .9 g
  Dietary Fiber . . . . .1 g
  Sugars . . . . .2 g
Protein . . . . .3 g

Egg Salad

Serves 4   Serving size: 1/4 recipe

1 **cup** egg substitute	1 **Tbsp** vinegar
1/4 **cup** canola mayonnaise	1/4 **tsp** pepper
1/8 **cup** minced green onion	1/2 **cup** shredded carrot
1 **Tbsp** mustard	

Cook egg substitute. In a medium bowl, combine all ingredients and mix until well blended. Refrigerate 2 hours before serving.

Exchanges/Choices

1 Lean Meat
1/2 Fat

Basic Nutritional Values

Calories 85
  Calories from Fat 40
Total Fat . . . . .4.5 g
  Saturated Fat . . . . .0.0 g
  Trans Fat . . . . .0.0 g
Cholesterol . . . . .0 mg
Sodium . . . . .255 mg
Total Carbohydrate . . .3 g
  Dietary Fiber . . . . .1 g
  Sugars . . . . .2 g
Protein . . . . .6 g

Peas and Cheese Salad

Serves 4   Serving size: 1/4 recipe

3 1/2 **Tbsp** canola mayonnaise

2 **tsp** prepared mustard

1/3 **tsp** basil leaves, crushed
Dash black pepper

2 **cups** frozen peas, thawed

2 **oz** fat-free cheddar cheese slices, diced

1 1/2 **oz** reduced-fat shredded sharp cheddar cheese

4 **oz** water chestnuts sliced, drained

5 **Tbsp** green onions, sliced

4 romaine lettuce leaves

In a large bowl, combine mayonnaise, mustard, basil, and pepper until blended. Stir in peas, cheese, water chestnuts, and green onions until well coated. Cover and chill at least 2 hours. To serve, spoon onto romaine leaves.

Exchanges/Choices

1 Starch
1 Lean Meat
1 Fat

Basic Nutritional Values

Calories 170
 Calories from Fat 65
Total Fat . . . . 7.0 g
 Saturated Fat . . . . 1.4 g
 Trans Fat . . . . 0.0 g
Cholesterol . . . . 10 mg
Sodium . . . . 460 mg
Total Carbohydrate . . . 17 g
 Dietary Fiber . . . . 6 g
 Sugars . . . . 7 g
Protein . . . . 11 g

New Orleans Chilled Rice

Serves 4   Serving size: 1/4 recipe

3/4 **cups** whole-grain rice

1 **Tbsp** Smart Balance Omega oil

1/2 **cup** chopped dill pickle

1/2 **cup** celery, diced

1/2 **cup** onion

1/2 **cup** shallots, chopped

1/2 medium red pepper, chopped

1/4 **cup** canola mayonnaise

1/4 **cup** fat-free plain yogurt

1/2 **Tbsp** vinegar

Cook rice according to package directions. In a large bowl, combine all other ingredients with the cooked rice; chill before serving.

Exchanges/Choices

2 Starch
2 Vegetable
1 Fat

Basic Nutritional Values

Calories 255
 Calories from Fat 70
Total Fat . . . . 8.0 g
 Saturated Fat . . . . 0.4 g
 Trans Fat . . . . 0.0 g
Cholesterol . . . . 0 mg
Sodium . . . . 345 mg
Total Carbohydrate . . . 39 g
 Dietary Fiber . . . . 2 g
 Sugars . . . . 5 g
Protein . . . . 5 g

Scallops Provençal

Serves 4   Serving size: 1/4 recipe

1 **Tbsp** Smart Balance
  Omega oil

1 medium zucchini

2 medium cloves garlic, minced

1/2 **tsp** dried thyme, crumbled

  Pepper, to taste

3/4 **lb** bay or sea scallops

12 cherry tomatoes, sliced

1/3 **cup** unsweetened apple juice

Heat the oil in a large nonstick skillet. Cook the zucchini, garlic, thyme, and pepper until the zucchini is crisp-tender. Rinse the scallops and pat dry. Add sliced tomatoes and apple juice to skillet. Add scallops and cook until scallops have turned white (4 minutes for bay scallops and 5 minutes for sea scallops) and the zucchini is tender, stirring occasionally.

Exchanges/Choices

1 Vegetable
2 Lean Meat

Basic Nutritional Values

Calories	130
Calories from Fat	40
Total Fat	4.5 g
Saturated Fat	0.4 g
Trans Fat	0.0 g
Cholesterol	35 mg
Sodium	175 mg
Total Carbohydrate	7 g
Dietary Fiber	1 g
Sugars	4 g
Protein	16 g

Stir-Fry Vegetables

Serves 4   Serving size: 1/4 recipe

1 **Tbsp** Smart Balance
  Omega oil

1 small onion, peeled,
  quartered, and thinly sliced

2 cloves garlic, minced

3/4 **cup** carrots, pared and thinly
  sliced

3/4 **cup** zucchini, thinly sliced

3/4 **cup** celery, thinly sliced

3/4 **cup** broccoli florets

1 **Tbsp** sodium-free chicken
  bouillon

1/4 **cup** water

2 **tsp** ground ginger

1/3 **cup** sliced water chestnuts

3 green onions, sliced

2 **tsp** light soy sauce

Heat oil in a large heavy skillet; sauté onion and garlic for 2 minutes. Add carrots, zucchini, celery, and broccoli; mix well. In a small bowl, combine bouillon and water to form a broth. Add broth and ginger to skillet; cover and cook 3 minutes. Add water chestnuts, green onions, and soy sauce. Stir until chestnuts and onions are heated through and vegetables are crisp-tender.

Exchanges/Choices

2 Vegetable
1/2 Fat

Basic Nutritional Values

Calories	85
Calories from Fat	35
Total Fat	4.0 g
Saturated Fat	0.3 g
Trans Fat	0.0 g
Cholesterol	0 mg
Sodium	140 mg
Total Carbohydrate	12 g
Dietary Fiber	3 g
Sugars	5 g
Protein	2 g

Apple Crisp

Serves 4   Serving size: 1/4 recipe

2 1/2 **cups** pared and sliced apples

3/8 **cup** Splenda

3/8 **cup** whole-wheat flour

3/8 **cup** dry oats

1 1/2 **Tbsp** cinnamon

1 1/2 **Tbsp** Smart Balance margarine

Arrange apples in a pan. Combine the Splenda, flour, oats, cinnamon, and margarine until the mixture is crumbly. Press mixture over apples and bake at 350°F for 45–50 minutes or until tops are browned. Serve warm.

Exchanges/Choices

1 1/2 Starch
1/2 Fruit
1/2 Fat

Basic Nutritional Values

Calories 150
 Calories from Fat 40
Total Fat . . . . 4.5 g
 Saturated Fat . . . . 1.1 g
 Trans Fat . . . . 0.0 g
Cholesterol . . . . 0 mg
Sodium . . . . 35 mg
Total Carbohydrate . . . 28 g
 Dietary Fiber . . . . 5 g
 Sugars . . . . 11 g
Protein . . . . 3 g

Sauerkraut Salad

Serves 4   Serving size: 1/4 recipe

1/3 **cup** vinegar

1/2 **cup** Splenda

1/2 **cup** diced celery

1/2 **cup** diced bell pepper

1/2 **cup** diced onion

1 1/2 **cups** sauerkraut, drained

Pour the vinegar over the Splenda in a saucepan and heat. Pour this mixture over the celery, peppers, and onion and then let cool. Add this mixture to the sauerkraut; toss together. Cover and chill for 3 hours before serving.

Exchanges/Choices

2 Vegetable

Basic Nutritional Values

Calories 40
 Calories from Fat 0
Total Fat . . . . 0.0 g
 Saturated Fat . . . . 0.0 g
 Trans Fat . . . . 0.0 g
Cholesterol . . . . 0 mg
Sodium . . . . 365 mg
Total Carbohydrate . . . 10 g
 Dietary Fiber . . . . 3 g
 Sugars . . . . 5 g
Protein . . . . 1 g

German Potato Salad

Serves 4   Serving size: 1/4 recipe

4	**cups** potatoes	1	**cup** water
4	slices turkey bacon	1/2	**cup** cider vinegar
1/2	**cup** chopped onions	2 1/2	**Tbsp** Splenda
2	**Tbsp** whole-wheat flour	1/16	**tsp** black pepper

Peel and dice the potatoes; place in boiling water. Cook until just soft. Fry bacon in a large skillet until crisp; remove and drain. Place the onions in the skillet and cook until tender. Slowly stir in flour; blend well. Add water and vinegar; cook, stirring, until bubbly and slightly thick. Stir in Splenda and pepper; simmer for 10 minutes. Crumble bacon. Carefully stir bacon and potatoes into hot mixture. Heat through, stirring gently to coat potato slices. Serve warm.

Exchanges/Choices
2 Starch

Basic Nutritional Values
Calories 160
  Calories from Fat 25
Total Fat . . . . 3.0 g
  Saturated Fat . . . . 0.8 g
  Trans Fat . . . . 0.0 g
Cholesterol . . . . 15 mg
Sodium . . . . 180 mg
Total Carbohydrate . . . 28 g
  Dietary Fiber . . . . 3 g
  Sugars . . . . 4 g
Protein . . . . 5 g

Baked Sole

Serves 4   Serving size: 1/4 recipe

4	**tsp** Smart Balance margarine	12	unsalted saltine crackers, crushed (about 1/2 cup)
1	**lb** sole fillets		Dash pepper
1/4	**cup** egg white substitute		

Preheat oven to 400°F. Melt margarine in a baking dish until golden brown (do not burn). Clean and pat fish dry. Dip fillets in egg white substitute and then coat thoroughly with cracker crumbs. Add to baking dish. Sprinkle with remaining cracker crumbs and pepper. Bake for 15–18 minutes or until fish flakes easily with a fork.

Exchanges/Choices
1/2 Starch
3 Lean Meat

Basic Nutritional Values
Calories 175
  Calories from Fat 55
Total Fat . . . . 6.0 g
  Saturated Fat . . . . 1.2 g
  Trans Fat . . . . 0.0 g
Cholesterol . . . . 60 mg
Sodium . . . . 220 mg
Total Carbohydrate . . . 7 g
  Dietary Fiber . . . . 0 g
  Sugars . . . . 0 g
Protein . . . . 24 g

Italian-Style Zucchini with Whole-Wheat Pasta

Serves 6   Serving size: 1/6 recipe

- **6 oz** whole-wheat pasta, macaroni or elbows
- **1** large onion, chopped
- **1** clove garlic, minced
- **1** medium carrot, thinly chopped
- **2 Tbsp** Smart Balance Omega oil
- **1** (**16-oz**) can Italian-style stewed tomatoes
- **1** zucchini, halved lengthwise and sliced in 1/4-inch pieces
- **1/2 tsp** fennel seeds, crushed
- **1/4 tsp** red pepper flakes

Exchanges/Choices

1 1/2 Starch
2 Vegetable
1/2 Fat

Basic Nutritional Values

Calories	185
Calories from Fat	45
Total Fat	5.0 g
Saturated Fat	0.5 g
Trans Fat	0.0 g
Cholesterol	0 mg
Sodium	255 mg
Total Carbohydrate	33 g
Dietary Fiber	5 g
Sugars	8 g
Protein	6 g

Cook the pasta according to package directions; drain and set aside. In a large skillet, cook the onion, garlic, and carrot in hot oil for 5 minutes or until tender. Add tomatoes, zucchini, fennel seeds, and red pepper flakes. Bring to a boil and reduce heat. Simmer uncovered for about 3 minutes. Stir in pasta and heat through.

Low-Fat Corn Bread

Serves 8   Serving size: 1/8 recipe

1/2	**cup** egg substitute		1 1/2	**cup** whole-wheat flour
1/2	**cup** Splenda		2/3	**cup** cornmeal
3/4	**cup** nonfat milk		1	**Tbsp** baking powder
1/2	**cup** unsweetened applesauce			Nonstick cooking spray

Beat together the egg substitute, Splenda, milk, and applesauce; set aside. In a separate bowl, sift and combine flour, cornmeal, and baking powder. Stir into egg mixture using as few strokes as possible. Spray an 8 × 8-inch baking pan with nonstick cooking spray. Bake at 400°F for 25–30 minutes or until a toothpick inserted near the middle comes out clean.

Exchanges/Choices

2 Starch

Basic Nutritional Values

Calories 150	
Calories from Fat 5	
Total Fat . . . . 0.5 g	
Saturated Fat . . . . 0.1 g	
Trans Fat . . . . 0.0 g	
Cholesterol . . . . 0 mg	
Sodium . . . . 180 mg	
Total Carbohydrate . . 30 g	
Dietary Fiber . . . . 4 g	
Sugars . . . . 4 g	
Protein . . . . 6 g	

Grilled Vegetable Wrap

Serves 4   Serving size: 1 wrap

2	medium zucchini, sliced into 1/4-inch strips		1	**tsp** no-added-salt lemon pepper seasoning
2	medium red onions, sliced into 1/4-inch strips		1	**tsp** ground cumin
1	medium red bell pepper, seeded and sliced into 1/4-inch strips			Pepper, season to taste
1	**cup** no-added-salt white beans		4	(**6-inch**) low-fat whole-wheat tortillas

Preheat broiler. Broil zucchini, onion, and pepper until browned and slightly soft. Place beans, lemon pepper, cumin, and pepper in a food processor or blender and process until smooth. Spread an equal amount of the bean mixture on each tortilla. Top the mixture with 1/4 vegetables strips. Roll up the tortillas and serve.

Exchanges/Choices

1 1/2 Starch
2 Vegetable
1/2 Fat

Basic Nutritional Values

Calories 180	
Calories from Fat 20	
Total Fat . . . . 2.5 g	
Saturated Fat . . . . 0.2 g	
Trans Fat . . . . 0.0 g	
Cholesterol . . . . 0 mg	
Sodium . . . . 100 mg	
Total Carbohydrate . . . 35 g	
Dietary Fiber . . . . 7 g	
Sugars . . . . 7 g	
Protein . . . . 8 g	

Bread Pudding

Serves 10   Serving size: 1/10 recipe

Nonstick cooking spray

2 cups stale whole-wheat bread, cut into 1/2-inch cubes

3/4 cup raisins

1/4 cup chopped walnuts

4 cups nonfat milk

3/4 cup Splenda

3/4 cup egg substitute

2 tsp ground cinnamon

2 tsp pure vanilla extract

1/4 cup Smart Balance margarine

Exchanges/Choices

1/2 Fat-Free Milk
1 Carbohydrate
1 Fat

Basic Nutritional Values

Calories 165
  Calories from Fat 55
Total Fat . . . . 6.0 g
  Saturated Fat . . . . 1.3 g
  Trans Fat . . . . 0.0 g
Cholesterol . . . . 0 mg
Sodium . . . . 175 mg
Total Carbohydrate . . . 21 g
  Dietary Fiber . . . . 2 g
  Sugars . . . . 14 g
Protein . . . . 8 g

Preheat oven to 325°F. Spray a shallow 1 1/2-quart casserole with nonstick cooking spray. Place bread cubes, raisins, and nuts in casserole. In a large bowl, combine milk, Splenda, egg substitute, cinnamon, and vanilla. Pour over bread mixture; mix well. Dot with margarine. Place casserole in a large baking pan; fill pan with hot water to a depth of 1 inch. Bake for 45–55 minutes or until a knife inserted halfway between center and edge of casserole comes out clean. Serve warm or cold.

Turkey Tetrazzini

Serves 4   Serving size: 1/4 recipe

4 **oz** thin whole-wheat noodles	1 1/2 **cup** cooked skinless lean turkey breast (trimmed of fat), diced
1/2 **cup** mushrooms	
1/4 **cup** Smart Balance margarine	1/4 **cups** fat-free mozzarella cheese
2 **Tbsp** whole-wheat flour	
1 **cup** nonfat milk	1/2 **cup** egg substitute
2 **tsp** sodium-free chicken bouillon	1/4 **cup** pimento
2 **Tbsp** lemon juice	

Exchanges/Choices

2 Starch
3 Lean Meat
1/2 Fat

Basic Nutritional Values

Calories 320	
Calories from Fat 90	
Total Fat. . . . . 10.0 g	
Saturated Fat . . . . 2.8 g	
Trans Fat. . . . . 0.0 g	
Cholesterol. . . . . 45 mg	
Sodium. . . . . 300 mg	
Total Carbohydrate . . . 30 g	
Dietary Fiber. . . . . 3 g	
Sugars . . . . 5 g	
Protein . . . . 28 g	

1. Cook noodles according to package directions; drain and set aside.

2. In a saucepan over medium heat, sauté mushrooms in 2 Tbsp margarine; remove and set aside. In the same saucepan over medium heat, add remaining margarine and flour. Cook and stir for 1 minute. Add nonfat milk and chicken bouillon. Stirring constantly, bring to a boil until thickened. Stir in lemon juice. Stir in turkey, noodles, cheese, egg substitute, mushrooms, and pimento. Pour into a casserole dish. Bake at 350°F for about 30 minutes.

Spaghetti with Meat Sauce
Serves 4   Serving size: 1/4 recipe

3/4 **lb** 96% lean ground beef

6 **oz** no-added-salt tomato paste

8 **oz** no-added-salt diced tomatoes

1 small zucchini, diced

1 medium onion, diced

1/2 **cup** dry red wine

1 **tsp** chopped oregano

1 **tsp** chopped basil

1 clove garlic, minced

Pepper, to taste

8 **oz** spaghetti

Brown the beef in a large frying pan and cook thoroughly; drain away excess fat. Stir in all remaining ingredients, except spaghetti, and bring to a boil. Reduce heat and simmer for about 30 minutes. Cook spaghetti according to package directions; drain. To serve, spoon sauce over spaghetti.

Exchanges/Choices

3 Starch
2 Vegetable
2 Lean Meat

Basic Nutritional Values

Calories 400
  Calories from Fat 45
Total Fat. . . . . .5.0 g
  Saturated Fat . . . . .1.7 g
  Trans Fat. . . . . .0.2 g
Cholesterol. . . . . .45 mg
Sodium. . . . . .95 mg
Total Carbohydrate . . .59 g
  Dietary Fiber. . . . . .6 g
  Sugars . . . . .7 g
Protein . . . . .28 g

Beef Stew
Serves 4   Serving size: 1/4 recipe

1 1/2 **lb** stew beef cubes (trimmed of fat)

1/4 **cup** whole-wheat flour

1 **Tbsp** Smart Balance margarine

3 **cups** water

3 **cups** cubed potato

2 **cups** diced carrot

1/2 **cup** diced bell pepper

1/2 **cup** diced celery

1/2 **cup** diced onion

1 **Tbsp** sodium-free beef bouillon

Coat meat with flour. Melt margarine in a deep skillet or large saucepan and brown meat thoroughly. Add water and heat to boiling. Reduce heat, cover, and simmer for 2 hours. Stir in remaining ingredients. If needed, add more water a 1/2 cup at a time. Simmer an additional 30 minutes, until vegetables are tender. If desired, stew can be thickened with flour.

Exchanges/Choices

2 Starch
1 Vegetable
3 Lean Meat
1/2 Fat

Basic Nutritional Values

Calories 355
  Calories from Fat 80
Total Fat. . . . . .9.0 g
  Saturated Fat . . . . .2.8 g
  Trans Fat. . . . . .0.0 g
Cholesterol. . . . . .85 mg
Sodium. . . . . .145 mg
Total Carbohydrate . . .38 g
  Dietary Fiber. . . . . .5 g
  Sugars . . . . .7 g
Protein . . . . .30 g

Pumpkin Spice Muffins

Serves 8   Serving size: 2 muffins

1 **cup** whole-wheat flour	1 **cup** canned pumpkin
3 **tsp** baking powder	1/2 **cup** nonfat milk
2 **tsp** ground cinnamon	1/4 **cup** unsweetened applesauce
2 **tsp** ground nutmeg	1/4 **cup** raisins or chopped nuts
1/4 **cup** egg substitute	
2 **Tbsp** Splenda	

Preheat oven to 400°F. Line sixteen muffin-pan cups with paper liners or spray with nonstick cooking spray. In a large bowl, stir together the flour, baking powder, cinnamon, and nutmeg. In a medium bowl, beat egg substitute with a whisk. Add Splenda, pumpkin, milk, and applesauce; stir until well blended. Stir in raisins. Stir into flour mixture until just blended. Fill muffin-pan cups 2/3 full. Bake 20–25 minutes until a wooden toothpick inserted in the center comes out clean. Remove muffins from muffin pans. Serve warm or at room temperature.

Exchanges/Choices

1 1/2 Carbohydrate

Basic Nutritional Values

Calories 95
 Calories from Fat 5
Total Fat . . . . 0.5 g
 Saturated Fat . . . . 0.2 g
 Trans Fat . . . . 0.0 g
Cholesterol . . . . 0 mg
Sodium . . . . 160 mg
Total Carbohydrate . . . 20 g
 Dietary Fiber . . . . 3 g
 Sugars . . . . 6 g
Protein . . . . 4 g

Chicken Pasta Salad

Serves 4   Serving size: 1/4 recipe

8 **oz** penne pasta	2 cloves garlic, minced
1/2 **cup** shredded carrots	1/2 **lb** cooked skinless, boneless chicken breasts, cubed
1/2 **cup** diced green onions	2 **Tbsp** reduced-fat grated Parmesan cheese
1/2 **cup** diced broccoli	
3 **Tbsp** cider vinegar	
1 **Tbsp** Smart Balance Omega Oil	

Cook pasta according to package directions. When pasta has cooked for about 3 minutes add carrots, green onions, and broccoli, and cook 5 more minutes. Drain and run under cool water. Combine the vinegar, oil, and garlic; mix with the pasta and chicken. Sprinkle with cheese and refrigerate 1 hour before serving.

Exchanges/Choices

3 Starch
3 Lean Meat

Basic Nutritional Values

Calories 370
 Calories from Fat 65
Total Fat . . . . 7.0 g
 Saturated Fat . . . . 1.4 g
 Trans Fat . . . . 0.0 g
Cholesterol . . . . 50 mg
Sodium . . . . 115 mg
Total Carbohydrate . . . 48 g
 Dietary Fiber . . . . 4 g
 Sugars . . . . 3 g
Protein . . . . 26 g

Tangerine Broccoli

Serves 4   Serving size: 1/4 recipe

2 **cups** broccoli florets

2 **Tbsp** cider vinegar

1/4 **tsp** ground ginger

1/4 **tsp** ground cinnamon

1/4 **cup** sugar-free tangerine or orange marmalade

Cook broccoli in a steamer basket in a medium saucepan over a small amount of simmering water, covered, for about 7 minutes. Meanwhile, in a small saucepan, stir together vinegar, ginger, cinnamon, and marmalade; cook over low heat until marmalade has melted. To serve, spoon an equal amount of the sauce over each broccoli serving.

Exchanges/Choices

1/2 Carbohydrate

Basic Nutritional Values

Calories 20
 Calories from Fat 0
Total Fat . . . . 0.0 g
 Saturated Fat . . . . 0.0 g
 Trans Fat . . . . 0.0 g
Cholesterol . . . . 0 mg
Sodium . . . . 10 mg
Total Carbohydrate . . . 7 g
 Dietary Fiber . . . . 1 g
 Sugars . . . . 3 g
Protein . . . . 1 g

Citrus Dijon Pork

Serves 4   Serving size: 1/4 recipe

3/4 **lb** boneless sirloin pork chops (trimmed of fat)

1 1/2 **cup** unsweetened orange juice

2 **Tbsp** Dijon mustard

1 **Tbsp** Splenda

1 1/2 **tsp** cornstarch

8 **oz** mushrooms, sliced

1/2 **cup** sliced green onions

2 **tsp** Smart Balance margarine

1 **(11-oz)** can mandarin orange segments in juice, drained

2 **Tbsp** slivered almonds, toasted

Thinly slice pork diagonally across the grain; set aside. Combine orange juice, mustard, Splenda, and cornstarch in a bowl; set aside. Cook mushrooms and green onions in margarine in a large skillet over medium-high heat. Remove from skillet. Add pork to skillet; cook until browned. Stir in mushrooms, onions, and orange juice mixture. Cook, stirring frequently, until thoroughly heated. Add oranges, toss until heated. Transfer to serving dish and sprinkle with almonds.

Exchanges/Choices

1 Fruit
3 Lean Meat

Basic Nutritional Values

Calories 180
 Calories from Fat 35
Total Fat . . . . 4.0 g
 Saturated Fat . . . . 0.8 g
 Trans Fat . . . . 0.0 g
Cholesterol . . . . 40 mg
Sodium . . . . 410 mg
Total Carbohydrate . . . 19 g
 Dietary Fiber . . . . 2 g
 Sugars . . . . 15 g
Protein . . . . 18 g

Skillet Green Bean Casserole

Serves 4   Serving size: 1/4 recipe

1 **tsp** Smart Balance Omega oil

8 **oz** mushrooms, cut into 1/4-inch slices

1 medium onion, minced

3 medium cloves garlic, minced

1 **tsp** minced thyme leaves Pinch cayenne

2 **cups** green beans, ends trimmed

2 **Tbsp** sodium-free chicken bouillon

1 **tsp** cornstarch

1 **Tbsp** water

3 **Tbsp** fat-free cream cheese Ground black pepper, to taste

2 **Tbsp** reduced-fat Parmesan cheese

Exchanges/Choices

1/2 Carbohydrate
2 Vegetable

Basic Nutritional Values

Calories 90
 Calories from Fat 15
Total Fat . . . . 1.5 g
 Saturated Fat . . . . 0.2 g
 Trans Fat . . . . 0.0 g
Cholesterol . . . . 0 mg
Sodium . . . . 90 mg
Total Carbohydrate . . . 15 g
 Dietary Fiber . . . . 3 g
 Sugars . . . . 5 g
Protein . . . . 5 g

1. Combine the oil, mushrooms, and onion in a 12-inch nonstick skillet. Cover and cook over medium-low heat, stirring occasionally, until the mushrooms release their liquid, 5–10 minutes. Uncover, increase to medium-high heat, and continue to cook, stirring often, until the mushrooms are browned, 2–5 minutes.

2. Stir in the garlic, thyme, and cayenne; cook until fragrant, about 30 seconds, and add the green beans. Increase to medium-high heat, cover, and cook until the green beans are tender, with a light crunch in the center, 6–9 minutes.

3. Push the green beans to one side of the skillet. Whisk the bouillon, cornstarch, and water together and then pour into the empty side of the skillet; bring to a simmer, about 30 seconds. Whisk the cream cheese into the sauce until smooth. Toss the sauce with the green beans and continue to cook, uncovered, until the green beans are tender and the sauce has thickened, 1–3 minutes. Sprinkle with pepper and Parmesan cheese before serving.

Whole-Wheat French Toast

Serves 4   Serving size: 1/4 recipe

1 1/2 cup egg substitute

1 cup nonfat milk

1 Tbsp Splenda

3 Tbsp Smart Balance
Omega oil

8 thick slices whole-wheat
bread

In a shallow bowl, beat together the egg substitute, milk, and Splenda with a whisk. Pour 1 Tbsp oil in the skillet and heat over medium heat. Dip the bread into the milk mixture one slice at a time. Place each dipped slice into the hot oil in the frying pan. Do not overlap or crowd the pieces. Fry for 2–3 minutes until golden brown and then turn over and continue frying until the second side is golden brown. Put the browned slices on an oven-safe plate and place in the 200°F oven to keep hot. Continue dipping and frying the remaining slices of bread. Add 1–2 Tbsp oil as needed.

Exchanges/Choices

2 Starch
1 Lean Meat
2 Fat

Basic Nutritional Values

Calories 285
  Calories from Fat 110
Total Fat . . . . 12.0 g
  Saturated Fat . . . . 1.2 g
  Trans Fat . . . . 0.0 g
Cholesterol . . . . 0 mg
Sodium . . . . 430 mg
Total Carbohydrate . . . 27 g
  Dietary Fiber . . . . 4 g
  Sugars . . . . 6 g
Protein . . . . 16 g

Meatloaf

Serves 4   Serving size: 1/4 recipe

1 Tbsp sodium-free beef
bouillon

1/4 cup water

1 lb 96% lean ground beef

1/2 cup quick-cooking oatmeal

1/4 cup egg substitute

1/3 cup finely chopped onions

In large bowl, thoroughly combine bouillon, water, ground beef, oatmeal, egg substitute, and onion. Firmly shape the mixture into a loaf. Bake at 350°F for about 1 1/4 hours.

Exchanges/Choices

1/2 Starch
4 Lean Meat

Basic Nutritional Values

Calories 200
  Calories from Fat 45
Total Fat . . . . 5.0 g
  Saturated Fat . . . . 2.1 g
  Trans Fat . . . . 0.3 g
Cholesterol . . . . 60 mg
Sodium . . . . 115 mg
Total Carbohydrate . . . 10 g
  Dietary Fiber . . . . 1 g
  Sugars . . . . 2 g
Protein . . . . 27 g

Cauliflower au Gratin

Serves 4   Serving size: 1/4 recipe

1 **lb** cauliflower	3/4 **cup** nonfat milk
1 **Tbsp** Smart Balance margarine	2 **Tbsp** fat-free shredded cheddar cheese
2 **Tbsp** whole-wheat flour	2 **Tbsp** reduced-fat cheddar cheese
1/2 **tsp** dry mustard	

Over a large pot of boiling water, break apart the cauliflower into bite-size pieces and steam until soft. Meanwhile, melt margarine in a saucepan over low heat. Blend in flour and dry mustard; cook over low heat until mixture is smooth and bubbly. Stir in milk and heat to boiling, stirring constantly, for 1 minute. Stir in cheeses over low heat until melted. Pour sauce over cooked cauliflower and serve.

Exchanges/Choices

1/2 Carbohydrate
1 Vegetable
1/2 Fat

Basic Nutritional Values

Calories 95
  Calories from Fat 30
Total Fat . . . . 3.5 g
  Saturated Fat . . . . 1.1 g
  Trans Fat . . . . 0.0 g
Cholesterol . . . . 5 mg
Sodium . . . . 145 mg
Total Carbohydrate . . . 12 g
  Dietary Fiber . . . . 3 g
  Sugars . . . . 5 g
Protein . . . . 6 g

Caribbean Ham Slice

Serves 6   Serving size: 1/6 recipe

1 **lb** lean ham steak	3 **tsp** cornstarch
2 medium oranges, sectioned	2 **Tbsp** rum
1/2 **cup** frozen orange juice concentrate	3 **Tbsp** honey
2/3 **tsp** ground cloves	1 **cup** pineapple chunks
1/4 **cup** Splenda	1/3 **cup** raisins

Slash edge of ham slice; place on the rack of a roasting pan. Bake for 30 minutes at 350°F. Meanwhile, peel and section oranges. In a saucepan, combine orange juice and cloves; bring to boiling. Reduce heat; simmer gently, uncovered, for 5 minutes. Combine Splenda and cornstarch; stir in rum and honey. Stir mixture into orange juice. Cook and stir until thickened and bubbly. Cook and stir for 1–2 more minutes. Stir in orange sections, pineapple chunks, and raisins. Heat through. Spoon over cooked ham.

This recipe is high in sodium.

Exchanges/Choices

2 1/2 Fruit
2 Lean Meat

Basic Nutritional Values

Calories 245
  Calories from Fat 30
Total Fat . . . . 3.5 g
  Saturated Fat . . . . 1.1 g
  Trans Fat . . . . 0.0 g
Cholesterol . . . . 35 mg
Sodium . . . . 965 mg
Total Carbohydrate . . . 39 g
  Dietary Fiber . . . . 2 g
  Sugars . . . . 34 g
Protein . . . . 16 g

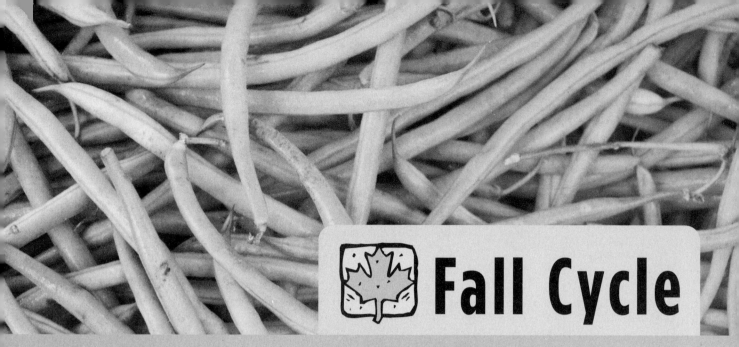

FEATURED RECIPES

Yogurt Muffins*

Sweet and Sour Beef

Chicken à la King

Mexican Corn Salad

Quick and Easy Chili*

Chicken Scaloppini

Western Omelet*

Turkey and Fruit Pasta Salad

Baked Boston Cod

German Red Cabbage

Haddock with Zucchini and Tomatoes

Homemade Stuffing

Chicken Flautas

Zucchini Carrot Muffins*

Creamy Beef and Green Beans

Chicken Noodle Casserole

Banana Bran Muffin*

Cheddar and Colby Quesadilla

Chicken Parmigiana

Low-Fat, Sugar-Free Eggnog

Pumpkin Spice Muffins*

Chicken and Black Bean Chili

Broiled Salmon

*Indicates that the recipe has been used previously.

1500 calorie MEAL PLAN FALL WEEK 2

	Sunday	Monday	Tuesday	Wednesday	Thursday	Friday	Saturday
Breakfast	**Yogurt Muffins*** 1/2 Tbsp jam 1 medium banana 1 cup nonfat milk 1/2 oz reduced-fat cheese 1 tsp margarine	1/2 cup shredded wheat 1/2 English muffin 1/2 large grapefruit 1 cup nonfat milk 2 tsp margarine	**Western Omelet*** 2 slices whole-grain bread 1 cup papaya 1 cup nonfat milk 1 1/2 tsp margarine	1 cup plain oatmeal 12 cherries 1 cup nonfat milk 1 1/2 tsp margarine	**Zucchini Carrot Muffins*** 9 small grapes 1 cup nonfat milk 1/2 tsp margarine	**Banana Bran Muffin*** 1/4 cup low-fat granola 1 cup nonfat milk 2 tsp margarine	**Pumpkin Spice Muffins*** 1/2 cup bran cereal 1/2 large grapefruit 1 cup nonfat milk 2 tsp margarine
Lunch	**Sweet and Sour Beef** (1/2 serving) 1 cup brown rice 9 small grapes 1/2 cup green beans	**Quick and Easy Chili*** 1/2 cup corn 1 dinner roll 2 tangerines 1/2 tsp margarine	**Turkey and Fruit Pasta Salad** (1/2 serving) 1 small dinner roll 1/3 cup cooked peas 2 dried apple rings 1/2 cup carrot sticks 3/4 tsp margarine	**Haddock with Zucchini and Tomatoes Homemade Stuffing** 1/2 cup corn 1 slice multigrain bread 3/4 cup mixed berries	**Creamy Beef and Green Beans** 2 pieces flatbread 1 1/4 cup strawberries 1/2 tsp margarine	**Cheddar and Colby Quesadilla** 1 1/2 cup popcorn 3/4 cup blueberries 1 1/2 tsp margarine	**Chicken and Black Bean Chili** 1/3 cup brown rice 1 small whole-wheat dinner roll 1 cup melon balls 1 tsp margarine
Snack A							
Snack B							
Dinner	**Chicken à la King** (1/2 serving) **Mexican Corn Salad** 3/4 cup blueberries 3/4 cup nonfat milk 2 cups vegetable salad 1 Tbsp light salad dressing	**Chicken Scaloppini** 2/3 cup cooked pasta 3/4 cup blackberries 1 cup nonfat milk 8 walnut halves	**Baked Boston Cod German Red Cabbage** 1 slice rye bread 3 oz potato 2 apricots 1 cup green beans 1 1/2 tsp margarine	**Chicken Flautas** 1/2 cup brown rice 1/2 cup fruit cocktail in water 1 cup nonfat milk 1/2 cup cooked kale 2 tsp margarine	**Chicken Noodle Casserole** 1 cup raspberries 1 cup nonfat milk 2 cups salad greens 2 Tbsp light salad dressing	**Chicken Parmigiana Low-Fat, Sugar-Free Eggnog** 1/2 cup cooked pasta 1/2 cup unsweetened peaches 1 cup nonfat milk 1 cup cooked Italian beans 1 tsp margarine 10 stuffed green olives	**Broiled Salmon** 1/2 cup butternut squash 3/4 cup mixed berries 1 cup nonfat milk 1 cup cauliflower and broccoli 1/2 tsp margarine

*Indicates that the recipe has been used previously.

	Sunday	Monday	Tuesday	Wednesday	Thursday	Friday	Saturday
Breakfast	**Yogurt Muffins*** 1/2 Tbsp jam 1 medium banana 1 cup nonfat milk 1/2 oz reduced-fat cheese 1 tsp margarine	1/2 cup shredded wheat 1/2 English muffin 1/2 large grapefruit 1 cup nonfat milk 1/4 cup egg substitute 2 tsp margarine	**Western Omelet*** 2 slices whole-grain bread 1 cup papaya 1 cup nonfat milk 1 1/2 tsp margarine	1 cup plain oatmeal 12 cherries 1 cup nonfat milk 1 oz Canadian bacon 2 tsp margarine	**Zucchini Carrot Muffins*** 9 small grapes 1 cup nonfat milk 1/4 cup egg substitute 1/2 tsp margarine	**Banana Bran Muffin*** 1/4 cup low-fat granola 1 cup nonfat milk 1 oz lean turkey sausage 2 tsp margarine	**Pumpkin Spice Muffins*** 1/2 cup bran cereal 1/2 large grapefruit 1 cup nonfat milk 1/4 cup low-fat cottage cheese 2 tsp margarine
Lunch	**Sweet and Sour Beef** (1/2 serving) 1 cup brown rice 9 small grapes 1/2 cup green beans 1 tsp margarine	**Quick and Easy Chili*** 1/2 cup corn 1 dinner roll 2 tangerines 1/2 tsp margarine	**Turkey and Fruit Pasta Salad** (1/2 serving) 1 small dinner roll 1/3 cup cooked peas 2 dried apple rings 1/2 cup carrot sticks 1 1/4 tsp margarine	**Haddock with Zucchini and Tomatoes Homemade Stuffing** 1/2 cup corn 1 slice multigrain bread 3/4 cup mixed berries 1 tsp margarine	**Creamy Beef and Green Beans** 2 pieces flatbread 1 1/4 cup strawberries 1 1/2 tsp margarine	**Cheddar and Colby Quesadilla** 1 1/2 cup popcorn 3/4 cup blueberries 1 1/2 tsp margarine	**Chicken and Black Bean Chili** 1/3 cup brown rice 1 small whole-wheat dinner roll 1 cup melon balls 2 tsp margarine
Snack A	4 walnut halves 1/2 cup unsweetened plums	3 macadamia nuts 1 cup cantaloupe	10 peanuts 1 medium banana	2 Brazil nuts 1 small orange	1 1/2 tsp peanut butter 1 small apple	1 Tbsp light salad dressing 3 dried plums	10 peanuts 1 small orange
Snack B	1 cup nonfat milk	6 oz fat-free yogurt	1 cup nonfat milk	1 cup nonfat milk	6 oz fat-free yogurt	1 cup nonfat milk	1 cup nonfat milk
Dinner	**Chicken à la King** (1/2 serving) **Mexican Corn Salad** 3/4 cup blueberries 1/2 cup nonfat milk 2 cups vegetable salad 1 Tbsp light salad dressing	**Chicken Scaloppini** 2/3 cup cooked pasta 3/4 cup blackberries 1 cup nonfat milk 8 walnut halves	**Baked Boston Cod German Red Cabbage** 1 slice rye bread 3 oz potato 2 apricots 1 cup green beans 1 1/2 tsp margarine	**Chicken Flautas** 1/2 cup brown rice 1/2 cup fruit cocktail in water 1 cup nonfat milk 1/2 cup cooked kale 2 tsp margarine	**Chicken Noodle Casserole** 1 cup raspberries 1 cup nonfat milk 2 cups salad greens 2 Tbsp light salad dressing	**Chicken Parmigiana Low-Fat, Sugar-Free Eggnog** 1/2 cup cooked pasta 1/2 cup unsweetened peaches 1 cup nonfat milk 1 cup cooked Italian beans 1 tsp margarine 10 stuffed green olives	**Broiled Salmon** 1/2 cup butternut squash 3/4 cup mixed berries 1 cup nonfat milk 1 cup cauliflower and broccoli 1/2 tsp margarine

*Indicates that the recipe has been used previously.

2000 calorie MEAL PLAN FALL WEEK 2

	Sunday	Monday	Tuesday	Wednesday	Thursday	Friday	Saturday
Breakfast	Yogurt Muffins* 1/2 Tbsp jam 1 medium banana 1 cup nonfat milk 1/2 oz reduced-fat cheese 1 tsp margarine	1/2 cup shredded wheat 1/2 English muffin 1/2 large grapefruit 1 cup nonfat milk 1/4 cup egg substitute 2 tsp margarine	Western Omelet* 2 slices whole-grain bread 1 cup papaya 1 cup nonfat milk 1 1/2 tsp margarine	1 cup plain oatmeal 12 cherries 1 cup nonfat milk 1 oz Canadian bacon 2 tsp margarine	Zucchini Carrot Muffins* 9 small grapes 1 cup nonfat milk 1/4 cup egg substitute 1/2 tsp margarine	Banana Bran Muffin* 1/4 cup low-fat granola 1 cup nonfat milk 1 oz lean turkey sausage 2 tsp margarine	Pumpkin Spice Muffins* 1/2 cup bran cereal 1/2 large grapefruit 1 cup nonfat milk 1/4 cup low-fat cottage cheese 2 tsp margarine
Lunch	Sweet and Sour Beef (1/2 serving) 1 cup brown rice 26 small grapes 1/2 cup green beans 1 tsp margarine	Quick and Easy Chili* 1/2 cup corn 1 dinner roll 2 tangerines 1 cup honeydew melon 1 1/2 tsp margarine	Turkey and Fruit Pasta Salad (1/2 serving) 1 small dinner roll 1/3 cup cooked peas 6 dried apple rings 1/2 cup carrot sticks 1 1/4 tsp margarine	Haddock with Zucchini and Tomatoes Homemade Stuffing 1/2 cup corn 1 slice multigrain bread 1 1/2 cup mixed berries 1/2 cup okra 1 tsp margarine	Creamy Beef and Green Beans 2 pieces flatbread 1 1/4 cup strawberries 1 kiwi fruit 1 1/2 tsp margarine	Cheddar and Colby Quesadilla 1 1/2 cup popcorn 1 1/2 cup blueberries 1 cup mixed raw vegetable sticks 1 1/2 tsp margarine	Chicken and Black Bean Chili 1/3 cup brown rice 1 small whole-wheat dinner roll 2 cups melon balls 2 tsp margarine
Snack A	1 cup carrot sticks 4 walnut halves 1/2 cup unsweetened plums	1 cup salad vegetables 1 Tbsp light salad dressing 1 cup cantaloupe	1 cup celery sticks 10 peanuts 1 medium banana	1 cup cherry tomatoes 2 Brazil nuts 1 small orange	1 cup raw celery 1 1/2 tsp peanut butter 1 small apple	1 cup green pepper slices 1 Tbsp light salad dressing 3 dried plums	1 cup cucumber slices 10 peanuts 1 small orange
Snack B	3/4 oz wheat crackers 1 1/2 tsp peanut butter 1 cup nonfat milk	3 graham crackers 3 macadamia nuts 6 oz fat-free yogurt	3 ginger snaps 1 1/2 tsp cashew butter 1 cup nonfat milk	1 small unfrosted brownie 1 cup nonfat milk	1 slice raisin bread 1 tsp margarine 6 oz fat-free yogurt	2 rice cakes 1 1/2 tsp almond butter 1 cup nonfat milk	1 mini bagel 1 tsp margarine 1 cup nonfat milk
Dinner	Chicken à la King (1/2 serving) Mexican Corn Salad 3/4 cup blueberries 1/2 cup nonfat milk 2 cups vegetable salad 1 Tbsp light salad dressing	Chicken Scaloppini 2/3 cup cooked pasta 3/4 cup blackberries 1 cup nonfat milk 8 walnut halves	Baked Boston Cod German Red Cabbage 1 slice rye bread 3 oz potato 2 apricots 1 cup green beans 1 1/2 tsp margarine	Chicken Flautas 1/2 cup brown rice 1/2 cup fruit cocktail in water 2 apricots 1 cup nonfat milk 1/2 cup cooked kale 2 tsp margarine	Chicken Noodle Casserole 1 cup raspberries 1 cup nonfat milk 2 cups salad greens 2 Tbsp light salad dressing	Chicken Parmigiana Low-Fat, Sugar-Free Eggnog 1/2 cup cooked pasta 1/2 cup unsweetened peaches 1 cup nonfat milk 1 cup cooked Italian beans 1 tsp margarine 10 stuffed green olives	Broiled Salmon 1/2 cup butternut squash 3/4 cup mixed berries 1 cup nonfat milk 1 cup cauliflower and broccoli 1/2 tsp margarine

*Indicates that the recipe has been used previously.

	Sunday	Monday	Tuesday	Wednesday	Thursday	Friday	Saturday
Breakfast	Yogurt Muffins* 1/2 Tbsp jam 1 medium banana 1 cup nonfat milk 1 1/2 oz reduced-fat cheese 1 tsp margarine	1/2 cup shredded wheat 1/2 English muffin 1/2 large grapefruit 1 cup nonfat milk 1/2 cup egg substitute 2 tsp margarine	Western Omelet* 1 1/2 slice whole-grain bread 1 cup papaya 1 cup nonfat milk 1 tsp margarine	1 cup plain oatmeal 12 cherries 1 cup nonfat milk 2 oz Canadian bacon 2 tsp margarine	Zucchini Carrot Muffins* 9 small grapes 1 cup nonfat milk 1/2 cup egg substitute 1/2 tsp margarine	Banana Bran Muffin* 1/4 cup low-fat granola 1 cup nonfat milk 2 oz lean turkey sausage 2 tsp margarine	Pumpkin Spice Muffins* 1/2 cup bran cereal 1/2 large grapefruit 1 cup nonfat milk 1/2 cup low-fat cottage cheese 2 tsp margarine
Lunch	Sweet and Sour Beef (1/2 serving) 1 cup brown rice 26 small grapes 1/2 cup green beans 1 tsp margarine	Quick and Easy Chili* 1/2 cup corn 1 dinner roll 2 tangerines 1 cup honeydew melon 1 1/2 tsp margarine	Turkey and Fruit Pasta Salad (1/2 serving) 1 small dinner roll 1/3 cup cooked peas 6 dried apple rings 1/2 cup carrot sticks 1 1/4 tsp margarine	Haddock with Zucchini and Tomatoes Homemade Stuffing 1/2 cup corn 1 slice multigrain bread 1 1/2 cup mixed berries 1/2 cup okra 1 tsp margarine	Creamy Beef and Green Beans 2 pieces flatbread 1 1/4 cup strawberries 1 kiwi fruit 1 1/2 tsp margarine	Cheddar and Colby Quesadilla 1 1/2 cup popcorn 1 1/2 cup blueberries 1 cup mixed raw vegetable sticks 1 1/2 tsp margarine	Chicken and Black Bean Chili 1/3 cup brown rice 1 small whole-wheat dinner roll 2 cups melon balls 2 tsp margarine
Snack A	1 cup carrot sticks 4 walnut halves 1/2 cup unsweetened plums	1 cup salad vegetables 1 Tbsp light salad dressing 1 cup cantaloupe	1 cup celery sticks 10 peanuts 1 medium banana	1 cup cherry tomatoes 2 Brazil nuts 1 small orange	1 cup raw celery 1 1/2 tsp peanut butter 1 small apple	1 cup green pepper slices 1 Tbsp light salad dressing 3 dried plums	1 cup cucumber slices 10 peanuts 1 small orange
Snack B	3/4 oz wheat crackers 1 1/2 tsp peanut butter 1 cup nonfat milk	3 graham crackers 3 macadamia nuts 6 oz fat-free yogurt	3 ginger snaps 1 1/2 tsp cashew butter 1 cup nonfat milk	1 small unfrosted brownie 1 cup nonfat milk	1 slice raisin bread 1 tsp margarine 6 oz fat-free yogurt	2 rice cakes 1 1/2 tsp almond butter 1 cup nonfat milk	1 mini bagel 1 tsp margarine 1 cup nonfat milk
Dinner	Chicken à la King (1/2 serving) Mexican Corn Salad 3/4 cup blueberries 1/2 cup nonfat milk 2 cups vegetable salad 1 Tbsp light salad dressing	Chicken Scaloppini 1 cup cooked pasta 3/4 cup blackberries 1 cup nonfat milk 8 walnut halves	Baked Boston Cod German Red Cabbage 1 slice rye bread 6 oz potato 2 apricots 1 cup green beans 1 1/2 tsp margarine	Chicken Flautas 3/4 cup brown rice 1/2 cup fruit cocktail in water 1 cup nonfat milk 1/2 cup cooked kale 2 tsp margarine	Chicken Noodle Casserole 1 slice oatmeal bread 1 cup raspberries 1 cup nonfat milk 2 cups salad greens 2 Tbsp light salad dressing	Chicken Parmigiana Low-Fat, Sugar-Free Eggnog 1/2 cup cooked pasta 1 slice Italian bread 1/2 cup unsweetened peaches 1 cup nonfat milk 1 cup cooked Italian beans 1 tsp margarine 10 stuffed green olives	Broiled Salmon 1/2 cup butternut squash 3/4 cup mixed berries 1 cup nonfat milk 1 cup cauliflower and broccoli 1/2 tsp margarine

*Indicates that the recipe has been used previously.

SHOPPING LIST FALL WEEK 2

VEGETABLES
____ bell peppers, green
____ bell peppers, red
____ broccoli
____ cabbage, red
____ carrots
____ cauliflower
____ celery
____ corn, frozen
____ garlic
____ green beans, frozen
____ kale
____ lettuce, romaine
____ mushrooms
____ okra
____ onions, yellow or white
____ onions, green
____ peas
____ potatoes
____ radishes
____ squash, butternut
____ tomatoes
____ tomatoes, plum
____ zucchini

MEATS
____ bacon, Canadian
____ beef flank steak
____ beef, ground, 96% lean
____ beef, stew cubes or sirloin cubes
____ Boston cod fillets
____ chicken breasts, boneless, skinless
____ haddock fillets
____ ham, extra-lean, lower-sodium
____ salmon steaks
____ sausage, turkey, lean
____ turkey breast

FRUITS
____ apples, tart
____ apricots
____ bananas
____ blackberries
____ blueberries
____ cherries
____ dried apple rings
____ grapefruit
____ grapes
____ honeydew melon
____ kiwi fruit
____ papaya
____ peaches, unsweetened
____ pineapple, chunks (canned light, fresh, or frozen)
____ plums
____ raisins
____ raspberries
____ strawberries
____ tangerines

DAIRY
____ egg substitute
____ egg whites
____ half and half, fat-free
____ milk, evaporated, fat-free
____ milk, nonfat
____ Smart Balance Light Spread
____ Smart Balance margarine
____ yogurt, fat-free, plain
____ yogurt, fat-free, vanilla

CHEESE
____ cheddar, fat-free, shredded
____ Colby and Monterey Jack, reduced-fat, shredded
____ Colby Jack, reduced-fat, shredded
____ cottage cheese, low-fat
____ Parmesan, reduced-fat, grated

BREAD, GRAINS, & PASTA
____ bread, multigrain
____ bread, rye
____ bread, whole-wheat, whole-grain
____ dinner rolls, small, whole-wheat
____ English muffin, whole-grain
____ flatbreads
____ noodles, whole-wheat, wide
____ pasta, macaroni, whole-wheat
____ rice, brown, whole-grain

BEANS

____ black beans, no-added-salt
____ Italian beans
____ kidney beans,
     no-added-salt, 15-oz can

NUTS

____ walnuts

CONDIMENTS

____ horseradish
____ hot sauce

SPICES & HERBS

____ basil
____ bay leaf
____ black pepper
____ cayenne pepper
____ chili powder, no-added-salt
____ cinnamon, ground
____ marjoram
____ nutmeg, ground
____ oregano
____ paprika
____ parsley
____ red pepper flakes
____ sage
____ tarragon
____ thyme

OTHER

____ applesauce, unsweetened
____ bread crumbs
____ cereal, bran
____ cereal, shredded wheat
____ croutons
____ fruit cocktail, in water
____ granola, low-fat
____ honey
____ jam
____ salsa, no-added-salt
____ juice, lemon or lime
____ juice, tomato,
     no-added-salt
____ molasses, dark
____ oats, old-fashioned
____ olives, green, stuffed
____ onion soup mix,
     1-oz envelope
____ pimentos
____ popcorn
____ pumpkin, canned
____ salad dressing, light
____ soy sauce, light
____ tomato sauce,
     no-added-salt, 8-oz can
____ tomatoes, diced,
     no-added-salt
____ tomatoes, stewed,
     no-added-salt, 14-oz can
____ tortillas, corn, 6-inch
____ tortillas, flour, 8-inch
____ vanilla extract
____ wheat germ
____ wine, red, dry
____ wine, white

STAPLES

____ baking powder
____ baking soda
____ bouillon, beef, sodium-free
____ bouillon, chicken,
     sodium-free
____ cornstarch
____ flour, all-purpose
____ flour, whole-wheat
____ nonstick cooking spray
____ Smart Balance Omega oil
____ Splenda
____ vinegar, white

Yogurt Muffins

Serves 4   Serving size: 1 muffin

2/3	**cup** all-purpose flour	
1/2	**tsp** baking powder	
1/4	**tsp** baking soda	
2	**Tbsp** Splenda	
6	**Tbsp** vanilla fat-free yogurt	

2 **Tbsp** Smart Balance Omega oil

1/2 **tsp** vanilla extract

2 egg whites

Nonstick cooking spray

Exchanges/Choices

1 1/2 Starch
1 Fat

Basic Nutritional Values

Calories 165	
Calories from Fat 65	
Total Fat . . . . 7.0 g	
Saturated Fat . . . . 0.5 g	
Trans Fat . . . . 0.0 g	
Cholesterol . . . . 0 mg	
Sodium . . . . 165 mg	
Total Carbohydrate . . . 20 g	
Dietary Fiber . . . . 1 g	
Sugars . . . . 3 g	
Protein . . . . 5 g	

Combine the flour, baking powder, baking soda, and Splenda in a medium bowl; make a well in center of mixture. Combine yogurt, oil, vanilla, and egg whites; add to dry ingredients, stirring just until dry ingredients are moistened. Spoon batter evenly into 4 muffin pan cups coated with cooking spray. Bake at 400°F for 30–36 minutes or until golden. Remove from pan immediately.

Sweet and Sour Beef

Serves 4   Serving size: 1/4 recipe

1 1/2 **lb** flank beef steak (trimmed of fat)

3 **Tbsp** Smart Balance Omega oil

1 medium onion, diced

8 **oz** pineapple chunks (fresh, frozen, or canned light)

1/4 **cup** Splenda

1/4 **cup** vinegar

1 **Tbsp** sodium-free beef bouillon

1 **Tbsp** light soy sauce

1 **Tbsp** cornstarch

1 **Tbsp** water

1 bell pepper, sliced and diced

2 medium tomato, sliced and diced

Exchanges/Choices

1/2 Fruit
2 Vegetable
5 Lean Meat
2 Fat

Basic Nutritional Values

Calories 400	
Calories from Fat 180	
Total Fat . . . . 20.0 g	
Saturated Fat . . . . 4.5 g	
Trans Fat . . . . 0.0 g	
Cholesterol . . . . 60 mg	
Sodium . . . . 215 mg	
Total Carbohydrate . . . 21 g	
Dietary Fiber . . . . 3 g	
Sugars . . . . 12 g	
Protein . . . . 35 g	

Cut beef into 2-inch strips; then cut the strips across the grain in 1/8-inch slices. Heat oil in a large skillet or wok over medium heat. Add beef and onion; cook and stir until beef is brown, about 3 minutes. Stir in the pineapple chunks, Splenda, vinegar, bouillon, 1/2 cup water, and soy sauce. Heat to boiling. Mix cornstarch and 1 Tbsp cold water in a small bowl. Stir into the beef mixture. Cook and stir 1 minute. Stir in the bell pepper and tomatoes. Cook and stir 1 minute. Serve over rice.

Chicken à la King

Serves 4   Serving size: 1/4 recipe

1/2 **cup** green bell pepper, chopped

1/4 **cup** mushroom, sliced

1/4 **cup** pimento, chopped

1   **Tbsp** Smart Balance margarine

1/4 **cup** whole-wheat flour

1   **cup** fat-free half and half

Dash pepper

Dash paprika

3/4 **lb** boneless, skinless chicken breasts, cooked and diced

4   slices whole-grain toast

Cook green pepper, mushrooms, and pimento in margarine for 5 minutes. Move the vegetables to the side of the pan and blend the flour into the pan drippings. Add half and half and cook until thick, stirring constantly. Add pepper and paprika. Add cooked chicken. Cook over low heat for a few minutes. Serve over toast.

Exchanges/Choices

1 1/2 Starch
4 Lean Meat

Basic Nutritional Values

Calories 295
   Calories from Fat 65
Total Fat . . . . 7.0 g
   Saturated Fat . . . . 2.2 g
   Trans Fat . . . . 0.0 g
Cholesterol . . . . 75 mg
Sodium . . . . 280 mg
Total Carbohydrate . . . 24 g
   Dietary Fiber . . . . 2 g
   Sugars . . . . 5 g
Protein . . . . 33 g

Mexican Corn Salad

Serves 4   Serving size: 1/4 recipe

10   **oz** frozen corn, thawed

1/2 **cup** no-added-salt salsa

1   green onion, sliced and diced

1/2 **cup** radishes, sliced and diced

4   romaine lettuce leaves

Combine frozen corn, salsa, green onion, and radishes. Spoon mixture evenly over lettuce leaves.

Exchanges/Choices

1 Starch

Basic Nutritional Values

Calories 80
   Calories from Fat 5
Total Fat . . . . 0.5 g
   Saturated Fat . . . . 0.1 g
   Trans Fat . . . . 0.0 g
Cholesterol . . . . 0 mg
Sodium . . . . 80 mg
Total Carbohydrate . . . 18 g
   Dietary Fiber . . . . 3 g
   Sugars . . . . 4 g
Protein . . . . 3 g

Quick and Easy Chili

Serves 6   Serving size: 1/6 recipe

Nonstick cooking spray

1 **lb** 96% lean ground beef

1/2 **cup** chopped onion (about 1 large)

1/2 **cup** chopped green bell pepper (about 2 small)

6 cloves garlic, minced

1 (**14-oz**) can no-added-salt stewed tomatoes, chopped and juice reserved

1 (**15-oz**) can no-added-salt kidney beans, rinsed and drained

1 (**8-oz**) can no-added-salt tomato sauce

1 (**1-oz**) envelope onion soup mix

1 **cup** water

1 **Tbsp** no-added-salt chili powder

1 **Tbsp** paprika

1 **tsp** hot sauce

Exchanges/Choices

1 Starch
2 Vegetable
2 Lean Meat
1/2 Fat

Basic Nutritional Values

Calories 240
  Calories from Fat 65
Total Fat . . . . 7.0 g
  Saturated Fat . . . . 2.5 g
  Trans Fat . . . . 0.4 g
Cholesterol . . . . 45 mg
Sodium . . . . 545 mg
Total Carbohydrate . . . 24 g
  Dietary Fiber . . . . 6 g
  Sugars . . . . 9 g
Protein . . . . 21 g

Lightly spray a Dutch oven with nonstick cooking spray; heat over medium-high heat. Add beef, onion, pepper, and garlic. Cook until meat is browned, stirring until it crumbles. Drain away fat. Return mixture to pan; add all remaining ingredients. Bring to a boil; cover, reduce heat, and simmer 20 minutes, stirring occasionally. To serve, ladle chili into bowls.

Chicken Scaloppini

Serves 4   Serving size: 1/4 recipe

2	**Tbsp**	Smart Balance light margarine
8	**oz**	mushrooms, sliced
1		small onion, minced
2		cloves garlic, minced
2	**cups**	no-added-salt diced tomatoes

		Pepper, to taste
1/4	**tsp**	crushed tarragon
1/4	**tsp**	crushed thyme
1/4	**tsp**	crushed marjoram
1	**lb**	boneless, skinless chicken breasts (trimmed of fat)

In a large nonstick skillet, heat 1 Tbsp margarine. Sauté mushrooms over high heat for 3 minutes, stirring. Add onion and garlic; continue to stir-fry for 5 minutes. Add tomatoes, pepper, tarragon, thyme, and marjoram; bring to boil. Reduce heat; cover and simmer for 20 minutes. Cut each chicken breast in half once, then in half again diagonally. Place each quarter between wax paper and hit with a mallet to flatten to 1/4-inch thickness. Heat remaining 1 Tbsp margarine in another skillet; sauté meat, a few pieces at a time, until cooked through and slightly golden, about 5 minutes. Sprinkle lightly with pepper. Remove and place on hot platter. Cover with sauce and serve immediately.

Exchanges/Choices

2 Vegetable
3 Lean Meat

Basic Nutritional Values

Calories	200
Calories from Fat	55
Total Fat	6.0 g
Saturated Fat	1.6 g
Trans Fat	0.0 g
Cholesterol	65 mg
Sodium	155 mg
Total Carbohydrate	11 g
Dietary Fiber	3 g
Sugars	6 g
Protein	27 g

Western Omelet

Serves 4   Serving size: 1/4 recipe

1	**cup** egg substitute	**1/2**	**cup** diced onion
2	**Tbsp** Smart Balance Light margarine	**1/2**	**cup** diced bell pepper
4	**oz** extra-lean, lower-sodium ham, cooked, sliced, and diced		

Make each omelet individually. Mix egg substitute until blended. Place margarine in a skillet and melt. When it just begins to brown, the skillet is the right temperature. Pour a single portion of egg into the skillet and cook quickly. Fold the ham, onions, and peppers into the omelet and cover. Repeat for additional omelets.

Exchanges/Choices

1 Vegetable
1 Lean Meat
1/2 Fat

Basic Nutritional Values

Calories 95
 Calories from Fat 25
Total Fat . . . . .3.0 g
 Saturated Fat . . . . .1.0 g
 Trans Fat . . . . .0.0 g
Cholesterol . . . . .15 mg
Sodium . . . . .390 mg
Total Carbohydrate . . .5 g
 Dietary Fiber . . . . .1 g
 Sugars . . . . .3 g
Protein . . . . .11 g

Turkey and Fruit Pasta Salad

Serves 4   Serving size: 1/4 recipe

8	**oz** whole-wheat macaroni	**1/4**	**cup** Smart Balance Omega oil
3/4	**lb** cooked turkey breast, chopped	**1**	**Tbsp** honey
2	medium onions, diced	**1/2**	**tsp** thyme
1/3	**cup** lemon or lime juice	**2**	medium plums, sliced
		1	**cup** strawberries

Cook pasta according to package directions. Drain pasta, rinse, and then drain again. In a large bowl, combine pasta with turkey and onions; toss to mix. In a separate bowl, combine the lemon or lime juice, oil, honey, and thyme. Cover and shake well to mix. Pour the dressing over the pasta and chill for at least 4 hours. Just before serving, stir in plums and strawberries.

Exchanges/Choices

2 1/2 Starch
1 Fruit
1 Vegetable
4 Lean Meat
1 1/2 Fat

Basic Nutritional Values

Calories 510
 Calories from Fat 145
Total Fat . . . . .16.0 g
 Saturated Fat . . . . .1.4 g
 Trans Fat . . . . .0.0 g
Cholesterol . . . . .70 mg
Sodium . . . . .55 mg
Total Carbohydrate . . .61 g
 Dietary Fiber . . . . .7 g
 Sugars . . . . .14 g
Protein . . . . .35 g

Baked Boston Cod

Serves 4   Serving size: 1/4 recipe

1 **lb** Boston cod fillets
  Pepper, to taste
1 tomato, peeled and chopped
1 1/2 **tsp** green onion, chopped
1/4 **tsp** basil, crushed
1/4 **tsp** oregano

1/4 **cup** reduced-fat shredded Colby and Monterey Jack cheese
1 **Tbsp** reduced-fat grated Parmesan cheese

Cut cod into serving-size pieces; place in a baking dish. Sprinkle with pepper to taste. Combine tomato, green onion, and seasonings; spoon over cod. Bake at 450°F for 8–10 minutes or until cod flakes easily when tested with a fork. Sprinkle with cheeses; bake until melted.

Exchanges/Choices

3 Lean Meat

Basic Nutritional Values

Calories 125
 Calories from Fat 20
Total Fat. . . . . .2.5 g
 Saturated Fat . . . . .1.2 g
 Trans Fat. . . . . .0.0 g
Cholesterol . . . . .55 mg
Sodium. . . . . .160 mg
Total Carbohydrate . . .2 g
 Dietary Fiber. . . . . .0 g
 Sugars . . . . .1 g
Protein . . . . .23 g

German Red Cabbage

Serves 4   Serving size: 1/4 recipe

3/4 large onion, chopped
2 **Tbsp** Smart Balance Light Spread
3/4 medium head red cabbage, finely sliced
1 bay leaf

1 clove garlic, minced
1 **Tbsp** vinegar
2 tart apples, peeled and sliced
1/2 **Tbsp** Splenda
2 **Tbsp** dry red wine

Brown the onion in the Smart Balance Light Spread. Add the cabbage and stir until it is also slightly browned. Add bay leaf, garlic, vinegar, 1/2 cup water, and apples. Cover and simmer for about 45 minutes or until the cabbage is tender. Add Splenda and wine; cook 5 minutes longer.

Exchanges/Choices

1/2 Fruit
3 Vegetable
1/2 Fat

Basic Nutritional Values

Calories 120
 Calories from Fat 25
Total Fat. . . . . .3.0 g
 Saturated Fat . . . . .0.8 g
 Trans Fat. . . . . .0.0 g
Cholesterol . . . . .0 mg
Sodium. . . . . .60 mg
Total Carbohydrate . . .23 g
 Dietary Fiber. . . . . .5 g
 Sugars . . . . .17 g
Protein . . . . .3 g

Haddock with Zucchini and Tomatoes

Serves 4   Serving size: 1/4 recipe

2 Tbsp Smart Balance Omega oil

2 medium cloves garlic, minced

1 tsp minced oregano leaves

1/8 tsp red pepper flakes

1/8 tsp black pepper

3 medium plum tomatoes, chopped into 1/2-inch pieces

2 medium zucchini, sliced 1/4-inch thick

3/4 lb haddock fillets

1/4 cup minced basil

Exchanges/Choices

1 Vegetable
2 Lean Meat
1 Fat

Basic Nutritional Values

Calories	160
Calories from Fat	70
Total Fat	8.0 g
Saturated Fat	0.7 g
Trans Fat	0.0 g
Cholesterol	50 mg
Sodium	70 mg
Total Carbohydrate . . .	6 g
Dietary Fiber	2 g
Sugars	3 g
Protein	18 g

1. Place the oven rack in the middle of the oven and preheat to 450°F.

2. Combine the oil, garlic, oregano, pepper flakes, and black pepper in a medium bowl. Put half of the oil mixture into another medium bowl and toss gently with the tomatoes. Add the zucchini to the first oil mixture and toss to coat.

3. Cut four 12-inch squares of aluminum foil and lay them flat. Place zucchini slices in the center of each foil square. Season the haddock fillets with pepper and place on top of the zucchini. Top fish with tomatoes. Tightly crimp the foil into packets.

4. Set the packets on a baking sheet and bake until the fish just flakes apart, about 20 minutes. Carefully open the packets and let cool briefly. Smooth out the edges of the foil and, using a spatula, gently push the fish, vegetables, and juices out onto warmed plates. Sprinkle with basil before serving.

Homemade Stuffing

Serves 4   Serving size: 1/4 recipe

1/4 **cup** minced onion

1/4 **cup** celery, sliced and diced

5 **tsp** Smart Balance margarine

2 **cups** croutons

1 **tsp** sage

1 **tsp** thyme

Mix all ingredients together. Bake at 350°F for approximately 45 minutes.

Exchanges/Choices

1 Starch
1/2 Fat

Basic Nutritional Values

Calories 100
 Calories from Fat 45
Total Fat. . . . . .5.0 g
 Saturated Fat . . . . .1.3 g
 Trans Fat. . . . . .0.0 g
Cholesterol. . . . . .0 mg
Sodium. . . . . .150 mg
Total Carbohydrate . . .13 g
 Dietary Fiber. . . . . .1 g
 Sugars . . . . .1 g
Protein . . . . .2 g

Chicken Flautas

Serves 4   Serving size: 1/4 recipe

3/4 **lb** boneless, skinless chicken breasts (trimmed of fat)

1 **Tbsp** sodium-free chicken bouillon

1 **cup** water

1 medium onion, chopped

1 medium green bell pepper, seeded and diced

1 **cup** canned no-added-salt tomatoes, diced and drained

4 (**8-inch**) flour tortillas

Exchanges/Choices

1 1/2 Starch
1 Vegetable
3 Lean Meat

Basic Nutritional Values

Calories 275
 Calories from Fat 55
Total Fat. . . . . .6.0 g
 Saturated Fat . . . . .1.5 g
 Trans Fat. . . . . .0.0 g
Cholesterol. . . . . .50 mg
Sodium. . . . . .365 mg
Total Carbohydrate . . .32 g
 Dietary Fiber. . . . . .3 g
 Sugars . . . . .5 g
Protein . . . . .23 g

1. Place the chicken in boiling water and cook until done. Shred the chicken. Combine bouillon and water; heat in a sauté pan over medium heat. Add onions and peppers; sauté for about 4 minutes. Add tomatoes and chicken; simmer for another 10 minutes. Remove from heat and drain off excess liquids.

2. Divide the chicken mixture among the tortillas, fold closed, and secure with toothpicks.

3. Place rolled tortillas on a baking sheet and bake at 365°F for 5–7 minutes. Remove from the oven and discard toothpicks.

Zucchini Carrot Muffins
Serves 8   Serving size: 1 muffin

- 3/4 **cup** rolled oats
- 2 1/2 **cups** whole-wheat flour
- 2/3 **cup** nonfat milk
- 1/2 **cup** wheat germ, toasted
- 3 **tsp** baking powder
- 3/4 **cup** Splenda
- 1 **Tbsp** ground cinnamon
- 2 **tsp** ground nutmeg
- 3 **Tbsp** Smart Balance Omega oil
- 3 egg whites, beaten
- 1 **cup** carrots, finely shredded
- 1/2 **cup** zucchini, stemmed and grated

Preheat oven to 350°F. Combine all ingredients and mix well; pour into muffin liners in muffin pans. Bake for about 1 hour. Let cool for about 30 minutes before removing.

Exchanges/Choices
2 1/2 Carbohydrate
1 1/2 Fat

Basic Nutritional Values
Calories	260
Calories from Fat	65
Total Fat	7.0 g
Saturated Fat	0.9 g
Trans Fat	0.0 g
Cholesterol	0 mg
Sodium	180 mg
Total Carbohydrate	42 g
Dietary Fiber	7 g
Sugars	5 g
Protein	11 g

Creamy Beef and Green Beans
Serves 4   Serving size: 1/4 recipe

- 1 **Tbsp** Smart Balance margarine
- 1 **lb** stew beef or sirloin cubes (trimmed of fat)
- 1/4 **cup** chopped onion
- 1 clove garlic, minced
- 1 **Tbsp** soy sauce
- 1 **Tbsp** dark molasses
- 1 **lb** frozen green beans
- 2 **Tbsp** cornstarch

Melt margarine in a large skillet. Brown the beef and let simmer until tender (sirloin cubes should cook for about 1 hour; stew beef cubes may take 3 hours). Drain fat and add onions. Stir in garlic, 1 1/2 cup water, soy sauce, and molasses; heat to boiling. Add green beans; bring to a boil. Blend the cornstarch into 1/4 cup water and slowly stir into the mixture. Cook, stirring constantly, until the mixture thickens and boils.

Exchanges/Choices
1/2 Carbohydrate
2 Vegetable
2 Lean Meat
1/2 Fat

Basic Nutritional Values
Calories	200
Calories from Fat	65
Total Fat	7.0 g
Saturated Fat	2.0 g
Trans Fat	0.0 g
Cholesterol	55 mg
Sodium	300 mg
Total Carbohydrate	16 g
Dietary Fiber	3 g
Sugars	6 g
Protein	20 g

Chicken Noodle Casserole

Serves 4   Serving size: 1/4 recipe

1 lb boneless, skinless chicken breasts (trimmed of fat)	**1/4 cup** fat-free plain yogurt
4 oz wide whole-wheat noodles	**1/2 cup** nonfat milk
1/2 cup sliced mushrooms	**2 Tbsp** reduced-fat Parmesan cheese
1/2 cup fat-free cottage cheese	**1/4 cup** dry bread crumbs

Place chicken breasts in boiling water and thoroughly cook. Cook noodles according to package directions. Drain. When chicken has cooled to touch, cut it into small cubes. Combine noodles, chicken, mushrooms, cottage cheese, yogurt, milk, and Parmesan cheese in a casserole dish. Bake uncovered at 350°F for about 45 minutes or until hot and bubbly. Sprinkle with bread crumbs for the last 10 minutes of baking.

Exchanges/Choices

2 Starch
3 Lean Meat

Basic Nutritional Values

Calories 275
 Calories from Fat 35
Total Fat . . . . 4.0 g
 Saturated Fat . . . . 1.3 g
 Trans Fat . . . . 0.0 g
Cholesterol . . . . 70 mg
Sodium . . . . 250 mg
Total Carbohydrate . . . 27 g
 Dietary Fiber . . . . 3 g
 Sugars . . . . 4 g
Protein . . . . 34 g

Banana Bran Muffin
Serves 8   Serving size: 1 muffin

2/3 **cup** bran cereal

2/3 **cup** plain fat-free yogurt

5/8 **cup** whole-wheat flour

5 **Tbsp** Splenda

1 **tsp** ground cinnamon

1/2 **tsp** baking soda

3/16 **tsp** ground nutmeg

2 **cups** bananas, mashed

1/4 **cup** unsweetened applesauce

1/2 **cup** egg substitute, beaten

1. Preheat oven to 375°F. Place paper liners in muffin pan cups.

2. In a medium bowl, mix cereal and yogurt. Let stand for 5 minutes or until cereal is softened and breaks up.

3. Meanwhile, in a small bowl, combine the flour, Splenda, cinnamon, baking soda, and nutmeg; set aside.

4. Stir banana, applesauce, and egg substitute into cereal mixture. Stir in flour mixture until moistened. Fill muffin cups to about 2/3 full. Bake for 20–25 minutes or until muffins are lightly browned on top. Remove from pan and let cool on a wire rack before serving.

Exchanges/Choices
1 Starch
1 Fruit

Basic Nutritional Values
Calories 120
  Calories from Fat 5
Total Fat. . . . . .0.5 g
  Saturated Fat . . . . .0.2 g
  Trans Fat. . . . . .0.0 g
Cholesterol . . . . .0 mg
Sodium. . . . . .135 mg
Total Carbohydrate . . .27 g
  Dietary Fiber. . . . . .5 g
  Sugars . . . . .11 g
Protein . . . . .5 g

Cheddar and Colby Quesadilla
Serves 4   Serving size: 1/4 recipe

4 **oz** shredded fat-free cheddar cheese

4 **oz** shredded reduced-fat Colby Jack cheese

1 medium tomato, diced

1 small onion, diced

12 **(6-inch)** corn tortillas

Divide the ingredients evenly among 6 tortillas. Top each filled tortilla with another tortilla. Place quesadillas on a baking sheet or large piece of foil. Broil until hot and the cheese is melted, turning over once.

Exchanges/Choices
2 1/2 Starch
1 Vegetable
2 Lean Meat
1/2 Fat

Basic Nutritional Values
Calories 320
  Calories from Fat 70
Total Fat. . . . . .8.0 g
  Saturated Fat . . . . .2.5 g
  Trans Fat. . . . . .0.0 g
Cholesterol . . . . .20 mg
Sodium. . . . . .475 mg
Total Carbohydrate . . .41 g
  Dietary Fiber. . . . . .5 g
  Sugars . . . . .5 g
Protein . . . . .22 g

Chicken Parmigiana
Serves 4   Serving size: 1/4 recipe

1 **lb** boneless, skinless chicken breasts (trimmed of fat)

3 **Tbsp** grated reduced-fat Parmesan cheese

1/4 **cup** bread crumbs

1 **tsp** oregano

1 **tsp** parsley flakes

1/4 **tsp** paprika

1/4 **tsp** red pepper flakes

Nonstick cooking spray

Place chicken breasts in boiling water and thoroughly cook. Combine cheese, bread crumbs, oregano, parsley, paprika, and red pepper flakes. Place chicken in a shallow baking pan sprayed with nonstick cooking spray. Coat the tops of the chicken with the bread crumb and cheese mixture. Bake for 20–25 minutes at 400°F until cooked through.

Exchanges/Choices
1/2 Starch
3 Lean Meat

Basic Nutritional Values
Calories 180
  Calories from Fat 40
Total Fat . . . . .4.5 g
  Saturated Fat . . . . .1.4 g
  Trans Fat . . . . .0.0 g
Cholesterol . . . . .70 mg
Sodium . . . . .195 mg
Total Carbohydrate . . .7 g
  Dietary Fiber . . . . .0 g
  Sugars . . . . .0 g
Protein . . . . .26 g

Low-Fat, Sugar-Free Eggnog
Serves 8   Serving size: 1/8 recipe

3 **cups** nonfat milk

1 **cup** fat-free evaporated milk

2 **Tbsp** cornstarch

1/2 **cup** Splenda

1/2 **cup** egg substitute

2 **tsp** pure vanilla extract

1/4 **tsp** ground cinnamon

1/8 **tsp** ground nutmeg

1. Mix together 1 cup nonfat milk, evaporated milk, cornstarch, and Splenda in small saucepan. Heat, stirring constantly, for 1 minute.

2. Beat egg substitute in a medium bowl. Mix about half of the milk mixture into the egg substitute; then add to remaining milk in the saucepan.

3. Cook over very low heat until slightly thickened, about 1–2 minutes, stirring constantly. Remove from heat. Stir in vanilla and cinnamon. Cool to room temperature; refrigerate until chilled or until serving time.

4. Stir 2 cups chilled nonfat milk into custard-like mixture, serving in small glasses or punch cups. Sprinkle tops lightly with nutmeg.

Exchanges/Choices
1/2 Fat-Free Milk
1/2 Carbohydrate

Basic Nutritional Values
Calories 85
  Calories from Fat 0
Total Fat . . . . .0.0 g
  Saturated Fat . . . . .0.1 g
  Trans Fat . . . . .0.0 g
Cholesterol . . . . .5 mg
Sodium . . . . .115 mg
Total Carbohydrate . . .12 g
  Dietary Fiber . . . . .0 g
  Sugars . . . . .10 g
Protein . . . . .7 g

Pumpkin Spice Muffins

Serves 8   Serving size: 2 muffins

1 **cup** whole-wheat flour	2 **Tbsp** Splenda
3 **tsp** baking powder	1 **cup** canned pumpkin
2 **tsp** ground cinnamon	1/2 **cup** nonfat milk
2 **tsp** ground nutmeg	1/4 **cup** unsweetened applesauce
1/4 **cup** egg substitute	1/4 **cup** raisins or chopped nuts

Preheat oven to 400°F. Line sixteen muffin-pan cups with paper liners or spray with nonstick cooking spray. In a large bowl, stir together the flour, baking powder, cinnamon, and nutmeg. In a medium bowl, beat egg substitute with a whisk. Add Splenda, pumpkin, milk, and applesauce; stir until well blended. Stir in raisins. Stir into flour mixture until just blended. Fill muffin-pan cups 2/3 full. Bake 20–25 minutes until a wooden toothpick inserted in the center comes out clean. Remove muffins from muffin pans. Serve warm or at room temperature.

Exchanges/Choices

1 1/2 Carbohydrate

Basic Nutritional Values

Calories 95
 Calories from Fat 5
Total Fat. . . . . 0.5 g
 Saturated Fat . . . . 0.2 g
 Trans Fat. . . . . 0.0 g
Cholesterol . . . . 0 mg
Sodium. . . . . 160 mg
Total Carbohydrate . . . 20 g
 Dietary Fiber. . . . . 3 g
 Sugars . . . . 6 g
Protein . . . . 4 g

Chicken and Black Bean Chili

Serves 4   Serving size: 1/4 recipe

2 **Tbsp** sodium-free chicken bouillon	1/2 **cup** diced onion
1 **cup** water	1/2 **cup** diced carrots
1/2 **lb** boneless, skinless chicken breasts (trimmed of fat)	1 clove garlic, minced
	1 bay leaf
1 1/3 **cup** canned no-added-salt black beans, rinsed and drained	1 1/2 **cup** no-added-salt tomato juice
	2 **Tbsp** chili powder
1/2 **cup** diced red bell pepper	1/4 **tsp** cayenne pepper

Heat bouillon and water in a large saucepan. Add chicken and sauté until it is no longer pink, about 3 minutes. Remove the chicken and rinse to cool. Then shred the chicken or dice into very small pieces. Return to pan. Stir in all remaining ingredients. Bring to a boil, reduce heat, and simmer for 20 minutes. Remove from heat and discard bay leaf.

Exchanges/Choices

1 Starch
2 Vegetable
2 Lean Meat

Basic Nutritional Values

Calories 200
 Calories from Fat 20
Total Fat. . . . . 2.5 g
 Saturated Fat . . . . 0.5 g
 Trans Fat. . . . . 0.0 g
Cholesterol . . . . 35 mg
Sodium. . . . . 95 mg
Total Carbohydrate . . . 28 g
 Dietary Fiber. . . . . 6 g
 Sugars . . . . 9 g
Protein . . . . 18 g

Broiled Salmon

Serves 4   Serving size: 1/4 recipe

1 **lb** salmon steak
(about 3/4 inch thick)

1 **cup** white wine

Black pepper, to taste

2 **tsp** Smart Balance margarine

1 **cup** dry bread crumbs

2 **Tbsp** horseradish

2 green onions, minced

Arrange salmon steaks in a baking dish just large enough to hold them in one layer. Brush salmon lightly with the wine and season with pepper. Pour remaining wine around the steaks and broil about 4 inches from the heat for 4–5 minutes or until almost cooked through. While steaks are cooking, stir together the margarine, bread crumbs, horseradish, and green onion. Pat the crumb mixture evenly on the steaks and broil for 2–4 more minutes or until just cooked through and bread crumbs are golden.

Exchanges/Choices

1 1/2 Starch
3 Lean Meat
1 1/2 Fat

Basic Nutritional Values

Calories 335
  Calories from Fat 115
Total Fat. . . . . 13.0 g
  Saturated Fat . . . . 2.5 g
  Trans Fat. . . . . 0.0 g
Cholesterol . . . . 75 mg
Sodium. . . . . 295 mg
Total Carbohydrate . . . 21 g
  Dietary Fiber . . . . 2 g
  Sugars . . . . 3 g
Protein . . . . 28 g

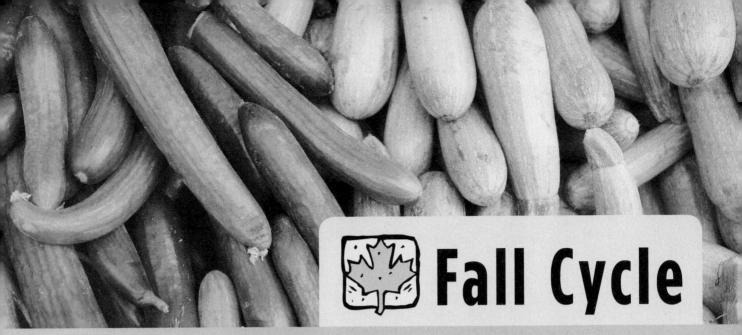

FEATURED RECIPES

Zucchini Carrot Muffins*

Pizza Muffins*

Beef Pot Roast

Apple Oatmeal Squares*

Confetti Cottage Cheese Salad

Low-Fat Corn Bread*

Spiced Chicken with Apples

Mexican Corn Salad*

Whole-Wheat Cornmeal Muffin*

Bean and Cheese Enchiladas

Oven-Poached Salmon

Far East Cabbage Salad*

Whole-Wheat French Toast*

Asian Beef, Noodles, and Vegetables

Baked Chicken Florida

Buttermilk Biscuits*

Carrots in Sherry Wine*

Pumpkin Spice Muffins*

Turkey Sausage Sandwich

Tangerine Broccoli*

Crunchy Baked Trout

Baked Apples*

Whole-Wheat Blueberry Muffins*

Curried Chicken Salad

Beef Tips with Onions

Blackberry Cobbler*

Deli Turkey Sandwich

Macaroni Salad

Chicken Marengo

Mashed Potatoes*

*Indicates that the recipe has been used previously.

1500 calorie MEAL PLAN   FALL WEEK 3

	Sunday	Monday	Tuesday	Wednesday	Thursday	Friday	Saturday
Breakfast	Zucchini Carrot Muffins* 1 small nectarine 1/2 cup nonfat milk 1/2 tsp margarine	Apple Oatmeal Squares* 1/2 cup shredded wheat 1 cup nonfat milk 6 walnut halves	Whole-Wheat Cornmeal Muffin (2)* 1/2 cup unsweetened applesauce 1 cup nonfat milk	Whole-Wheat French Toast* 1/2 cup unsweetened plums 1 cup nonfat milk	Pumpkin Spice Muffins* 1/2 Tbsp jam 1/2 cup mango 1 cup nonfat milk 1 tsp margarine 6 almonds	Baked Apples* Whole-Wheat Blueberry Muffins (2 muffins)* 1 cup nonfat milk 1/2 tsp margarine	Blackberry Cobbler* 1/2 whole-grain English muffin 1 cup nonfat milk 1 tsp margarine
Lunch	Pizza Muffins* 1/2 cup sugar-free pudding 1 medium banana 1 1/2 tsp peanut butter	Confetti Cottage Cheese Salad (2 servings) Low-Fat Corn Bread* 3/4 cup blueberries 1 cup mixed vegetable sticks 1 tsp margarine	Bean and Cheese Enchiladas 1 cup papaya 1 cup tomatoes and cucumbers 1 oz reduced-fat cheese	Asian Beef, Noodles, and Vegetables (2 servings) 2 fortune cookies 1/2 cup unsweetened mandarin oranges	Turkey Sausage Sandwich Tangerine Broccoli* 1 medium ear corn on the cob 17 small grapes 1/2 cup steamed collard greens 1/2 tsp margarine	Curried Chicken Salad (1/2 serving) 3/4 cup brown rice 1 cup salad greens 1 tsp light salad dressing	Deli Turkey Sandwich Macaroni Salad 1 fresh fig 1/2 cup steamed green beans
Snack A							
Snack B							
Dinner	Beef Pot Roast 1 medium peach 1 cup nonfat milk 1 cup salad greens 2 tsp light salad dressing	Spiced Chicken with Apples Mexican Corn Salad* 1 slice whole-grain bread 1 cup nonfat milk 1 cup cooked spinach 2 tsp margarine	Oven-Poached Salmon Far East Cabbage Salad* 1/2 cup wild rice 1 small dinner roll 1 cup honeydew melon 1 cup nonfat milk 1/2 cup steamed asparagus 1/2 tsp margarine	Baked Chicken Florida Buttermilk Biscuits* Carrots in Sherry Wine* 1/2 cup green peas 1 1/4 cup strawberries 1 cup nonfat milk	Crunchy Baked Trout 1 medium baked sweet potato 3/4 cup blueberries 1 cup nonfat milk 1 cup steamed asparagus	Beef Tips with Onions 1/3 cup cooked pasta 1/2 cup pineapple 1 cup nonfat milk 1 cup steamed carrots and broccoli 1 1/2 tsp margarine	Chicken Marengo Mashed Potatoes* 1 slice rye bread 2 small plums 1 cup nonfat milk 1/2 tsp margarine

*Indicates that the recipe has been used previously.

	Sunday	Monday	Tuesday	Wednesday	Thursday	Friday	Saturday
Breakfast	Zucchini Carrot Muffins* 1 small nectarine 1/2 cup nonfat milk 1/4 cup egg substitute 1/2 tsp margarine	Apple Oatmeal Squares* 1/2 cup shredded wheat 1 cup nonfat milk 1 oz Canadian bacon 6 walnut halves	Whole-Wheat Cornmeal Muffin (2)* 1/2 cup unsweetened applesauce 1 cup nonfat milk 1 oz lean beef sausage	Whole-Wheat French Toast* 1/2 cup unsweetened plums 1 cup nonfat milk	Pumpkin Spice Muffins* 1/2 Tbsp jam 1/2 cup mango 1 cup nonfat milk 1 oz lean ham 1 tsp margarine 6 almonds	Baked Apples* Whole-Wheat Blueberry Muffins (2 muffins)* 1 cup nonfat milk 1/4 cup egg substitute 1/2 tsp margarine	Blackberry Cobbler* 1/2 whole-grain English muffin 1 cup nonfat milk 1/4 cup low-fat cottage cheese 1 tsp margarine
Lunch	Pizza Muffins* 1/2 cup sugar-free pudding 1 medium banana 1 Tbsp peanut butter	Confetti Cottage Cheese Salad (2 servings) Low-Fat Corn Bread* 3/4 cup blueberries 1 cup mixed vegetable sticks 2 tsp margarine	Bean and Cheese Enchiladas 1 cup papaya 1 cup tomatoes and cucumbers 1 oz reduced-fat cheese 2 Tbsp avocado	Asian Beef, Noodles, and Vegetables (2 servings) 2 fortune cookies 1/2 cup unsweetened mandarin oranges 6 almonds	Turkey Sausage Sandwich Tangerine Broccoli* 1 medium ear corn on the cob 17 small grapes 1/2 cup steamed collard greens 1/2 tsp margarine	Curried Chicken Salad (1/2 serving) 3/4 cup brown rice 1 cup salad greens 2 tsp light salad dressing	Deli Turkey Sandwich Macaroni Salad 1 fresh fig 1/2 cup steamed green beans 1 tsp margarine
Snack A	4 pecans 3/4 cup pineapple	6 almonds 12 cherries	5 hazelnuts 1/2 large pear	2 Tbsp fat-free whipped topping 1 cup raspberries	16 pistachios 3 dates	2 Brazil nuts 12 cherries	6 almonds 4 apricots
Snack B	1 cup nonfat milk	1 cup nonfat milk	6 oz fat-free yogurt	1 cup nonfat milk	1 cup nonfat milk	6 oz fat-free yogurt	1 cup nonfat milk
Dinner	Beef Pot Roast 1 medium peach 1 cup nonfat milk 1 cup salad greens 2 tsp light salad dressing	Spiced Chicken with Apples Mexican Corn Salad* 1 slice whole-grain bread 1 cup nonfat milk 1 cup cooked spinach 2 tsp margarine	Oven-Poached Salmon Far East Cabbage Salad* 1/2 cup wild rice 1 small dinner roll 1 cup honeydew melon 1 cup nonfat milk 1/2 cup steamed asparagus 1/2 tsp margarine	Baked Chicken Florida Buttermilk Biscuits* Carrots in Sherry Wine* 1/2 cup green peas 1 1/4 cup strawberries 1 cup nonfat milk 1/2 tsp margarine	Crunchy Baked Trout 1 medium baked sweet potato 3/4 cup blueberries 1 cup nonfat milk 1 cup steamed asparagus	Beef Tips with Onions 1/3 cup cooked pasta 1/2 cup pineapple 1 cup nonfat milk 1 cup steamed carrots and broccoli 1 1/2 tsp margarine	Chicken Marengo Mashed Potatoes* 1 slice rye bread 2 small plums 1 cup nonfat milk 1/2 tsp margarine

*Indicates that the recipe has been used previously.

2000 calorie MEAL PLAN FALL WEEK 3

	Sunday	Monday	Tuesday	Wednesday	Thursday	Friday	Saturday
Breakfast	**Zucchini Carrot Muffins*** 1 small nectarine 1/2 cup nonfat milk 1/4 cup egg substitute 1/2 tsp margarine	**Apple Oatmeal Squares*** 1/2 cup shredded wheat 1 cup nonfat milk 1 oz Canadian bacon 6 walnut halves	**Whole-Wheat Cornmeal Muffin (2)*** 1/2 cup unsweetened applesauce 1 cup nonfat milk 1 oz lean beef sausage	**Whole-Wheat French Toast*** 1/2 cup unsweetened plums 1 cup nonfat milk	**Pumpkin Spice Muffins*** 1/2 Tbsp jam 1/2 cup mango 1 cup nonfat milk 1 oz lean ham 1 tsp margarine 6 almonds	**Baked Apples*** **Whole-Wheat Blueberry Muffins** **(2 muffins)*** 1 cup nonfat milk 1/4 cup egg substitute 1/2 tsp margarine	**Blackberry Cobbler*** 1/2 whole-grain English muffin 1 cup nonfat milk 1/4 cup low-fat cottage cheese 1 tsp margarine
Lunch	**Pizza Muffins*** 1/2 cup sugar-free pudding 1 large banana 1 Tbsp peanut butter	**Confetti Cottage Cheese Salad (2 servings)** **Low-Fat Corn Bread*** 1 1/2 cup blueberries 2 cups mixed vegetable sticks 2 tsp margarine	**Bean and Cheese Enchiladas** 2 cups papaya 1 cup tomatoes and cucumbers 1 oz reduced-fat cheese 2 Tbsp avocado	**Asian Beef, Noodles, and Vegetables (2 servings)** 2 fortune cookies 1 cup unsweetened mandarin oranges 6 almonds	**Turkey Sausage Sandwich** **Tangerine Broccoli*** 1 medium ear corn on the cob 17 small grapes 1 cup cantaloupe 1 cup steamed collard greens 1/2 tsp margarine	**Curried Chicken Salad** (1/2 serving) 3/4 cup brown rice 2 cups salad greens 2 tsp light salad dressing	**Deli Turkey Sandwich** **Macaroni Salad** 3 fresh figs 1 cup steamed green beans 1 tsp margarine
Snack A	1 cup carrot sticks 4 pecans 3/4 cup pineapple	1 cup celery sticks 1 1/2 tsp cashew butter 12 cherries	1 cup mixed vegetables 5 hazelnuts 1/2 large pear	1 cup broccoli 1 Tbsp light salad dressing 1 cup raspberries	1 cup green bell pepper slices 1 Tbsp light salad dressing 3 dates	1 cup green bell pepper slices 1 Tbsp light salad dressing 12 cherries	1 cup cucumber slices 1 Tbsp light salad dressing 4 apricots
Snack B	1/2 whole-grain English muffin 1 tsp margarine 1 cup nonfat milk	8 animal crackers 6 almonds 1 cup nonfat milk	1/2 (6-inch) pita bread 2 tsp tahini (sesame paste) 6 oz fat-free yogurt	3/4 oz pretzels 1 Tbsp pine nuts 1 cup nonfat milk	1 cup oven-baked French fries 16 pistachios 1 cup nonfat milk	1/4 cup low-fat granola 2 Brazil nuts 6 oz fat-free yogurt	3/4 oz pretzels 6 almonds 1 cup nonfat milk
Dinner	**Beef Pot Roast** 1 medium peach 1 cup nonfat milk 1 cup salad greens 2 tsp light salad dressing	**Spiced Chicken with Apples** **Mexican Corn Salad*** 1 slice whole-grain bread 1 cup nonfat milk 1 cup cooked spinach 2 tsp margarine	**Oven-Poached Salmon** **Far East Cabbage Salad*** 1/2 cup wild rice 1 small dinner roll 1 cup honeydew melon 1 cup nonfat milk 1/2 cup steamed asparagus 1/2 tsp margarine	**Baked Chicken Florida** **Buttermilk Biscuits*** **Carrots in Sherry Wine*** 1/2 cup green peas 1 1/4 cup strawberries 1 cup nonfat milk 1/2 tsp margarine	**Crunchy Baked Trout** 1 medium baked sweet potato 3/4 cup blueberries 1 cup nonfat milk 1 cup steamed asparagus	**Beef Tips with Onions** 1/3 cup cooked pasta 1/2 cup pineapple 1 cup nonfat milk 1 cup steamed carrots and broccoli 1 1/2 tsp margarine	**Chicken Marengo** **Mashed Potatoes*** 1 slice rye bread 2 small plums 1 cup nonfat milk 1/2 tsp margarine

*Indicates that the recipe has been used previously.

	Sunday	Monday	Tuesday	Wednesday	Thursday	Friday	Saturday
Breakfast	Zucchini Carrot Muffins* 1 small nectarine 1/2 cup nonfat milk 1/2 cup egg substitute 1/2 tsp margarine	Apple Oatmeal Squares* 1/2 cup shredded wheat 1 cup nonfat milk 1 oz Canadian bacon 6 walnut halves	Whole-Wheat Cornmeal Muffin (2)* 1/2 cup unsweetened applesauce 1 cup nonfat milk 2 oz lean beef sausage	Whole-Wheat French Toast* 1/2 cup unsweetened plums 1 cup nonfat milk 1/4 cup egg substitute	Pumpkin Spice Muffins* 1/2 Tbsp jam 1/2 cup mango 1 cup nonfat milk 2 oz lean ham 1 tsp margarine 6 almonds	Baked Apples* Whole-Wheat Blueberry Muffins (2 muffins)* 1 cup nonfat milk 1/2 cup egg substitute 1/2 tsp margarine	Blackberry Cobbler* 1/2 whole-grain English muffin 1 cup nonfat milk 1/2 cup low-fat cottage cheese 1 tsp margarine
Lunch	Pizza Muffins* 1/2 cup sugar-free pudding 1 large banana 1 Tbsp peanut butter	Confetti Cottage Cheese Salad (2 servings) Low-Fat Corn Bread* 1 1/2 cup blueberries 2 cups mixed vegetable sticks 2 tsp margarine	Bean and Cheese Enchiladas 2 cups papaya 1 cup tomatoes and cucumbers 1 oz reduced-fat cheese 2 Tbsp avocado	Asian Beef, Noodles, and Vegetables (2 servings) 2 fortune cookies 1 cup unsweetened mandarin oranges 6 almonds	Turkey Sausage Sandwich Tangerine Broccoli* 1 medium ear corn on the cob 17 small grapes 1 cup cantaloupe 1 cup steamed collard greens 1/2 tsp margarine	Curried Chicken Salad (1/2 serving) 3/4 cup brown rice 2 cups salad greens 2 tsp light salad dressing	Deli Turkey Sandwich Macaroni Salad 3 fresh figs 1 cup steamed green beans 1 tsp margarine
Snack A	1 cup carrot sticks 4 pecans 3/4 cup pineapple	1 cup celery sticks 1 1/2 tsp cashew butter 12 cherries	1 cup mixed vegetables 5 hazelnuts 1/2 large pear	1 cup broccoli 1 Tbsp light salad dressing 1 cup raspberries	1 cup green bell pepper slices 1 Tbsp light salad dressing 3 dates	1 cup green bell pepper slices 1 Tbsp light salad dressing 12 cherries	1 cup cucumber slices 1 Tbsp light salad dressing 4 apricots
Snack B	1/2 whole-grain English muffin 1 tsp margarine 1 cup nonfat milk	8 animal crackers 6 almonds 1 cup nonfat milk	1/2 (6-inch) pita bread 2 tsp tahini (sesame paste) 6 oz fat-free yogurt	3/4 oz pretzels 1 Tbsp pine nuts 1 cup nonfat milk	1 cup oven-baked French fries 16 pistachios 1 cup nonfat milk	1/4 cup low-fat granola 2 Brazil nuts 6 oz fat-free yogurt	3/4 oz pretzels 6 almonds 1 cup nonfat milk
Dinner	Beef Pot Roast 1 slice multigrain bread 1 medium peach 1 cup nonfat milk 1 cup salad greens 2 tsp light salad dressing	Spiced Chicken with Apples Mexican Corn Salad* 2 slices whole-grain bread 1 cup nonfat milk 1 cup cooked spinach 2 tsp margarine	Oven-Poached Salmon Far East Cabbage Salad* 1/2 cup wild rice 1 small dinner roll 1 cup honeydew melon 1 cup nonfat milk 1/2 cup steamed asparagus 1/2 tsp margarine	Baked Chicken Florida Buttermilk Biscuits* Carrots in Sherry Wine* 1 cup green peas 1 1/4 cup strawberries 1 cup nonfat milk 1/2 tsp margarine	Crunchy Baked Trout 1 medium baked sweet potato 3/4 cup blueberries 1 cup nonfat milk 1 cup steamed asparagus	Beef Tips with Onions 1/3 cup cooked pasta 1/2 cup pineapple 1 cup nonfat milk 1 cup steamed carrots and broccoli 1 1/2 tsp margarine	Chicken Marengo Mashed Potatoes* 2 slices rye bread 2 small plums 1 cup nonfat milk 1/2 tsp margarine

*Indicates that the recipe has been used previously.

SHOPPING LIST

VEGETABLES

_____ asparagus
_____ bell peppers, green
_____ broccoli
_____ cabbage
_____ carrots
_____ celery
_____ collard greens
_____ corn kernels, frozen
_____ corn on the cob
_____ cucumbers
_____ garlic
_____ green beans
_____ lettuce, romaine
_____ mushrooms
_____ onions, green
_____ onions, red
_____ onions, white
_____ onions, yellow
_____ peas
_____ potatoes
_____ potatoes, sweet
_____ radishes
_____ spinach
_____ tomatoes
_____ zucchini

MEATS

_____ bacon, Canadian
_____ beef, rump roast, lean
_____ beef, sirloin, boneless
_____ beef, stew or sirloin cubes, lean
_____ chicken breasts, boneless, skinless
_____ ham, lean
_____ salmon fillets
_____ sausage, beef, lean
_____ trout fillets
_____ turkey breast, deli-style sliced, light
_____ turkey breast, lean, ground

FRUITS

_____ apples
_____ apples, tart
_____ avocado
_____ bananas
_____ blackberries
_____ blueberries
_____ cantaloupe
_____ figs
_____ grapes, green, seedless
_____ honeydew melon
_____ lemons
_____ mango
_____ nectarines
_____ oranges, mandarin
_____ papaya
_____ peaches
_____ pineapple
_____ plums
_____ raisins
_____ strawberries

DAIRY

_____ buttermilk, fat-free
_____ egg substitute
_____ egg whites
_____ milk, nonfat
_____ Smart Balance margarine
_____ yogurt, fat-free, plain

CHEESE

_____ cheese, any kind, reduced-fat
_____ cottage cheese, fat-free
_____ cottage cheese, low-fat
_____ Mexican cheese blend, reduced-fat, shredded
_____ mozzarella, fat-free, shredded
_____ mozzarella, reduced-fat, shredded

BREAD, GRAINS, & PASTA

_____ bread, rye
_____ bread, whole-grain, whole-wheat
_____ buns, hamburger, whole-grain
_____ dinner rolls, whole-wheat
_____ English muffins, whole-grain or multigrain
_____ noodles, rice
_____ pasta, macaroni, whole-wheat
_____ rice, brown, whole-grain
_____ rice, wild

BEANS

_____ refried beans, fat-free (vegetarian), 16-oz can

NUTS

_____ almonds
_____ walnuts

CONDIMENTS

_____ canola mayonnaise
_____ mustard, Dijon
_____ soy sauce, light

SPICES & HERBS

_____ allspice
_____ basil
_____ bay leaf
_____ black pepper
_____ chili powder
_____ chives
_____ cilantro
_____ cinnamon, ground
_____ curry powder
_____ dill weed
_____ garlic powder
_____ ginger, ground
_____ marjoram
_____ mint leaves
_____ nutmeg, ground
_____ oregano
_____ parsley
_____ pumpkin pie spice
_____ sage
_____ tarragon, fresh
_____ thyme

OTHER

_____ applesauce, unsweetened
_____ biscuit mix
_____ bread crumbs, dry
_____ cereal, shredded wheat
_____ enchilada sauce, red, 10-oz can
_____ fortune cookies
_____ juice, apple
_____ juice, cranberry
_____ juice, lemon
_____ juice, orange concentrate, frozen
_____ marmalade, tangerine or orange, sugar-free
_____ peanut butter
_____ pimentos
_____ preserves or jam, sugar-free
_____ pudding mix, sugar-free, any flavor
_____ pumpkin, canned
_____ salad dressing, light
_____ salsa, no-added-salt
_____ sesame seeds
_____ spaghetti sauce, no-added-salt
_____ taco sauce, red
_____ tomatoes, diced, no-added-salt, 16-oz can
_____ tortillas, flour, 8-inch
_____ wheat germ
_____ wine, sherry, dry cooking
_____ wine, white

STAPLES

_____ baking powder
_____ baking soda
_____ bouillon, beef, sodium-free
_____ bouillon, chicken, sodium-free
_____ cornmeal, yellow
_____ cornstarch
_____ flour, all-purpose
_____ flour, whole-wheat
_____ nonstick cooking spray
_____ oats, old-fashioned
_____ Smart Balance Omega oil
_____ Splenda
_____ vinegar, cider

Zucchini Carrot Muffins

Serves 8   Serving size: 1 muffin

3/4 **cup** rolled oats	2 **tsp** ground nutmeg
2 1/2 **cups** whole-wheat flour	3 **Tbsp** Smart Balance Omega oil
2/3 **cup** nonfat milk	3 egg whites, beaten
1/2 **cup** wheat germ, toasted	1 **cup** carrots, finely shredded
3 **tsp** baking powder	1/2 **cup** zucchini, stemmed and grated
3/4 **cup** Splenda	
1 **Tbsp** ground cinnamon	

Preheat oven to 350°F. Combine all ingredients and mix well; pour into muffin liners in muffin pans. Bake for about 1 hour. Let cool for about 30 minutes before removing.

Exchanges/Choices

2 1/2 Carbohydrate
1 1/2 Fat

Basic Nutritional Values

Calories 260
 Calories from Fat 65
Total Fat . . . . 7.0 g
 Saturated Fat . . . . 0.9 g
 Trans Fat . . . . 0.0 g
Cholesterol . . . . 0 mg
Sodium . . . . 180 mg
Total Carbohydrate . . . 42 g
 Dietary Fiber . . . . 7 g
 Sugars . . . . 5 g
Protein . . . . 11 g

Pizza Muffins

Serves 4   Serving size: 1 muffin

4 light multigrain English muffins	4 **oz** reduced-fat shredded mozzarella cheese
1 **cup** no-salt-added spaghetti sauce	1/4 **cup** sliced mushrooms
4 **oz** fat-free shredded mozzarella cheese	1 small onion, sliced into thin rings
	4 green bell pepper rings

1. Preheat the oven to 400°F.

2. Split the English muffins in half and put on a baking sheet, cut sides up. Spread spaghetti sauce over muffins. Top with 1 ounce of each of the cheeses. Top with mushrooms, onion rings, and pepper rings. Place pizzas in oven and bake for about 5 minutes or until cheese melts.

This recipe is high in sodium.

Exchanges/Choices

2 Starch
2 Vegetable
2 Lean Meat

Basic Nutritional Values

Calories 305
 Calories from Fat 65
Total Fat . . . . 7.0 g
 Saturated Fat . . . . 2.4 g
 Trans Fat . . . . 0.0 g
Cholesterol . . . . 15 mg
Sodium . . . . 660 mg
Total Carbohydrate . . . 42 g
 Dietary Fiber . . . . 12 g
 Sugars . . . . 8 g
Protein . . . . 25 g

Beef Pot Roast

Serves 4   Serving size: 1/4 recipe

1 1/4 **lb** lean beef rump roast
(trimmed of fat)

3 **Tbsp** whole-wheat flour

1 **Tbsp** Smart Balance
Omega oil

Pepper, to taste

1/3 large onion, sliced

2 large potatoes, quartered

2 medium carrots, julienned

Exchanges/Choices

2 Starch
1 Vegetable
3 Lean Meat

Basic Nutritional Values

Calories 320
  Calories from Fat 65
Total Fat . . . . .7.0 g
  Saturated Fat . . . . .2.2 g
  Trans Fat . . . . .0.0 g
Cholesterol . . . . .75 mg
Sodium . . . . .85 mg
Total Carbohydrate . . .37 g
  Dietary Fiber . . . . .5 g
  Sugars . . . . .5 g
Protein . . . . .28 g

1. Preheat oven to 350°F. Dust roast on all sides with 1 Tbsp flour. Heat oil in a Dutch oven over medium-high heat. Put roast in Dutch oven and brown on all sides. Sprinkle with pepper. Remove roast; place a low wire rack in Dutch oven. Put roast on rack.

2. Place onion slices on top and around roast. Cover and bake for 2 hours. Add potatoes and carrots; cook 1 more hour. Remove from oven. Slice meat, put on a warmed platter, and surround with vegetables. Keep warm.

3. Add enough water to juices in Dutch oven to make 2 cups. Put an additional 1/3 cup water in a small bowl; add 2 Tbsp flour and whisk until smooth. Stir into juices in the Dutch oven and cook, stirring constantly, until gravy is bubbly. Simmer 2–3 minutes; stir occasionally. Serve gravy on the side with the sliced pot roast.

Apple Oatmeal Squares

Serves 6   Serving Size: 1/6 recipe

1/2 **cup** nonfat milk

1/4 **cup** Splenda

2 **Tbsp** Smart Balance margarine

1 1/2 **cup** dry oats

2 1/2 **cup** unsweetened applesauce

1 **tsp** cinnamon

1/2 **cup** raisins

Nonstick cooking spray

Heat the milk, Splenda, and margarine to a boil, stirring constantly so they don't burn. Stir in the oats, applesauce, cinnamon, and raisins. Heat without stirring until bubbles appear at the edges. Remove from heat and spread evenly in a pan lightly sprayed with nonstick cooking spray. Bake at 350°F for 30 minutes. Cut into 2-inch squares.

Exchanges/Choices

1 Starch
1 Fruit
1/2 Fat

Basic Nutritional Values

Calories 160
 Calories from Fat 40
Total Fat . . . . 4.5 g
 Saturated Fat . . . . 1.1 g
 Trans Fat . . . . 0.0 g
Cholesterol . . . . 0 mg
Sodium . . . . 45 mg
Total Carbohydrate . . . 27 g
 Dietary Fiber . . . . 3 g
 Sugars . . . . 12 g
Protein . . . . 4 g

Confetti Cottage Cheese Salad

Serves 4   Serving size: 1/4 recipe

1/4 **cup** grated carrot

1/4 **cup** chopped chives

1/4 **cup** chopped parsley

1/4 **cup** grated bell pepper

16 **oz** fat-free cottage cheese

Combine carrot, chives, parsley, and bell pepper. Sprinkle mixture over cottage cheese. Chill before serving.

Exchanges/Choices

1/2 Fat-Free Milk
1 Lean Meat

Basic Nutritional Values

Calories 90
 Calories from Fat 0
Total Fat . . . . 0.0 g
 Saturated Fat . . . . 0.0 g
 Trans Fat . . . . 0.0 g
Cholesterol . . . . 5 mg
Sodium . . . . 420 mg
Total Carbohydrate . . . 7 g
 Dietary Fiber . . . . 1 g
 Sugars . . . . 4 g
Protein . . . . 15 g

Low-Fat Corn Bread
Serves 8　　Serving size: 1/8 recipe

1/2　**cup** egg substitute

1/2　**cup** Splenda

3/4　**cup** nonfat milk

1/2　**cup** unsweetened applesauce

1 1/2　**cup** whole-wheat flour

2/3　**cup** cornmeal

1　**Tbsp** baking powder

　　Nonstick cooking spray

Beat together the egg substitute, Splenda, milk, and applesauce; set aside. In a separate bowl, sift and combine flour, cornmeal, and baking powder. Stir into egg mixture using as few strokes as possible. Spray an 8 × 8-inch baking pan with nonstick cooking spray. Bake at 400°F for 25–30 minutes or until a toothpick inserted near the middle comes out clean.

Exchanges/Choices

2 Starch

Basic Nutritional Values

Calories 150
　Calories from Fat 5
Total Fat. . . . . .0.5 g
　Saturated Fat . . . . .0.1 g
　Trans Fat. . . . . .0.0 g
Cholesterol . . . . .0 mg
Sodium. . . . . .180 mg
Total Carbohydrate . . .30 g
　Dietary Fiber. . . . . .4 g
　Sugars . . . . .4 g
Protein . . . . .6 g

Spiced Chicken with Apples
Serves 4　　Serving size: 1/4 recipe

1　**Tbsp** Smart Balance margarine

1　**lb** boneless, skinless chicken breasts (trimmed of fat)

1　medium apple, cored and sliced

1　**cup** apple juice

1　**Tbsp** Splenda

1　**Tbsp** cornstarch

1　**Tbsp** sodium-free chicken bouillon

1/2　**cup** water

1/8　**tsp** cinnamon

1/8　**tsp** nutmeg

Preheat oven to 350°F. In a large skillet, melt the margarine; add chicken and brown it. Drain off any remaining fat. Add apple slices. Combine apple juice, Splenda, cornstarch, bouillon, water, cinnamon, and nutmeg. Pour over chicken and apple slices; bring to a boil. Reduce heat, cover, and simmer 10 minutes. Cook, uncovered, for 5 more minutes.

Exchanges/Choices

1 Fruit
3 Lean Meat

Basic Nutritional Values

Calories 210
　Calories from Fat 45
Total Fat. . . . . .5.0 g
　Saturated Fat . . . . .1.4 g
　Trans Fat. . . . . .0.0 g
Cholesterol . . . . .65 mg
Sodium. . . . . .85 mg
Total Carbohydrate . . .16 g
　Dietary Fiber. . . . . .1 g
　Sugars . . . . .11 g
Protein . . . . .24 g

Mexican Corn Salad

Serves 4   Serving size: 1/4 recipe

10 oz frozen corn, thawed

1/2 cup no-added-salt salsa

1 green onion, sliced and diced

1/2 cup radishes, sliced and diced

4 romaine lettuce leaves

Combine frozen corn, salsa, green onion, and radishes. Spoon mixture evenly over lettuce leaves.

Exchanges/Choices

1 Starch

Basic Nutritional Values

Calories 80
 Calories from Fat 5
Total Fat . . . . 0.5 g
 Saturated Fat . . . . 0.1 g
 Trans Fat . . . . 0.0 g
Cholesterol . . . . 0 mg
Sodium . . . . 80 mg
Total Carbohydrate . . . 18 g
 Dietary Fiber . . . . 3 g
 Sugars . . . . 4 g
Protein . . . . 3 g

Whole-Wheat Cornmeal Muffin

Serves 8   Serving size: 1 muffin

2/3 **cup** yellow cornmeal

2/3 **cup** whole-wheat flour

1 **Tbsp** Splenda

2 **tsp** baking powder

2/3 **cup** nonfat milk

1/4 **cup** egg substitute

2 **Tbsp** Smart Balance
     Omega oil

Preheat oven to 400°F. Place paper liners in muffin trays. Thoroughly mix dry ingredients. Combine milk, egg substitute, and oil; add to dry ingredients. Stir until dry ingredients are just moistened. Batter will be lumpy. Fill muffin tins 2/3 full. Bake until slightly browned, about 20 minutes.

Exchanges/Choices

1 Carbohydrate
1 Fat

Basic Nutritional Values

Calories 120
  Calories from Fat 35
Total Fat . . . . 4.0 g
  Saturated Fat . . . . 0.3 g
  Trans Fat . . . . 0.0 g
Cholesterol . . . . 0 mg
Sodium . . . . 115 mg
Total Carbohydrate . . . 18 g
  Dietary Fiber . . . . 2 g
  Sugars . . . . 1 g
Protein . . . . 4 g

Bean and Cheese Enchiladas

Serves 4   Serving size: 1 enchilada

Nonstick cooking spray

1 medium onion, chopped

16 oz fat-free (vegetarian) refried beans

1/2 cup red taco sauce

1/8 tsp garlic powder

4 (8-inch) tortillas

1 (10-oz) can red enchilada sauce

1/2 cup reduced-fat Mexican cheese blend, shredded

Exchanges/Choices

2 Starch
3 Vegetable
1 Lean Meat
1 Fat

Basic Nutritional Values

Calories 325
 Calories from Fat 80
Total Fat . . . . 9.0 g
 Saturated Fat . . . . 2.7 g
 Trans Fat . . . . 1.0 g
Cholesterol . . . . 10 mg
Sodium . . . . 1410 mg
Total Carbohydrate . . 48 g
 Dietary Fiber . . . . 6 g
 Sugars . . . . 4 g
Protein . . . . 14 g

1. Preheat oven to 350°F.

2. Spray a large skillet with nonstick cooking spray and put over medium-high heat; sauté onions until tender. Add beans, taco sauce, and garlic powder. Bring to a boil, reduce heat to a simmer, and cook until bean mixture is smooth and bubbling. Remove from heat; keep warm.

3. While beans cook, place tortillas between paper towels and heat for 10–20 seconds in the microwave or until tortillas are soft.

4. Pour half of the enchilada sauce in a baking dish.

5. Place about 1/3 cup of the bean filling on each tortilla and roll to enclose filling. Place tortillas seam side down in the baking dish. Pour remaining enchilada sauce over enchiladas. Sprinkle with cheese and bake, uncovered, for 20–25 minutes or until heated through and cheese is melted.

This recipe is high in sodium.

Oven-Poached Salmon

Serves 4   Serving size: 1/4 recipe

Nonstick cooking spray

3/4 **lb** salmon fillets

Pepper, to taste

2 **Tbsp** cider vinegar

6 sprigs tarragon or dill

3 lemons

2 **Tbsp** minced tarragon or dill leaves

1. Preheat oven to 250°F.

2. Spray three sheets of heavy-duty foil with nonstick cooking spray. Remove any bones from the salmon. Pat the salmon dry with paper towels and season both sides with pepper to taste. Lay the salmon fillets skin-side down on top of the foil. Sprinkle with vinegar; lay the herb sprigs on top. Slice two lemons and arrange slices on top of the herbs. Crimp the foil down over the fish into a tight packet.

3. Lay the foil-wrapped fish directly on the oven rack and bake for about 45–60 minutes, until the thickest part reads 135–140°F and the fish has turned from pink to orange. Remove fish from oven, open the foil packets, and discard lemon slices and herb sprigs. Let the salmon cool at room temperature on the foil for 30 minutes. Pour off any accumulated liquid, reseal the salmon in the foil, and refrigerate until cold, about 1 hour. (Poached salmon can be refrigerated for up to 2 days. Let the salmon sit at room temperature for 30 minutes before serving.)

4. To serve, unwrap the salmon and brush away any gelled poaching liquid. Sprinkle the salmon with minced tarragon or dill. Cut the remaining lemon into wedges and serve on the side.

Exchanges/Choices

3 Lean Meat

Basic Nutritional Values

Calories 145
  Calories from Fat 65
Total Fat . . . . 7.0 g
  Saturated Fat . . . . 1.3 g
  Trans Fat . . . . 0.0 g
Cholesterol . . . . 60 mg
Sodium . . . . 45 mg
Total Carbohydrate . . . 0 g
  Dietary Fiber . . . . 0 g
  Sugars . . . . 0 g
Protein . . . . 18 g

Far East Cabbage Salad

Serves 4   Serving size: 1/4 recipe

2 Tbsp lemon juice

2 tsp Splenda

4 cups shredded cabbage

2/3 medium red onion, diced

4 Tbsp diced mint leaves

4 Tbsp chopped cilantro

2 Tbsp Smart Balance
    Omega oil

In a bowl, stir together the lemon juice and Splenda until dissolved. Add all other ingredients and toss well until mixed.

Exchanges/Choices

1 Vegetable
1 1/2 Fat

Basic Nutritional Values

Calories 90
  Calories from Fat 65
Total Fat . . . . 7.0 g
  Saturated Fat . . . . 0.5 g
  Trans Fat . . . . 0.0 g
Cholesterol . . . . 0 mg
Sodium . . . . 15 mg
Total Carbohydrate . . . 7 g
  Dietary Fiber . . . . 2 g
  Sugars . . . . 4 g
Protein . . . . 1 g

Whole-Wheat French Toast
Serves 4   Serving size: 1/4 recipe

1 1/2 **cup** egg substitute

1 **cup** nonfat milk

1 **Tbsp** Splenda

3 **Tbsp** Smart Balance
Omega oil

8 thick slices whole-wheat
bread

In a shallow bowl, beat together the egg substitute, milk, and Splenda with a whisk. Pour 1 Tbsp oil in the skillet and heat over medium heat. Dip the bread into the milk mixture one slice at a time. Place each dipped slice into the hot oil in the frying pan. Do not overlap or crowd the pieces. Fry for 2–3 minutes until golden brown and then turn over and continue frying until the second side is golden brown. Put the browned slices on an oven-safe plate and place in the 200°F oven to keep hot. Continue dipping and frying the remaining slices of bread. Add 1–2 Tbsp oil as needed.

Exchanges/Choices

2 Starch
1 Lean Meat
2 Fat

Basic Nutritional Values

Calories 285
  Calories from Fat 110
Total Fat . . . . 12.0 g
  Saturated Fat . . . . 1.2 g
  Trans Fat . . . . 0.0 g
Cholesterol . . . . 0 mg
Sodium . . . . 430 mg
Total Carbohydrate . . . 27 g
  Dietary Fiber . . . . 4 g
  Sugars . . . . 6 g
Protein . . . . 16 g

Asian Beef, Noodles, and Vegetables
Serves 4   Serving size: 1/4 recipe

1 **tsp** Smart Balance
Omega Oil

1/2 **lb** boneless sirloin beef
(trimmed of fat)

1/2 **cup** sliced mushrooms

1 medium carrot, cut into thin
strips

2 medium cloves garlic, minced

2 **Tbsp** sodium-free beef
bouillon

1 **cup** water

1 **cup** asparagus, cut into
1/2-inch pieces

1 **tsp** light soy sauce

2 **oz** rice noodles

4 **oz** frozen chopped spinach

In a large skillet, heat the oil and add beef; cook over medium-high heat for about 3 minutes or until browned. Add mushrooms, carrot, and garlic; cook for a few more minutes, stirring occasionally. Add bouillon, water, asparagus, and soy sauce; bring to a boil. Then add the noodles and spinach. Simmer, covered, for about 10 minutes or until noodles are tender.

Exchanges/Choices

1 Starch
1 Vegetable
1 Lean Meat
1/2 Fat

Basic Nutritional Values

Calories 175
  Calories from Fat 35
Total Fat . . . . 4.0 g
  Saturated Fat . . . . 1.0 g
  Trans Fat . . . . 0.1 g
Cholesterol . . . . 20 mg
Sodium . . . . 140 mg
Total Carbohydrate . . . 20 g
  Dietary Fiber . . . . 3 g
  Sugars . . . . 4 g
Protein . . . . 15 g

Baked Chicken Florida

Serves 4   Serving size: 1/4 recipe

1 **Tbsp** sodium-free chicken bouillon

1 1/4 **cup** water

1/4 **cup** lemon juice

1 clove garlic, minced

1/4 **tsp** tarragon leaves, crushed

1 **lb** boneless, skinless chicken breast (trimmed of fat)

1 **Tbsp** cornstarch

In a large bowl, combine bouillon, water, lemon juice, garlic, and tarragon to make a marinade. Arrange the chicken in a shallow baking pan and pour marinade on top. Refrigerate for at least 2 hours, turning the pieces of chicken occasionally. Bake at 375°F for 1 hour or until the chicken is fork-tender. Baste frequently; then transfer chicken to a serving dish. Pour remaining marinade into a saucepan; add cornstarch. Stirring constantly, heat to boiling and then simmer until sauce is smooth throughout. Spoon sauce over the chicken and serve.

Exchanges/Choices

3 Lean Meat

Basic Nutritional Values

Calories 140
  Calories from Fat 25
Total Fat . . . . 3.0 g
  Saturated Fat . . . . 0.8 g
  Trans Fat . . . . 0.0 g
Cholesterol . . . . 65 mg
Sodium . . . . 65 mg
Total Carbohydrate . . . 4 g
  Dietary Fiber . . . . 0 g
  Sugars . . . . 1 g
Protein . . . . 24 g

Buttermilk Biscuits

Serves 6   Serving size: 1 biscuit

1 **cup** all-purpose flour

1 **Tbsp** Splenda

1 1/2 **tsp** baking powder

1/4 **tsp** baking soda

3 1/3 **Tbsp** Smart Balance margarine

1/2 **cup** fat-free buttermilk

Preheat oven to 450°F. In a medium bowl, combine flour, Splenda, baking powder, and baking soda. With a pastry blender, cut in margarine until mixture resembles coarse crumbs. Stir in buttermilk. Place on a lightly floured surface; knead 3–4 times and roll or pat to a 1/2- to 3/4-inch thickness. Cut with a 2 1/2-inch biscuit cutter dipped in flour. Bake on an ungreased baking sheet for 12–15 minutes or until golden brown.

Exchanges/Choices

1 Starch
1 Fat

Basic Nutritional Values

Calories 135
  Calories from Fat 45
Total Fat . . . . 5.0 g
  Saturated Fat . . . . 1.4 g
  Trans Fat . . . . 0.0 g
Cholesterol . . . . 0 mg
Sodium . . . . 215 mg
Total Carbohydrate . . . 19 g
  Dietary Fiber . . . . 1 g
  Sugars . . . . 3 g
Protein . . . . 3 g

Carrots in Sherry Wine

Serves 4   Serving size: 1/4 recipe

2 cups baby carrots

2 Tbsp Smart Balance Light margarine

1/2 cup dry cooking sherry

Combine all ingredients and cook carrots over medium heat until tender.

Exchanges/Choices

2 Vegetable
1/2 Fat

Basic Nutritional Values

Calories 70
  Calories from Fat 20
Total Fat . . . . 2.5 g
  Saturated Fat . . . . 0.8 g
  Trans Fat . . . . 0.0 g
Cholesterol . . . . 0 mg
Sodium . . . . 85 mg
Total Carbohydrate . . . 8 g
  Dietary Fiber . . . . 2 g
  Sugars . . . . 4 g
Protein . . . . 1 g

THURSDAY

Pumpkin Spice Muffins

Serves 8   Serving size: 2 muffins

1 **cup** whole-wheat flour	1 **cup** canned pumpkin
3 **tsp** baking powder	1/2 **cup** nonfat milk
2 **tsp** ground cinnamon	1/4 **cup** unsweetened applesauce
2 **tsp** ground nutmeg	
1/4 **cup** egg substitute	1/4 **cup** raisins or chopped nuts
2 **Tbsp** Splenda	

Preheat oven to 400°F. Line sixteen muffin-pan cups with paper liners or spray with nonstick cooking spray. In a large bowl, stir together the flour, baking powder, cinnamon, and nutmeg. In a medium bowl, beat egg substitute with a whisk. Add Splenda, pumpkin, milk, and applesauce; stir until well blended. Stir in raisins. Stir into flour mixture until just blended. Fill muffin-pan cups 2/3 full. Bake 20–25 minutes until a wooden toothpick inserted in the center comes out clean. Remove muffins from muffin pans. Serve warm or at room temperature.

Exchanges/Choices

1 1/2 Carbohydrate

Basic Nutritional Values

Calories 95
  Calories from Fat 5
Total Fat . . . . .0.5 g
  Saturated Fat . . . . 0.2 g
  Trans Fat . . . . 0.0 g
Cholesterol . . . . 0 mg
Sodium . . . . 160 mg
Total Carbohydrate . . . 20 g
  Dietary Fiber . . . . 3 g
  Sugars . . . . 6 g
Protein . . . . 4 g

Turkey Sausage Sandwich
Serves 4   Serving size: 1 sandwich

Nonstick cooking spray

3/4 **lb** lean ground turkey breast

4 egg white

2 **Tbsp** water

1 **tsp** dried basil

1 **tsp** dried sage

1 **tsp** dried oregano

1/2 **tsp** allspice

1/2 **tsp** ground nutmeg

1/2 **tsp** dill weed

1/2 **tsp** garlic powder

1/4 **tsp** chili powder

4 romaine lettuce leaves

4 **Tbsp** canola mayonnaise

4 whole-grain buns

Exchanges/Choices
1 1/2 Starch
2 Lean Meat
1/2 Fat

Basic Nutritional Values
Calories 235
  Calories from Fat 65
Total Fat. . . . . .7.0 g
  Saturated Fat . . . . .0.6 g
  Trans Fat. . . . . .0.0 g
Cholesterol . . . . .40 mg
Sodium. . . . . .340 mg
Total Carbohydrate . . .24 g
  Dietary Fiber. . . . . .4 g
  Sugars . . . . .5 g
Protein . . . . .20 g

1. Preheat the broiler and lightly spray a broiler pan with nonstick cooking spray.

2. In a medium bowl, thoroughly combine turkey, egg white, water, basil, sage, oregano, allspice, nutmeg, dill, garlic powder, and chili powder. Form into four equal patties and place on the broiler pan.

3. Broil about 2–4 inches from the heat for about 10 minutes. Flip the patties over and broil for another 5–10 minutes until the patties are no longer pink in the center.

4. Serve the patties with a lettuce leaf and 1 Tbsp mayonnaise on whole-grain buns.

Tangerine Broccoli

Serves 4   Serving size: 1/4 recipe

2 **cups** broccoli florets

2 **Tbsp** cider vinegar

1/4 **tsp** ground ginger

1/4 **tsp** ground cinnamon

1/4 **cup** sugar-free tangerine or orange marmalade

Cook broccoli in a steamer basket in a medium saucepan over a small amount of simmering water, covered, for about 7 minutes. Meanwhile, in a small saucepan, stir together vinegar, ginger, cinnamon, and marmalade; cook over low heat until marmalade has melted. To serve, spoon an equal amount of the sauce over each broccoli serving.

Exchanges/Choices

1/2 Carbohydrate

Basic Nutritional Values

Calories 20
 Calories from Fat 0
Total Fat . . . . 0.0 g
 Saturated Fat . . . . 0.0 g
 Trans Fat . . . . 0.0 g
Cholesterol . . . . 0 mg
Sodium . . . . 10 mg
Total Carbohydrate . . . 7 g
 Dietary Fiber . . . . 1 g
 Sugars . . . . 3 g
Protein . . . . 1 g

Crunchy Baked Trout

Serves 4   Serving size: 1/4 recipe

4 **tsp** Smart Balance Omega oil

1 medium clove garlic, minced

1 **lb** trout fillets

1/4 **cup** dry bread crumbs

2 **Tbsp** sesame seeds

Pepper, to taste

Preheat oven to 400°F. In a small saucepan, heat the oil. Add garlic and sauté until just browned. Using a brush, coat the insides of the trout with the oil-garlic mixture and then sprinkle with bread crumbs, sesame seeds, and pepper. Bake on the middle rack for 5 minutes or until fish flakes with a fork.

Exchanges/Choices

1/2 Starch
3 Lean Meat
2 Fat

Basic Nutritional Values

Calories 265
 Calories from Fat 135
Total Fat . . . . 15.0 g
 Saturated Fat . . . . 2.0 g
 Trans Fat . . . . 0.0 g
Cholesterol . . . . 65 mg
Sodium . . . . 110 mg
Total Carbohydrate . . . 6 g
 Dietary Fiber . . . . 1 g
 Sugars . . . . 0 g
Protein . . . . 25 g

Baked Apples

Serves 4   Serving size: 1/4 recipe

4 medium tart baking apples (Jonathan, York, or Rome Beauty), peeled and cored

1/4 cup Splenda

2 1/2 Tbsp Smart Balance margarine

3 Tbsp sugar-free preserves (any kind)

1 tsp pumpkin pie spice

3 Tbsp raisins

3/4 cup water

1. Preheat oven to 350°F.

2. With the tip of a knife, make six 1/4-inch deep cuts in each apple, from top to halfway down. Place the apples in an 8 × 8 × 2-inch baking dish.

3. In a small bowl, combine the Splenda, margarine, fruit preserves, and spice. Stir in raisins.

4. Stuff each apple with one-fourth of the mixture. Pour water into the bottom of the baking dish; cover with foil and seal tightly. Bake for 50–60 minutes or until fork-tender. Remove foil and gently transfer apples to four small dessert bowls. Spoon a little of the juice from the bottom of the pan over each apple.

Exchanges/Choices

2 Fruit
1 Fat

Basic Nutritional Values

Calories	150
Calories from Fat	55
Total Fat	6.0 g
Saturated Fat	1.6 g
Trans Fat	0.0 g
Cholesterol	0 mg
Sodium	60 mg
Total Carbohydrate	28 g
Dietary Fiber	3 g
Sugars	23 g
Protein	0 g

Whole-Wheat Blueberry Muffins

Serves 12   Serving size: 1 muffin

1 cup whole-wheat flour

5 1/2 Tbsp Splenda

1 tsp baking powder

6 Tbsp nonfat milk

3 Tbsp Smart Balance margarine

1/2 cup egg substitute

1/2 cup blueberries

Preheat oven to 400°F. In a medium bowl, combine flour, Splenda, and baking powder. In a small bowl, beat milk, margarine, and egg substitute; stir into dry ingredients until just moist. Fold in blueberries and spoon batter into 12 paper-lined muffin cups. Bake for 20–25 minutes or until golden brown. Serve immediately.

Exchanges/Choices

1/2 Starch
1/2 Fat

Basic Nutritional Values

Calories	70
Calories from Fat	20
Total Fat	2.5 g
Saturated Fat	0.7 g
Trans Fat	0.0 g
Cholesterol	0 mg
Sodium	75 mg
Total Carbohydrate	9 g
Dietary Fiber	1 g
Sugars	2 g
Protein	3 g

Curried Chicken Salad

Serves 4   Serving size: 1/4 recipe

1 **lb** boneless, skinless chicken breasts (trimmed of fat)

1/4 **cup** canola mayonnaise

3 **Tbsp** orange juice concentrate, frozen

3 **tsp** curry powder

1 **cup** diced peaches

1 **cup** diced celery

1 **cup** seedless green grapes

1/2 **cup** raisins

4 romaine lettuce leaves

Place chicken breasts in boiling water and thoroughly cook. Transfer chicken to the refrigerator to cool while preparing the other ingredients. In a large bowl, combine mayonnaise, orange juice, and curry powder until well blended. When cool to the touch, cut chicken into small chunks. Gently stir in chicken, diced peaches, celery, grapes, and raisins. Chill in the refrigerator. Spoon chicken mixture onto lettuce leaves on individual plates.

Exchanges/Choices

2 1/2 Fruit
4 Lean Meat

Basic Nutritional Values

Calories 315
  Calories from Fat 70
Total Fat . . . . 8.0 g
  Saturated Fat . . . . 0.9 g
  Trans Fat . . . . 0.0 g
Cholesterol . . . . 65 mg
Sodium . . . . 180 mg
Total Carbohydrate . . . 36 g
  Dietary Fiber . . . . 3 g
  Sugars . . . . 30 g
Protein . . . . 26 g

Beef Tips with Onions

Serves 4   Serving size: 1/4 recipe

1 **Tbsp** Smart Balance Omega oil

1 **lbs** lean stew beef or sirloin cubes (trimmed of fat)

1 **Tbsp** sodium-free beef bouillon

1 **Tbsp** soy sauce

1 clove garlic, minced

4 **oz** cranberry juice

2 medium onions, sliced thick

2 **Tbsp** cornstarch

Heat oil in a large skillet. Brown beef in oil on all sides. Stir in 1/2 cup water, bouillon, soy sauce, garlic, and cranberry juice. Heat to boiling. Cover, reduce heat, and simmer for 1 hour or until meat is tender (sirloin cubes should take about 1 hour; stew beef cubes may take 3 hours). When meat is tender, add onion slices. Blend cornstarch with 1/4 cup water; stir gradually into the meat mixture until it thickens and boils. Boil, stir 1 minute more, and serve.

Exchanges/Choices

1 Carbohydrate
3 Lean Meat
1/2 Fat

Basic Nutritional Values

Calories 220
  Calories from Fat 70
Total Fat . . . . 8.0 g
  Saturated Fat . . . . 1.6 g
  Trans Fat . . . . 0.0 g
Cholesterol . . . . 55 mg
Sodium . . . . 270 mg
Total Carbohydrate . . . 18 g
  Dietary Fiber . . . . 1 g
  Sugars . . . . 8 g
Protein . . . . 19 g

Blackberry Cobbler
Serves 4   Serving size: 1/4 recipe

Nonstick cooking spray

1/2 **cup** Splenda

1 **Tbsp** cornstarch

2 **cups** sliced blackberries,
fresh or frozen

2 **Tbsp** water

1 **cup** biscuit mix

1/4 **cup** nonfat milk

Preheat oven to 425°F. Spray a round casserole dish with nonstick cooking spray. Mix 1/2 cup Splenda and cornstarch in saucepan, stir in blackberries and water. Heat to boiling, stirring constantly. Boil and stir 1 minute. Pour mixture into casserole dish. Mix biscuit mix according to package directions and drop dough by the spoonful onto the hot blackberry mixture. Bake until golden brown, about 20 minutes. Serve with milk.

Exchanges/Choices
2 Carbohydrate
1 Fat

Basic Nutritional Values
Calories 195
  Calories from Fat 40
Total Fat . . . . 4.5 g
  Saturated Fat . . . . 1.2 g
  Trans Fat . . . . 1.2 g
Cholesterol . . . . 0 mg
Sodium . . . . 410 mg
Total Carbohydrate . . . 34 g
  Dietary Fiber . . . . 5 g
  Sugars . . . . 9 g
Protein . . . . 5 g

Deli Turkey Sandwich
Serves 4   Serving size: 1 sandwich

1/2 **lb** deli-style light turkey

4 romaine lettuce leaves

2 small tomatoes, sliced

4 **Tbsp** canola mayonnaise

8 slices whole-grain bread

Evenly divide turkey, lettuce, tomato slices, and mayonnaise between slices of bread.

This recipe is high in sodium.

Exchanges/Choices
2 Starch
2 Lean Meat

Basic Nutritional Values
Calories 245
  Calories from Fat 65
Total Fat . . . . 7.0 g
  Saturated Fat . . . . 0.5 g
  Trans Fat . . . . 0.0 g
Cholesterol . . . . 25 mg
Sodium . . . . 1135 mg
Total Carbohydrate . . . 30 g
  Dietary Fiber . . . . 6 g
  Sugars . . . . 7 g
Protein . . . . 17 g

Macaroni Salad

Serves 4   Serving size: 1/4 recipe

4 **oz** whole-wheat macaroni

1/4 **cup** canola mayonnaise

1/4 **cup** fat-free plain yogurt

1/4 **cup** diced celery

1/4 **cup** sliced green onion

1 **Tbsp** sliced pimento

2 **tsp** Dijon mustard

1/2 **tsp** dill weed, crushed

1/4 **tsp** marjoram, crushed

1/4 **tsp** pepper

1 **cup** cut green beans, cooked

Cook macaroni according to package directions; drain. In a medium bowl, combine mayonnaise, yogurt, celery, green onion, pimento, mustard, dill, marjoram, and pepper until well blended. Add macaroni and green beans; gently toss until well coated. Cover and chill at least 2 hours before serving.

Exchanges/Choices

1 1/2 Starch
1 Fat

Basic Nutritional Values

Calories 150
 Calories from Fat 45
Total Fat . . . . 5.0 g
 Saturated Fat . . . . 0.1 g
 Trans Fat . . . . 0.0 g
Cholesterol . . . . 0 mg
Sodium . . . . 160 mg
Total Carbohydrate . . . 23 g
 Dietary Fiber . . . . 3 g
 Sugars . . . . 2 g
Protein . . . . 5 g

Chicken Marengo

Serves 4   Serving size: 1/4 recipe

2 **Tbsp** Smart Balance
 Omega oil

1 **lb** boneless, skinless chicken
 breasts (trimmed of fat)

1/2 **cup** small white onions,
 peeled and diced

1/4 **cup** sliced mushrooms

1 clove garlic, minced

2 **Tbsp** whole-wheat flour

1 **(16-oz)** can no-added-salt
 diced tomatoes

1/4 **cup** white wine

2 **Tbsp** chopped parsley

1 bay leaf

1/8 **tsp** black pepper

1/8 **tsp** thyme

Heat the oil in a large skillet over medium-high heat; add chicken and brown. Remove chicken and set aside. Add onions, mushrooms, and garlic; sauté until golden. Stir in flour. Cook and stir for 1 minute. Add tomatoes, wine, parsley, bay leaf, pepper, and thyme. Stirring constantly over medium heat, bring to a boil; add chicken. Reduce heat to low, cover, and simmer for 40–45 minutes or until chicken is tender. Remove bay leaf before serving.

Exchanges/Choices

2 Vegetable
3 Lean Meat
1 Fat

Basic Nutritional Values

Calories 240
 Calories from Fat 90
Total Fat . . . . 10.0 g
 Saturated Fat . . . . 1.3 g
 Trans Fat . . . . 0.0 g
Cholesterol . . . . 65 mg
Sodium . . . . 135 mg
Total Carbohydrate . . . 11 g
 Dietary Fiber . . . . 3 g
 Sugars . . . . 5 g
Protein . . . . 26 g

Mashed Potatoes

Serves 4   Serving size: 1/4 recipe

2 cups peeled, diced potatoes

1/4 cup nonfat milk

5 tsp Smart Balance margarine

Pepper, to taste

Peel the potatoes and cut into cubes; place in a large pan. Cover with water, bring to a boil, and then simmer for approximately 45 minutes, until potatoes are tender. Mash potatoes until no lumps remain, slowly adding milk and margarine to make potatoes smoother and fluffy. Season with pepper and serve.

Exchanges/Choices

1 Starch
1/2 Fat

Basic Nutritional Values

Calories 85
  Calories from Fat 35
Total Fat . . . . 4.0 g
  Saturated Fat . . . . 1.1 g
  Trans Fat . . . . 0.0 g
Cholesterol . . . . 0 mg
Sodium . . . . 50 mg
Total Carbohydrate . . . 12 g
  Dietary Fiber . . . . 1 g
  Sugars . . . . 2 g
Protein . . . . 1 g

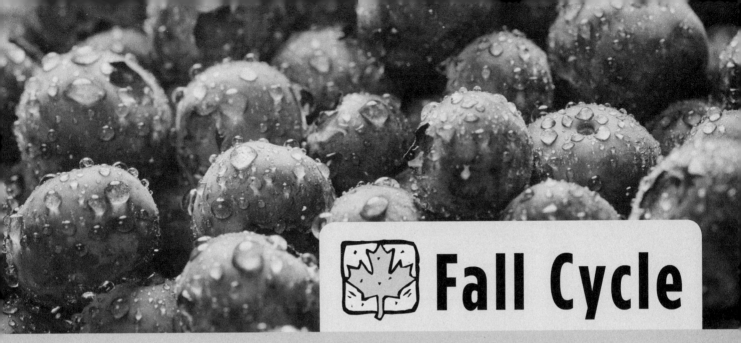

Fall Cycle

FEATURED RECIPES

Banana Walnut Bread*

Vegetarian Chili

Gratin of Broccoli

Chicken with Glazed Apples

Whole-Wheat Blueberry Muffins*

Shrimp and Peppers

Baked Squash*

Baked Sweet Potato Fries*†

Veal Parmesan Hoagie*

Bread Pudding*

Tabbouleh

Chicken Milanese

Broccoli Floret Salad*

Cinnamon Apple Yogurt*

Fried Bananas*

Turkey Sausage Sandwich*

Broccoli Slaw*

Buttered Parsley Potatoes*

Caribbean Tilapia

Buttermilk Biscuits*

Fruit Salad Medley*

Snap Peas and Shrimp Penne

Pepper Steak*

Carrot Cake*

Gram's Gingerbread*

Pork Cutlets with Melons

Green Beans and Red Peppers*

Spicy Seasoned Chicken

All-Natural High-Fiber Peach Squares*

Granola, Oats, Blackberry, and Raspberry Bake*

Roast Beef and Swiss Roll-Up*

Tasty Baked Chicken

Summer Pasta Salad

*Indicates that the recipe has been used previously.

†This recipe is used as a snack, but its ingredients are in the shopping list.

1500 calorie MEAL PLAN FALL WEEK 4

	Sunday	Monday	Tuesday	Wednesday	Thursday	Friday	Saturday
Breakfast	Banana Walnut **Bread** (2 slices)* 1/2 cup oatmeal 1 cup nonfat milk 1 tsp margarine	Whole-Wheat **Blueberry Muffins** (2 muffins)* 1/4 cup granola 12 cherries 1 cup nonfat milk 1 tsp margarine	Bread Pudding* 1/2 English muffin 1/2 cup unsweetened peaches 1/2 cup nonfat milk 1 tsp margarine	Cinnamon Apple **Yogurt*** **Fried Bananas*** 1 slice oatmeal bread 1/2 tsp margarine	Fruit Salad Medley* 1/2 cup grits 1 cup nonfat milk 1 tsp margarine 4 pecans	Gram's Gingerbread* 1/2 cup unsweetened applesauce 1 cup nonfat milk 20 peanuts	Granola, Oats, Blackberry, and Raspberry Bake* 3/4 cup grits 1 cup nonfat milk 1 1/2 tsp margarine
Lunch	Vegetarian Chili 1 6-inch tortilla 1 small orange 1 Tbsp avocado	Shrimp and Peppers Baked Squash* 3/4 cup brown rice 1/2 cup unsweetened applesauce	Tabbouleh 1 small pita pocket 1/3 cup hummus	Turkey Sausage Sandwich* Broccoli Slaw* Buttered Parsley Potatoes* 3 ginger snaps 1 cup honeydew melon	Snap Peas and Shrimp Penne 1 cup cantaloupe 1 oz reduced-fat cheese 5 hazelnuts	Pork Cutlets with Melons Green Beans and Red Peppers* 2/3 cup brown rice 1 small dinner roll 1 1/2 tsp margarine	Roast Beef and Swiss Roll-Up* 1 medium ear corn on the cob 2 small plums
Snack A							
Snack B							
Dinner	Gratin of Broccoli Chicken with Glazed Apples 1 large baked sweet potato 1 cup nonfat milk 2 tsp margarine	Veal Parmesan Hoagie* 1 cup nonfat milk 5 peanuts	Chicken Milanese Broccoli Floret Salad* 3/4 cup blueberries 1/2 cup nonfat milk 1/2 cup steamed carrots 1 1/2 tsp margarine	Caribbean Tilapia Buttermilk Biscuits* 1/2 cup wild rice 1/2 cup fruit cocktail in water 1 cup nonfat milk 1/2 cup cooked zucchini	Pepper Steak* Carrot Cake* 1/2 cup steamed spinach 1 tsp margarine	Spicy Seasoned Chicken All-Natural High-Fiber Peach Squares* 1 small dinner roll 1/2 cup nonfat milk 1 cup cooked spinach with tomatoes 1 tsp margarine	Tasty Baked Chicken Summer Pasta Salad 1 cup raspberries 1 cup nonfat milk 1/2 cup steamed broccoli 1 1/2 tsp margarine

*Indicates that the recipe has been used previously.

	Sunday	Monday	Tuesday	Wednesday	Thursday	Friday	Saturday
Breakfast	**Banana Walnut Bread** (2 slices)* 1/2 cup oatmeal 1 cup nonfat milk 1 tsp margarine	**Whole-Wheat Blueberry Muffins** (2 muffins)* 1/4 cup granola 12 cherries 1 cup nonfat milk 1 oz Canadian bacon 1 tsp margarine	**Bread Pudding*** 1/2 English muffin 1/2 cup unsweetened peaches 1/2 cup nonfat milk 1 oz low-fat turkey sausage 1 tsp margarine	**Cinnamon Apple Yogurt*** **Fried Bananas*** 1 slice oatmeal bread 1 oz lean beef sausage 1/2 tsp margarine	**Fruit Salad Medley*** 1/2 cup grits 1 cup nonfat milk 1 oz lean ham 1 tsp margarine 4 pecans	**Gram's Gingerbread*** 1/2 cup unsweetened applesauce 1 cup nonfat milk 1/4 cup egg substitute 20 peanuts	**Granola, Oats, Blackberry, and Raspberry Bake*** 3/4 cup grits 1 cup nonfat milk 1 oz lean meat (your choice) 1 1/2 tsp margarine
Lunch	**Vegetarian Chili** 1 6-inch tortilla 1 small orange 1 oz reduced-fat cheese 2 Tbsp avocado	**Shrimp and Peppers Baked Squash*** 3/4 cup brown rice 1/2 cup unsweetened applesauce 10 peanuts	**Tabbouleh** 1 small pita pocket 1/3 cup hummus 16 pistachios	**Turkey Sausage Sandwich*** **Broccoli Slaw*** **Buttered Parsley Potatoes*** 3 ginger snaps 1 cup honeydew melon 5 peanuts	**Snap Peas and Shrimp Penne** 1 cup cantaloupe 1 oz reduced-fat cheese 10 hazelnuts	**Pork Cutlets with Melons** **Green Beans and Red Peppers*** 2/3 cup brown rice 1 small dinner roll 1 1/2 tsp margarine	**Roast Beef and Swiss Roll-Up*** 1 medium ear corn on the cob 2 small plums 1 oz avocado
Snack A	2 Brazil nuts 17 grapes	4 walnut halves 1 cup raspberries	6 cashews 1 medium banana	1 1/2 tsp almond butter 1 small apple	3 macadamia nuts 2 Tbsp dried cranberries	1 Tbsp sunflower seeds 3/4 cup blueberries	6 cashews 3/4 cup unsweetened mandarin oranges
Snack B	1 cup nonfat milk	6 oz fat-free yogurt	1 cup nonfat milk	1 cup nonfat milk	6 oz fat-free yogurt	1 cup nonfat milk	6 oz fat-free yogurt
Dinner	**Gratin of Broccoli Chicken with Glazed Apples** 1 large baked sweet potato 1 cup nonfat milk 2 tsp margarine	**Veal Parmesan Hoagie*** 1 cup nonfat milk 5 peanuts	**Chicken Milanese Broccoli Floret Salad*** 3/4 cup blueberries 1/2 cup nonfat milk 1/2 cup steamed carrots 1 1/2 tsp margarine	**Caribbean Tilapia Buttermilk Biscuits*** 1/2 cup wild rice 1/2 cup fruit cocktail in water 1 cup nonfat milk 1/2 cup cooked zucchini 1/2 tsp margarine	**Pepper Steak*** **Carrot Cake*** 1/2 cup steamed spinach 1 tsp margarine	**Spicy Seasoned Chicken** **All-Natural High-Fiber Peach Squares*** 1 small dinner roll 1/2 cup nonfat milk 1 cup cooked spinach with tomatoes 1 tsp margarine	**Tasty Baked Chicken Summer Pasta Salad** 1 cup raspberries 1 cup nonfat milk 1/2 cup steamed broccoli 1 1/2 tsp margarine

*Indicates that the recipe has been used previously.

2000 calorie MEAL PLAN FALL WEEK 4

	Sunday	Monday	Tuesday	Wednesday	Thursday	Friday	Saturday
Breakfast	**Banana Walnut Bread** (2 slices)* 1/2 cup oatmeal 1 cup nonfat milk 1 tsp margarine	**Whole-Wheat Blueberry Muffins** (2 muffins)* 1/4 cup granola 12 cherries 1 cup nonfat milk 1 oz Canadian bacon 1 tsp margarine	**Bread Pudding*** 1/2 English muffin 1/2 cup unsweetened peaches 1/2 cup nonfat milk 1 oz low-fat turkey sausage 1 tsp margarine	**Cinnamon Apple Yogurt*** **Fried Bananas*** 1 slice oatmeal bread 1 oz lean beef sausage 1/2 tsp margarine	**Fruit Salad Medley*** 1/2 cup grits 1 cup nonfat milk 1 oz lean ham 1 tsp margarine 4 pecans	**Gram's Gingerbread*** 1/2 cup unsweetened applesauce 1 cup nonfat milk 1/4 cup egg substitute 20 peanuts	**Granola, Oats, Blackberry, and Raspberry Bake*** 3/4 cup grits 1 cup nonfat milk 1 oz lean meat (your choice) 1 1/2 tsp margarine
Lunch	**Vegetarian Chili** 1 6-inch tortilla 1 medium orange 1/2 cup steamed collard greens 1 oz reduced-fat cheese 2 Tbsp avocado	**Shrimp and Peppers Baked Squash*** 3/4 cup brown rice 1 cup unsweetened applesauce 10 peanuts	**Tabbouleh** 1 small pita pocket 1/3 cup hummus 2 medium figs 1 cup mixed vegetable sticks 16 pistachios	**Turkey Sausage Sandwich*** **Broccoli Slaw*** **Buttered Parsley Potatoes*** 3 ginger snaps 2 cups honeydew melon 5 peanuts	**Snap Peas and Shrimp Penne** 2 cups cantaloupe 1/2 cup steamed broccoli 1 oz reduced-fat cheese 10 hazelnuts	**Pork Cutlets with Melons** **Green Beans and Red Peppers*** 2/3 cup brown rice 1 small dinner roll 1 kiwi fruit 1 1/2 tsp margarine	**Roast Beef and Swiss Roll-Up*** 1 medium ear corn on the cob 2 small plums 1 oz avocado
Snack A	1 cup carrot sticks 2 Brazil nuts 17 grapes	1 cup celery sticks 4 walnut halves 1 cup raspberries	1 cup grape tomatoes 6 cashews 1 medium banana	1 cup broccoli 1 Tbsp light salad dressing 1 small apple	1 cup cauliflower 1 Tbsp light salad dressing 2 Tbsp dried cranberries	1 cup green pepper slices 1 Tbsp light salad dressing 3/4 cup blueberries	1 cup cucumber slices 1 Tbsp light salad dressing 3/4 cup unsweetened mandarin oranges
Snack B	1 slice rye bread 1 1/2 tsp almond butter 1 cup nonfat milk	**Baked Sweet Potato Fries*** 6 oz fat-free yogurt	2 rice cakes 1 1/2 tsp peanut butter 1 cup nonfat milk	3/4 oz baked potato chips 6 almonds 1 cup nonfat milk	1/4 cup low-fat granola 3 macadamia nuts 6 oz fat-free yogurt	1 slice whole-wheat toast 1 tsp margarine 1 cup nonfat milk	3 ginger snaps 6 cashews 6 oz fat-free yogurt
Dinner	**Gratin of Broccoli Chicken with Glazed Apples** 1 large baked sweet potato 1 cup nonfat milk 2 tsp margarine	**Veal Parmesan Hoagie*** 1 cup nonfat milk 5 peanuts	**Chicken Milanese Broccoli Floret Salad*** 3/4 cup blueberries 1/2 cup nonfat milk 1/2 cup steamed carrots 1 1/2 tsp margarine	**Caribbean Tilapia Buttermilk Biscuits*** 1/2 cup wild rice 1/2 cup fruit cocktail in water 1 cup nonfat milk 1/2 cup cooked zucchini 1/2 tsp margarine	**Pepper Steak*** **Carrot Cake*** 1/2 cup steamed spinach 1 tsp margarine	**Spicy Seasoned Chicken** **All-Natural High-Fiber Peach Squares*** 1 small dinner roll 1/2 cup nonfat milk 1 cup cooked spinach with tomatoes 1 tsp margarine	**Tasty Baked Chicken Summer Pasta Salad** 1 cup raspberries 1 cup nonfat milk 1/2 cup steamed broccoli 1 1/2 tsp margarine

*Indicates that the recipe has been used previously.

	Sunday	Monday	Tuesday	Wednesday	Thursday	Friday	Saturday
Breakfast	Banana Walnut Bread (2 slices)* 1/2 cup oatmeal 1 cup nonfat milk 1/4 cup egg substitute 1 tsp margarine	Whole-Wheat Blueberry Muffins (2 muffins)* 1/4 cup granola 12 cherries 1 cup nonfat milk 2 oz Canadian bacon 1 tsp margarine	Bread Pudding* 1/2 English muffin 1/2 cup unsweetened peaches 1/2 cup nonfat milk 2 oz low-fat turkey sausage 1 tsp margarine	Cinnamon Apple Yogurt* Fried Bananas* 1 slice oatmeal bread 2 oz lean beef sausage 1/2 tsp margarine	Fruit Salad Medley* 1/2 cup grits 1 cup nonfat milk 1 oz lean ham 1 tsp margarine 4 pecans	Gram's Gingerbread* 1/2 cup unsweetened applesauce 1 cup nonfat milk 1/2 cup egg substitute 20 peanuts	Granola, Oats, Blackberry, and Raspberry Bake* 3/4 cup grits 1 cup nonfat milk 2 oz lean meat (your choice) 1 1/2 tsp margarine
Lunch	Vegetarian Chili 1 6-inch tortilla 1 medium orange 1/2 cup steamed collard greens 1 oz reduced-fat cheese 2 Tbsp avocado	Shrimp and Peppers Baked Squash* 3/4 cup brown rice 1 cup unsweetened applesauce 10 peanuts	Tabbouleh 1 small pita pocket 1/3 cup hummus 2 medium figs 1 cup mixed vegetable sticks 16 pistachios	Turkey Sausage Sandwich* Broccoli Slaw* Buttered Parsley Potatoes* 3 ginger snaps 2 cups honeydew melon 5 peanuts	Snap Peas and Shrimp Penne 2 cups cantaloupe 1/2 cup steamed broccoli 1 oz reduced-fat cheese 10 hazelnuts	Pork Cutlets with Melons Green Beans and Red Peppers* 2/3 cup brown rice 1 small dinner roll 1 kiwi fruit 1 1/2 tsp margarine	Roast Beef and Swiss Roll-Up* 1 medium ear corn on the cob 2 small plums 1 oz avocado
Snack A	1 cup carrot sticks 2 Brazil nuts 17 grapes	1 cup celery sticks 4 walnut halves 1 cup raspberries	1 cup grape tomatoes 6 cashews 1 medium banana	1 cup broccoli 1 Tbsp light salad dressing 1 small apple	1 cup cauliflower 1 Tbsp light salad dressing 2 Tbsp dried cranberries	1 cup green pepper slices 1 Tbsp light salad dressing 3/4 cup blueberries	1 cup cucumber slices 1 Tbsp light salad dressing 3/4 cup unsweetened mandarin oranges
Snack B	1 slice rye bread 1 1/2 tsp almond butter 1 cup nonfat milk	Baked Sweet Potato Fries* 6 oz fat-free yogurt	2 rice cakes 1 1/2 tsp peanut butter 1 cup nonfat milk	3/4 oz baked potato chips 6 almonds 1 cup nonfat milk	1/4 cup low-fat granola 3 macadamia nuts 6 oz fat-free yogurt	1 slice whole-wheat toast 1 tsp margarine 1 cup nonfat milk	3 ginger snaps 6 cashews 6 oz fat-free yogurt
Dinner	Gratin of Broccoli Chicken with Glazed Apples 1 large baked sweet potato 1 small whole-grain dinner roll 1 cup nonfat milk 2 tsp margarine	Veal Parmesan Hoagie* 3/4 oz pretzels 1 cup nonfat milk 5 peanuts	Chicken Milanese Broccoli Floret Salad* 1 slice oatmeal bread 3/4 cup blueberries 1/2 cup nonfat milk 1/2 cup steamed carrots 1 1/2 tsp margarine	Caribbean Tilapia Buttermilk Biscuits* 1 cup wild rice 1/2 cup fruit cocktail in water 1 cup nonfat milk 1/2 cup cooked zucchini 1/2 tsp margarine	Pepper Steak* Carrot Cake* 1/2 cup corn 1/2 cup steamed spinach 1 tsp margarine	Spicy Seasoned Chicken All-Natural High-Fiber Peach Squares* 2 small dinner rolls 1/2 cup nonfat milk 1 cup cooked spinach with tomatoes 1 tsp margarine	Tasty Baked Chicken Summer Pasta Salad 1 slice whole-grain bread 1 cup raspberries 1 cup nonfat milk 1/2 cup steamed broccoli 1 1/2 tsp margarine

*Indicates that the recipe has been used previously.

VEGETABLES

_____ bell peppers, green
_____ bell peppers, red
_____ bell peppers, yellow
_____ broccoli
_____ carrots
_____ celery
_____ collard greens
_____ corn on the cob
_____ cucumbers
_____ garlic
_____ green beans
_____ lettuce, romaine
_____ onion, purple
_____ onions, yellow or white
_____ onions, green
_____ onions, red
_____ potatoes
_____ potatoes, sweet
_____ spinach
_____ squash, winter
_____ squash, yellow summer
_____ sugar snap peas
_____ tomatoes
_____ zucchini

MEATS

_____ bacon, Canadian
_____ beef round steak, lean
_____ chicken breasts, boneless, skinless
_____ ham, lean
_____ pork chops, boneless sirloin
_____ roast beef, deli-style
_____ sausage, beef, lean
_____ sausage, turkey, low-fat
_____ shrimp
_____ tilapia fillets
_____ turkey breast, ground
_____ veal, round steak

FRUITS

_____ apples
_____ avocados
_____ bananas
_____ blackberries
_____ blueberries
_____ cantaloupe
_____ cherries
_____ figs
_____ honeydew melon
_____ kiwi fruit
_____ lemon
_____ oranges
_____ peaches
_____ pineapple, chunks
_____ pineapple, crushed
_____ plums
_____ raisins
_____ raspberries
_____ strawberries

DAIRY

_____ buttermilk, fat-free
_____ egg substitute
_____ egg whites
_____ milk, nonfat
_____ Smart Balance Light margarine
_____ Smart Balance margarine
_____ yogurt, fat-free, plain
_____ yogurt, fat-free, vanilla

CHEESE

_____ cheddar, fat-free, shredded
_____ mozzarella, fat-free, shredded
_____ Parmesan, reduced-fat, grated
_____ Swiss, reduced-fat, sliced

BREAD, GRAINS, & PASTA

_____ bread, oatmeal
_____ bread, whole-grain, whole-wheat
_____ bulgur
_____ dinner rolls, small, whole-wheat
_____ English muffins
_____ pasta, penne, whole-wheat
_____ pasta, spirals, whole-wheat
_____ pita pocket breads, whole-wheat
_____ rice, brown, whole-grain
_____ rice, wild
_____ sub/hoagie buns, whole-grain

BEANS

____ kidney beans, no-added-salt, 16-oz can

NUTS

____ dates
____ hazelnuts
____ peanuts
____ pecans
____ pistachios
____ walnuts

CONDIMENTS

____ canola mayonnaise
____ horseradish
____ pickled watermelon rind
____ soy sauce, light

SPICES & HERBS

____ allspice
____ basil
____ bay leaf
____ black pepper
____ cayenne pepper
____ chili powder
____ cinnamon, ground
____ cream of tartar
____ cumin, ground
____ cumin seed
____ curry powder
____ dill weed
____ garlic powder
____ ginger, ground
____ mint leaves
____ nutmeg, ground
____ oregano
____ parsley
____ red pepper flakes
____ sage
____ turmeric, ground

OTHER

____ applesauce, unsweetened
____ fruit cocktail in water
____ ginger snaps
____ granola, low-fat
____ grits
____ hummus
____ jelly, apple, sugar-free
____ molasses
____ oats, old-fashioned
____ pasta sauce, red, light
____ preserves, apricot, sugar-free
____ pure vanilla extract
____ salad dressing, Catalina, light
____ salad dressing, Italian, light
____ tomato paste, no-added-salt
____ tomatoes, diced, no-added-salt
____ tomatoes, peeled, no-added-salt, 10-oz can
____ tomatoes, stewed, no-added-salt, 8-oz can
____ tortillas, corn, 6-inch
____ tuna, packed in water, 4-oz can
____ water chestnuts, 8-oz can

STAPLES

____ baking powder
____ baking soda
____ bouillon, beef, sodium-free
____ bouillon, chicken, sodium-free
____ cornstarch
____ flour, all-purpose
____ flour, whole-wheat
____ juice, apple, unsweetened
____ juice, lemon
____ juice, lime
____ juice, orange
____ nonstick cooking spray
____ Smart Balance Omega oil
____ Splenda
____ Splenda Brown Sugar Blend
____ vinegar, cider
____ vinegar, wine
____ wine, white, dry

Banana Walnut Bread

Serves 18   Serving size: 1 slice

Nonstick cooking spray

3 ripe bananas

1/2 **cup** egg substitute

3/4 **cup** Splenda

1/2 **cup** Smart Balance margarine

1 1/2 **cups** whole-wheat flour

1 **tsp** baking soda

1 **tsp** cream of tartar

1/4 **cup** shelled walnuts, crushed

Preheat oven to 350°F. Spray a 9 × 5 × 3-inch loaf pan with nonstick cooking spray. Mash the bananas and egg substitute together by hand or with an electric mixer. Add the Splenda and margarine, mixing by hand or electric mixer. Add remaining ingredients and blend well. Pour into the loaf pan and bake for 50 minutes. When done, a toothpick inserted in the center will come out clean. Let cool for 10 minutes before turning it out. Let cool completely. Makes one 9-inch loaf.

Exchanges/Choices

1/2 Starch
1/2 Fruit
1 Fat

Basic Nutritional Values

Calories 105
  Calories from Fat 45
Total Fat . . . . 5.0 g
  Saturated Fat . . . . 1.3 g
  Trans Fat . . . . 0.0 g
Cholesterol . . . . 0 mg
Sodium . . . . 125 mg
Total Carbohydrate . . . 13 g
  Dietary Fiber . . . . 2 g
  Sugars . . . . 4 g
Protein . . . . 3 g

Vegetarian Chili

Serves 4   Serving size: 1/4 recipe

2 **tsp** Smart Balance Omega oil

1 medium onion, chopped

1 medium green bell pepper, chopped

1 medium clove garlic, minced

1 **cup** water

1 **cup** no-added-salt canned diced tomatoes

1/2 **cup** uncooked bulgur

1 **Tbsp** ground cumin

1 **Tbsp** chili powder

1 **Tbsp** lemon juice

1 **(16-oz)** can no-added-salt kidney beans

In a pan over medium heat, heat the oil and coat the bottom of the pan. Cook onion, bell pepper, and garlic for 8–10 minutes or until the bell peppers are soft, stirring frequently. Reduce heat to prevent burning. Stir in the remaining ingredients except kidney beans. Reduce heat and simmer, covered, for 45–50 minutes or until bulgur is done and flavors have blended. Stir in beans and simmer, uncovered, for 10 minutes.

Exchanges/Choices

2 Starch
1 Vegetable
1 Lean Meat

Basic Nutritional Values

Calories 230
  Calories from Fat 35
Total Fat . . . . 4.0 g
  Saturated Fat . . . . 0.3 g
  Trans Fat . . . . 0.0 g
Cholesterol . . . . 0 mg
Sodium . . . . 70 mg
Total Carbohydrate . . . 42 g
  Dietary Fiber . . . . 14 g
  Sugars . . . . 7 g
Protein . . . . 11 g

Gratin of Broccoli

Serves 4   Serving size: 1/4 recipe

1 **Tbsp** Smart Balance Light margarine

2 **Tbsp** whole-wheat flour

1/2 **cup** nonfat milk

4 **oz** fat-free shredded cheddar cheese

1 **Tbsp** lemon juice

1 **Tbsp** nutmeg

1 **lb** broccoli florets

Pepper, to taste

Melt margarine. Blend in flour and stir until mixture becomes smooth and bubbly. Add milk and cheese; continue stirring until mixture comes to a boil and begins to thicken. Stir in lemon juice and nutmeg. Meanwhile, in a separate pot, cook broccoli in boiling water and drain; season with pepper. Cover broccoli with sauce.

Exchanges/Choices

2 Vegetable
1 Lean Meat

Basic Nutritional Values

Calories	115
Calories from Fat	20
Total Fat	2.5 g
Saturated Fat	0.8 g
Trans Fat	0.0 g
Cholesterol	5 mg
Sodium	350 mg
Total Carbohydrate	11 g
Dietary Fiber	4 g
Sugars	4 g
Protein	14 g

Chicken with Glazed Apples

Serves 4   Serving size: 1/4 recipe

1 **Tbsp** Smart Balance Omega oil

1 **lb** boneless, skinless chicken breasts (trimmed of fat)

2 **cups** apples, cut and cored

1/4 **cup** unsweetened apple juice

1/2 **tsp** ground nutmeg

Pepper, to taste

1/4 **cup** sugar-free apple jelly

Heat oil in a skillet. Cook chicken in oil, about 15 minutes or until done, turning once. Stir in apples and apple juice. Cook about 4 minutes longer, until apples are tender. Sprinkle chicken with nutmeg and pepper. Stir in jelly; cook, stirring constantly, until jelly is melted.

Exchanges/Choices

1 Fruit
3 Lean Meat

Basic Nutritional Values

Calories	210
Calories from Fat	55
Total Fat	6.0 g
Saturated Fat	1.1 g
Trans Fat	0.0 g
Cholesterol	65 mg
Sodium	60 mg
Total Carbohydrate	16 g
Dietary Fiber	2 g
Sugars	11 g
Protein	24 g

Whole-Wheat Blueberry Muffins

Serves 12   Serving size: 1 muffin

1	**cup** whole-wheat flour	3	**Tbsp** Smart Balance margarine
5 1/2	**Tbsp** Splenda	1/2	**cup** egg substitute
1	**tsp** baking powder	1/2	**cup** blueberries
6	**Tbsp** nonfat milk		

Preheat oven to 400°F. In a medium bowl, combine flour, Splenda, and baking powder. In a small bowl, beat milk, margarine, and egg substitute; stir into dry ingredients until just moist. Fold in blueberries and spoon batter into 12 paper-lined muffin cups. Bake for 20–25 minutes or until golden brown. Serve immediately.

Exchanges/Choices

1/2 Starch
1/2 Fat

Basic Nutritional Values

Calories 70
  Calories from Fat 20
Total Fat . . . . 2.5 g
  Saturated Fat . . . . 0.7 g
  Trans Fat . . . . 0.0 g
Cholesterol . . . . 0 mg
Sodium . . . . 75 mg
Total Carbohydrate . . . 9 g
  Dietary Fiber . . . . 1 g
  Sugars . . . . 2 g
Protein . . . . 3 g

Shrimp and Peppers

Serves 4   Serving size: 1/4 recipe

1	**Tbsp** Smart Balance Omega oil	2	medium cloves garlic, minced
2	medium onions, each cut into 8 slices	3/4	**lb** uncooked shrimp, peeled and deveined
2	**cups** red and yellow bell peppers, cut into 1/2-inch slices	1/4	**cup** lime juice (about 2–3 medium limes)
			Red pepper flakes, to taste

Heat oil in a large nonstick skillet. Over medium heat, sauté the onions, pepper, and garlic. Stir in the shrimp and lime juice; season with red pepper flakes. Cook for about 7–8 minutes or until shrimp turns pink, stirring frequently.

Exchanges/Choices

2 Vegetable
2 Lean Meat

Basic Nutritional Values

Calories 140
  Calories from Fat 40
Total Fat . . . . 4.5 g
  Saturated Fat . . . . 0.5 g
  Trans Fat . . . . 0.0 g
Cholesterol . . . . 120 mg
Sodium . . . . 145 mg
Total Carbohydrate . . . 12 g
  Dietary Fiber . . . . 2 g
  Sugars . . . . 5 g
Protein . . . . 14 g

Baked Squash

Serves 4   Serving size: 1/4 recipe

1 winter squash
(about 1 1/4 lb)

2 **Tbsp** Smart Balance
margarine, melted

1/8 **tsp** black pepper

Exchanges/Choices

1/2 Starch
1 Fat

Basic Nutritional Values

Calories 75
  Calories from Fat 45
Total Fat . . . . 5.0 g
  Saturated Fat . . . . 1.4 g
  Trans Fat . . . . 0.0 g
Cholesterol . . . . 0 mg
Sodium . . . . 45 mg
Total Carbohydrate . . . 8 g
  Dietary Fiber . . . . 3 g
  Sugars . . . . 3 g
Protein . . . . 1 g

Cut squash in half, clean out seeds, brush cut surfaces with melted margarine, and bake cut side down on a cookie sheet at 350°F for 30 minutes. Turn squash cut side up and continue baking until squash is tender when pierced with a pointed knife. Baking time ranges from 45 minutes to 1 hour. Cut through skin into serving-size pieces and season to taste with pepper. Any kind of winter squash can be used, such as acorn, Hubbard, butternut, or buttercup.

If you're on the 2,000- or 2,200-calorie meal plan, you'll also prepare the **Baked Sweet Potato Fries** for your evening (B) snack. You can find that recipe on pages 76 and 248.

Veal Parmesan Hoagie

Serves 4   Serving size: 1 hoagie

1 **Tbsp** Smart Balance
margarine

3/4 **lb** veal round steak

2 **Tbsp** reduced-fat Parmesan
cheese

4 whole-wheat buns

1 **cup** light red pasta sauce

2 **Tbsp** shredded fat-free
mozzarella cheese

Exchanges/Choices

2 Starch
1 Vegetable
3 Lean Meat
1/2 Fat

Basic Nutritional Values

Calories 340
  Calories from Fat 70
Total Fat . . . . 8.0 g
  Saturated Fat . . . . 2.3 g
  Trans Fat . . . . 0.0 g
Cholesterol . . . . 70 mg
Sodium . . . . 660 mg
Total Carbohydrate . . . 41 g
  Dietary Fiber . . . . 6 g
  Sugars . . . . 10 g
Protein . . . . 27 g

Melt margarine in a shallow baking dish. Place veal in a baking dish and sprinkle with Parmesan cheese. Bake at 350°F for 20 minutes; turn meat over and bake another 20 minutes, until tender. Place the veal on the buns, pour pasta sauce over meat, and top with mozzarella cheese. Return to oven for 3–4 minutes to heat the sauce and melt the cheese.

This recipe is high in sodium.

Bread Pudding

Serves 10   Serving size: 1/10 recipe

Nonstick cooking spray

2 **cups** stale whole-wheat bread, cut into 1/2-inch cubes

3/4 **cup** raisins

1/4 **cup** chopped walnuts

4 **cups** nonfat milk

3/4 **cup** Splenda

3/4 **cup** egg substitute

2 **tsp** ground cinnamon

2 **tsp** pure vanilla extract

1/4 **cup** Smart Balance margarine

Preheat oven to 325°F. Spray a shallow 1 1/2-quart casserole with nonstick cooking spray. Place bread cubes, raisins, and nuts in casserole. In a large bowl, combine milk, Splenda, egg substitute, cinnamon, and vanilla. Pour over bread mixture; mix well. Dot with margarine. Place casserole in a large baking pan; fill pan with hot water to a depth of 1 inch. Bake for 45–55 minutes or until a knife inserted halfway between center and edge of casserole comes out clean. Serve warm or cold.

Exchanges/Choices

1/2 Fat-Free Milk
1 Carbohydrate
1 Fat

Basic Nutritional Values

Calories 165
  Calories from Fat 55
Total Fat . . . . 6.0 g
  Saturated Fat . . . . 1.3 g
  Trans Fat . . . . 0.0 g
Cholesterol . . . . 0 mg
Sodium . . . . 175 mg
Total Carbohydrate . . . 21 g
  Dietary Fiber . . . . 2 g
  Sugars . . . . 14 g
Protein . . . . 8 g

Tabbouleh

Serves 4   Serving size: 1/4 recipe

1 **cup** bulgur wheat

2 **cups** water

1 **Tbsp** sodium-free chicken bouillon

1/4 **cup** lemon juice

1/2 **tsp** pepper

1 **cup** cucumber, peeled and diced

1 medium tomato, chopped

1/2 **cup** green onion, finely chopped

1/2 **cup** shredded carrot

1/2 **cup** chopped parsley

1 **Tbsp** mint leaves

4 romaine lettuce leaves

1 **(4-oz)** can tuna packed in water, drained

3/4 **cup** plain fat-free yogurt

Place bulgur in a large bowl. In a small saucepan over medium heat, bring water and bouillon to a boil. Pour over bulgur. Stir and let stand for 1 hour. Drain well and discard liquid; add lemon juice and pepper. Mix well. Add cucumber, tomato, green onions, carrot, parsley, and mint, stirring until well blended. Cover and chill at least 1 hour or overnight. Just before serving, fluff with a fork. For each serving, mound 1/4 of the mixture on lettuce leaves. Top with 1/4 of the tuna and 1/4 of the yogurt.

Exchanges/Choices

2 Starch
1 Vegetable
1 Lean Meat

Basic Nutritional Values

Calories 220
  Calories from Fat 10
Total Fat . . . . 1.0 g
  Saturated Fat . . . . 0.2 g
  Trans Fat . . . . 0.0 g
Cholesterol . . . . 10 mg
Sodium . . . . 590 mg
Total Carbohydrate . . . 40 g
  Dietary Fiber . . . . 9 g
  Sugars . . . . 7 g
Protein . . . . 16 g

Chicken Milanese

Serves 4   Serving size: 1/4 recipe

1/2 **cup** chopped onions	1/4 **tsp** black pepper
1 clove garlic, minced	1 1/4 **cup** water
2 **tsp** Smart Balance Omega oil	4 **Tbsp** white wine
1 **lb** boneless, skinless chicken breasts (trimmed of fat)	2 **Tbsp** no-added-salt tomato paste
2 **cups** sliced carrots	2 **Tbsp** cornstarch
2/3 **cup** sliced celery	2 **Tbsp** minced parsley
	2 **tsp** grated lemon peels

1. Sauté onion and garlic in oil for 3 minutes or until onion begins to soften. Add chicken, carrots, celery, and pepper.

2. In a small bowl, mix 1 cup water, wine, and tomato paste until blended; pour over chicken and vegetables. Over high heat, bring to a boil; reduce heat to low, cover, and simmer for 50 minutes or until chicken and vegetables are tender. Transfer chicken and vegetables to a platter; cover and keep warm.

3. In a small bowl, stir 1/4 cup water and cornstarch until smooth. Stir into chicken and vegetables. Stirring constantly over medium heat, bring to a boil; let boil for 1 minute. Stir in parsley and grated lemon peels. Spoon sauce over chicken and vegetables and serve.

Exchanges/Choices

3 Vegetable
3 Lean Meat

Basic Nutritional Values

Calories	210
Calories from Fat	45
Total Fat	5.0 g
Saturated Fat	1.0 g
Trans Fat	0.0 g
Cholesterol	65 mg
Sodium	125 mg
Total Carbohydrate	14 g
Dietary Fiber	3 g
Sugars	4 g
Protein	25 g

Broccoli Floret Salad

Serves 4   Serving size: 1/4 recipe

2 cups fresh or frozen broccoli florets, cut small

2 Tbsp chopped parsley

1 Tbsp basil

1 medium red pepper, thinly sliced

Black pepper, to taste

1 small purple onion, diced

2/3 cup light Italian salad dressing

Combine all ingredients (except dressing) in a large bowl. Add dressing. Stir well and chill for 2 hours before serving.

Exchanges/Choices

1/2 Carbohydrate
1 Vegetable
1/2 Fat

Basic Nutritional Values

Calories 80
  Calories from Fat 25
Total Fat . . . . 3.0 g
  Saturated Fat . . . . 0.3 g
  Trans Fat . . . . 0.0 g
Cholesterol . . . . 0 mg
Sodium . . . . 480 mg
Total Carbohydrate . . . 12 g
  Dietary Fiber . . . . 2 g
  Sugars . . . . 9 g
Protein . . . . 2 g

Cinnamon Apple Yogurt

Serves 4   Serving size: 1/4 serving

2 cups vanilla fat-free yogurt	**4 tsp** Splenda
1/2 cup unsweetened applesauce	**2 tsp** ground cinnamon

Spoon 1/2 cup yogurt into each of four dessert dishes. Top each with 2 Tbsp applesauce, 1 tsp Splenda, and 1/2 tsp cinnamon.

Exchanges/Choices

1 Carbohydrate

Basic Nutritional Values

Calories	90
Calories from Fat	0
Total Fat	0.0 g
Saturated Fat	0.0 g
Trans Fat	0.0 g
Cholesterol	0 mg
Sodium	65 mg
Total Carbohydrate	18 g
Dietary Fiber	0 g
Sugars	14 g
Protein	4 g

Fried Bananas

Serves 4   Serving size: 1 banana

4 small bananas (or plantains)	**1 Tbsp** Splenda
1/4 cup nonfat milk	**1/4 cup** whole-wheat flour
1/4 cup egg substitute	**1/4 cup** Smart Balance Omega oil

Peel the bananas and cut diagonally into half-inch-thick slices. Mix milk, egg substitute, Splenda, and flour until smooth. Heat oil in large skillet over medium heat. Dip each banana slice into batter and then drop into oil. Fry until browned, about 2 minutes on each side. Drain on paper towels. Serve warm or at room temperature.

Exchanges/Choices

1/2 Starch
1 1/2 Fruit
1 1/2 Fat

Basic Nutritional Values

Calories	190
Calories from Fat	65
Total Fat	7.0 g
Saturated Fat	0.6 g
Trans Fat	0.0 g
Cholesterol	0 mg
Sodium	40 mg
Total Carbohydrate	30 g
Dietary Fiber	4 g
Sugars	14 g
Protein	4 g

Turkey Sausage Sandwich

Serves 4   Serving size: 1 sandwich

Nonstick cooking spray
3/4 **lb** lean ground turkey breast
1 egg white
2 **Tbsp** water
1 **tsp** dried basil
1 **tsp** dried sage
1 **tsp** dried oregano
1/2 **tsp** allspice

1/2 **tsp** ground nutmeg
1/2 **tsp** dill weed
1/2 **tsp** garlic powder
1/4 **tsp** chili powder
4 romaine lettuce leaves
4 **Tbsp** canola mayonnaise
4 whole-grain buns

Exchanges/Choices

1 1/2 Starch
2 Lean Meat
1/2 Fat

Basic Nutritional Values

Calories 235
  Calories from Fat 65
Total Fat . . . . 7.0 g
  Saturated Fat . . . . 0.6 g
  Trans Fat . . . . 0.0 g
Cholesterol . . . . 40 mg
Sodium . . . . 340 mg
Total Carbohydrate . . . 24 g
  Dietary Fiber . . . . 4 g
  Sugars . . . . 5 g
Protein . . . . 20 g

1. Preheat the broiler and lightly spray a broiler pan with nonstick cooking spray.

2. In a medium bowl, thoroughly combine turkey, egg white, water, basil, sage, oregano, allspice, nutmeg, dill, garlic powder, and chili powder. Form into four equal patties and place on the broiler pan.

3. Broil about 2–4 inches from the heat for about 10 minutes. Flip the patties over and broil for another 5–10 minutes until the patties are no longer pink in the center.

4. Serve the patties with a lettuce leaf and 1 Tbsp mayonnaise on whole-grain buns.

Broccoli Slaw

Serves 4   Serving size: 1/4 recipe

1/4 **cup** fat-free plain yogurt

1/4 **cup** canola mayonnaise

3 **Tbsp** cider vinegar

2 **tsp** Splenda

1 **(8-oz)** can sliced water chestnuts, drained and rinsed, coarsely chopped

1/2 **cup** finely diced red onion

2 **cups** broccoli, finely chopped

Pepper, to taste

Exchanges/Choices

2 Vegetable
1 Fat

Basic Nutritional Values

Calories 100
  Calories from Fat 40
Total Fat . . . . 4.5 g
  Saturated Fat . . . . 0.0 g
  Trans Fat . . . . 0.0 g
Cholesterol . . . . 0 mg
Sodium . . . . 120 mg
Total Carbohydrate . . . 12 g
  Dietary Fiber . . . . 3 g
  Sugars . . . . 5 g
Protein . . . . 2 g

Whisk together yogurt, mayonnaise, vinegar, and Splenda in a large bowl. Add water chestnuts, onion, and broccoli; toss to coat. Cover and refrigerate for up to 2 days.

Buttered Parsley Potatoes

Serves 4   Serving size: 1/4 recipe

2 **cups** quartered potato

2 **Tbsp** Smart Balance Light margarine, melted

1/4 **cup** chopped parsley

Exchanges/Choices

1 Starch
1/2 Fat

Basic Nutritional Values

Calories 85
  Calories from Fat 20
Total Fat . . . . 2.5 g
  Saturated Fat . . . . 0.8 g
  Trans Fat . . . . 0.0 g
Cholesterol . . . . 0 mg
Sodium . . . . 50 mg
Total Carbohydrate . . . 14 g
  Dietary Fiber . . . . 1 g
  Sugars . . . . 1 g
Protein . . . . 1 g

Peel the potatoes. Cut into quarters and boil in water until tender. Just before serving, toss with margarine and parsley.

Caribbean Tilapia

Serves 4   Serving size: 1/4 recipe

1/4 **cup** onion, thinly sliced

1/4 **cup** green bell pepper, thinly sliced

1 clove garlic, minced

2 **Tbsp** Smart Balance margarine

1 **lb** tilapia fillets
   Pepper, to taste

1 **(8-oz)** can no-added-salt stewed tomatoes

2 **Tbsp** lime juice

Sauté onion, green pepper, and garlic in margarine; remove from skillet and set aside. Place fish in skillet; season with pepper. Spoon tomatoes and sautéed vegetables over fillets. Sprinkle with lime juice. Bring to a boil and then simmer, covered, for 5 minutes or until fish flakes easily when tested with a fork.

Exchanges/Choices

1 Vegetable
3 Lean Meat
1/2 Fat

Basic Nutritional Values

Calories 175
 Calories from Fat 65
Total Fat . . . . .7.0 g
 Saturated Fat . . . . .2.3 g
 Trans Fat . . . . .0.0 g
Cholesterol . . . . .75 mg
Sodium . . . . .90 mg
Total Carbohydrate . . . 6 g
 Dietary Fiber . . . . .1 g
 Sugars . . . . .2 g
Protein . . . . .23 g

Buttermilk Biscuits

Serves 6   Serving size: 1 biscuit

1 **cup** all-purpose flour

1 **Tbsp** Splenda

1 1/2 **tsp** baking powder

1/4 **tsp** baking soda

3 1/3 **Tbsp** Smart Balance margarine

1/2 **cup** fat-free buttermilk

Preheat oven to 450°F. In a medium bowl combine flour, Splenda, baking powder, and baking soda. With a pastry blender, cut in margarine until mixture resembles coarse crumbs. Stir in buttermilk. Place on a lightly floured surface; knead 3–4 times and roll or pat to a 1/2- to 3/4-inch thickness. Cut with a 2 1/2-inch biscuit cutter dipped in flour. Bake on an ungreased baking sheet for 12–15 minutes or until golden brown.

Exchanges/Choices

1 Starch
1 Fat

Basic Nutritional Values

Calories 135
 Calories from Fat 45
Total Fat . . . . .5.0 g
 Saturated Fat . . . . .1.4 g
 Trans Fat . . . . .0.0 g
Cholesterol . . . . .0 mg
Sodium . . . . .215 mg
Total Carbohydrate . . . 19 g
 Dietary Fiber . . . . .1 g
 Sugars . . . . .3 g
Protein . . . . .3 g

Fruit Salad Medley

Serves 4   Serving size: 1/4 recipe

1/2 **cup** strawberries, sliced

1/4 **cup** Splenda

1/2 **cup** blueberries (or canned light)

1 banana, sliced

3 **tsp** lemon juice

2 oranges, peeled and sliced crosswise

1/2 **cup** blackberries (or canned light)

1/2 **cup** pineapple (fresh, frozen, or canned light chunks)

1/2 **cup** orange juice

Sprig mint leaves

Exchanges/Choices

2 Fruit

Basic Nutritional Values

Calories 120
  Calories from Fat 5
Total Fat . . . . .0.5 g
  Saturated Fat . . . . .0.1 g
  Trans Fat . . . . .0.0 g
Cholesterol . . . . .0 mg
Sodium . . . . .0 mg
Total Carbohydrate . . .29 g
  Dietary Fiber . . . . .5 g
  Sugars . . . . .21 g
Protein . . . . .2 g

In a medium bowl, stir together half of the strawberries and half of the Splenda; set aside. In a 2-quart serving bowl, add blueberries and layer bananas on top; sprinkle with lemon juice. Add a layer of strawberries with remaining Splenda, then oranges and blackberries. Arrange pineapple tidbits around outer edge. Layer remaining strawberry slices around pineapple tidbits. Pour orange juice over all the fruit. Cover and chill for 1 hour. Just before serving, top with mint leaves.

Snap Peas and Shrimp Penne

Serves 4   Serving size: 1/4 recipe

1/2 **cup** dry white wine

2 **Tbsp** lemon juice

1 **Tbsp** lime juice

3/4 **lb** cooked shrimp, peeled and deveined

1 **cup** sugar snap peas

6 green onions, thinly sliced

1 **Tbsp** chopped parsley

1/2 **tsp** dried oregano

1/2 **tsp** ground black pepper

1 clove garlic, minced

1 bay leaf

8 **oz** penne pasta

Exchanges/Choices

3 Starch
1 Vegetable
1 Lean Meat

Basic Nutritional Values

Calories 295
  Calories from Fat 20
Total Fat . . . . .2.0 g
  Saturated Fat . . . . .0.2 g
  Trans Fat . . . . .0.0 g
Cholesterol . . . . .120 mg
Sodium . . . . .150 mg
Total Carbohydrate . . .48 g
  Dietary Fiber . . . . .3 g
  Sugars . . . . .4 g
Protein . . . . .21 g

Combine wine, lemon juice, and lime juice in a large skillet; bring to a boil. Add shrimp, peas, green onions, parsley, oregano, pepper, garlic, and bay leaf. Cook, stirring constantly, until peas are just tender and shrimp are pink, about 2 minutes. Remove bay leaf. Cook penne pasta according to package directions. Top pasta with shrimp sauce.

Pepper Steak

Serves 4   Serving size: 1/4 recipe

- **1 lb** lean round steak (trimmed of fat)
- **2 Tbsp** Smart Balance margarine
- **2 Tbsp** whole-wheat flour
- **1 (10-oz)** can no-added-salt peeled tomatoes
- **1 Tbsp** sodium-free beef bouillon
- **1** medium onion
- **2 cups** whole-grain rice, uncooked
- **1** medium green pepper

Cut steak into 1-inch thin strips and brown in a skillet with the margarine. Stir in flour. Drain tomatoes and reserve the liquid. Add water to the tomato liquid to make 4 cups total. Add the bouillon. Chop onion. Add onion and bouillon mixture to skillet; stir. Cover and cook over low heat for 1 hour or until meat is tender. Stir occasionally. Cook the rice according to package directions. Cut green pepper into thin strips. When meat is almost done, add peeled tomatoes and pepper strips to the skillet. Cover and heat for 5 more minutes. Serve over brown rice.

Exchanges/Choices

2 Starch
1 Vegetable
3 Lean Meat
1 Fat

Basic Nutritional Values

Calories 360
  Calories from Fat 100
Total Fat . . . . 11.0 g
  Saturated Fat . . . . 3.4 g
  Trans Fat . . . . 0.1 g
Cholesterol . . . . 75 mg
Sodium . . . . 115 mg
Total Carbohydrate . . . 35 g
  Dietary Fiber . . . . 4 g
  Sugars . . . . 6 g
Protein . . . . 29 g

Carrot Cake

Serves 6   Serving size: 1/6 recipe

- Nonstick cooking spray
- **1** cups whole-wheat flour
- **1 cup** Splenda
- **1 tsp** ground cinnamon
- **3/4 tsp** baking soda
- **1/2 cup** egg substitute
- **1 tsp** pure vanilla extract
- **1/4 cup** unsweetened applesauce
- **1/4 cup** fat-free plain yogurt
- **1 cup** carrot, pureed in a blender
- **1 cup** crushed pineapple (or canned light)
- Splenda, powdered (pulse in a food processor or coffee grinder until very fine)

Preheat oven to 350°F. Spray a 12-cup fluted tube pan with nonstick cooking spray. In a large bowl, mix flour, Splenda, cinnamon, and baking soda. Stir in egg substitute, vanilla, applesauce, and yogurt until well blended. Stir in carrot and pineapple. Pour into pan. Bake for 55 minutes or until a toothpick inserted 2 inches from edge comes out clean. Cool in pan on a wire rack for 20 minutes. Remove cake from pan. Allow cake to cool completely. To serve, lightly sprinkle with powdered Splenda.

Exchanges/Choices

2 Carbohydrate

Basic Nutritional Values

Calories 135
  Calories from Fat 0
Total Fat . . . . 0.0 g
  Saturated Fat . . . . 0.1 g
  Trans Fat . . . . 0.0 g
Cholesterol . . . . 0 mg
Sodium . . . . 220 mg
Total Carbohydrate . . . 28 g
  Dietary Fiber . . . . 4 g
  Sugars . . . . 11 g
Protein . . . . 6 g

Gram's Gingerbread

Serves 8   Serving size: 1 square

1/2 **cup** Splenda	1 1/2 **cup** whole-wheat flour
1/2 **cup** molasses	1 **tsp** ginger
1/4 **cup** unsweetened applesauce	1 **tsp** baking soda
1/2 **cup** egg substitute or egg whites, beaten	1/2 **cup** boiling water

Mix together all ingredients (except water); then add water. Mix thoroughly. Bake at 350°F until a toothpick inserted into the center comes out clean.

Exchanges/Choices

2 Carbohydrate

Basic Nutritional Values

Calories 155	
Calories from Fat 0	
Total Fat . . . . 0.0 g	
Saturated Fat . . . . 0.1 g	
Trans Fat . . . . 0.0 g	
Cholesterol . . . . 0 mg	
Sodium . . . . 195 mg	
Total Carbohydrate . . . 35 g	
Dietary Fiber . . . . 3 g	
Sugars . . . . 14 g	
Protein . . . . 5 g	

Pork Cutlets with Melons

Servings 4   Serving size: 1/4 recipe

1 **Tbsp** Smart Balance Omega oil	1 **Tbsp** grated ginger
3/4 **lb** boneless sirloin pork chops (trimmed of fat), cubed	3 **Tbsp** wine vinegar
	1 **tsp** cornstarch
1/2 onion, thinly sliced	3 **cups** melon (cantaloupe or honeydew), cubed
1 clove garlic, minced	1/2 **cup** pickled watermelon rind, diced

Heat oil in a large skillet over medium-high heat. Brown pork cubes, stirring, until slightly browned, about 4–5 minutes. Stir in onion, garlic, and ginger; cook and stir for 2–3 minutes. Mix together vinegar and cornstarch. Add to skillet. Cool and stir until sauce thickens. Stir in melon and watermelon rind (this condiment can be found in specialty stores or you can make it yourself). Heat through and serve.

Exchanges/Choices

1 Fruit
2 Lean Meat
1/2 Fat

Basic Nutritional Values

Calories 170	
Calories from Fat 55	
Total Fat . . . . 6.0 g	
Saturated Fat . . . . 0.7 g	
Trans Fat . . . . 0.0 g	
Cholesterol . . . . 40 mg	
Sodium . . . . 265 mg	
Total Carbohydrate . . . 14 g	
Dietary Fiber . . . . 1 g	
Sugars . . . . 11 g	
Protein . . . . 17 g	

Green Beans and Red Peppers

Serves 4   Serving size: 1/4 recipe

1/2	medium red bell pepper		16	oz frozen green beans
1/2	cup water		1/2	Tbsp Smart Balance Light margarine
1	Tbsp sodium-free chicken bouillon		1/4	tsp garlic powder

Cut bell pepper into strips. In a medium saucepan, combine water and bouillon to make a broth; bring to a boil. Add green beans. Cover and cook over medium heat for 8–12 minutes or until green beans are crisp-tender. Drain. Meanwhile, melt margarine in a small skillet. Add pepper strips and cook until just tender. In a serving bowl, combine green beans, pepper strips, and garlic powder; toss gently.

Exchanges/Choices

2 Vegetable

Basic Nutritional Values

Calories 45
 Calories from Fat 10
Total Fat . . . . 1.0 g
 Saturated Fat . . . . 0.2 g
 Trans Fat . . . . 0.0 g
Cholesterol . . . . 0 mg
Sodium . . . . 20 mg
Total Carbohydrate . . . 9 g
 Dietary Fiber . . . . 3 g
 Sugars . . . . 4 g
Protein . . . . 2 g

Spicy Seasoned Chicken

Serves 4   Serving size: 1/4 recipe

1	lb boneless, skinless chicken breasts (trimmed of fat)		1	Tbsp sodium-free chicken bouillon
1	tsp black pepper		1/2	cup water
1/2	tsp garlic powder		2	Tbsp lemon juice
5	Tbsp Splenda Brown Sugar Blend		1/3	tsp cayenne pepper
3 1/2	Tbsp light soy sauce		1	Tbsp cornstarch

Brown chicken in a skillet until fully cooked; remove from skillet and set aside. Combine all other ingredients in the skillet; simmer over low heat until mixture begins to thicken. Cut chicken into small strips and add to skillet. Serve hot.

Exchanges/Choices

1 1/2 Carbohydrate
3 Lean Meat

Basic Nutritional Values

Calories 225
 Calories from Fat 25
Total Fat . . . . 3.0 g
 Saturated Fat . . . . 0.8 g
 Trans Fat . . . . 0.0 g
Cholesterol . . . . 65 mg
Sodium . . . . 545 mg
Total Carbohydrate . . . 21 g
 Dietary Fiber . . . . 0 g
 Sugars . . . . 18 g
Protein . . . . 25 g

All-Natural High-Fiber Peach Squares

Serves 9   Serving Size: 1 square

3/4 **cup** fresh or frozen peaches, diced

1 **cup** Splenda

3/4 **cup** + 3/4 **Tbsp** whole-wheat flour

3/4 **cup** warm water

1 **cup** old-fashioned oats

1/4 **cup** Smart Balance margarine

1 **tsp** baking soda

1 **tsp** pure vanilla extract

1. Prepare the filling: bring the peaches, 1/2 cup Splenda, 3/4 Tbsp flour, and 3/4 cup water to a boil in a double boiler. Stir continuously until thickened.

2. Prepare the crumb base and topping: combine oats, margarine, 1/2 cup Splenda, 3/4 cup flour, baking soda, and vanilla; halve the mixture. Place half in the bottom of a 9-inch square baking dish. Layer the thickened filling on top. Add the remaining crumb base to the top.

3. Bake at 350°F for 30 minutes.

Exchanges/Choices

1 Starch
1 Fat

Basic Nutritional Values

Calories 125
  Calories from Fat 45
Total Fat . . . . 5.0 g
  Saturated Fat . . . . 1.2 g
  Trans Fat . . . . 0.0 g
Cholesterol . . . . 0 mg
Sodium . . . . 180 mg
Total Carbohydrate . . . 18 g
  Dietary Fiber . . . . 2 g
  Sugars . . . . 4 g
Protein . . . . 3 g

Granola, Oats, Blackberry, and Raspberry Bake

Serves 8   Serving size: 1/8 recipe

Blackberry Raspberry Filling

- 2 **Tbsp** Splenda
- 1 1/2 **Tbsp** whole-wheat flour
- 1 **tsp** ground cinnamon
- 1 **tsp** pure vanilla extract
- 3 **cups** fresh or frozen (partially thawed) blackberries
- 3 **cups** fresh or frozen (partially thawed) raspberries

     Nonstick cooking spray

Oats Topping

- 1 **cup** old-fashioned oats, uncooked
- 1/2 **cup** chopped dates

     Dash allspice

     Dash nutmeg

     Dash cinnamon

- 2 **Tbsp** Splenda
- 4 **Tbsp** Smart Balance Light margarine

Exchanges/Choices

1/2 Starch
1 Fruit
1/2 Fat

Basic Nutritional Values

Calories 150
  Calories from Fat 35
Total Fat . . . . 4.0 g
  Saturated Fat . . . . 0.9 g
  Trans Fat . . . . 0.0 g
Cholesterol . . . . 0 mg
Sodium . . . . 45 mg
Total Carbohydrate . . . 28 g
  Dietary Fiber . . . . 8 g
  Sugars . . . . 13 g
Protein . . . . 3 g

1.   To prepare the filling, mix Splenda, flour, cinnamon, and vanilla. Fold in berries until fruit is evenly coated. Spray an 8-inch glass baking dish with nonstick cooking spray; spoon filling into baking dish.

2.   Combine topping ingredients, mixing well. Sprinkle evenly over fruit filling. Preheat oven to 350°F. Bake for 35–40 minutes or until topping is golden and filling is bubbly. Serve warm.

Roast Beef and Swiss Roll-Up

Serves 4   Serving size: 3 roll-ups

1/2 lb deli-style roast beef

3 slices reduced-fat Swiss cheese

12 romaine lettuce leaves

2 small tomatoes, diced

12 (6-inch) corn tortillas

4 Tbsp horseradish (optional)

Place the tortillas on a flat surface and divide the roast beef evenly between the 12 tortillas. Cut the cheese into 12 slices and place one on each tortilla, followed by a lettuce leaf and some tomato. If desired, add horseradish. Roll up the tortillas and serve. If desired, warm roll-ups in the oven before serving.

Exchanges/Choices

2 Starch
1 Vegetable
2 Lean Meat
1/2 Fat

Basic Nutritional Values

Calories 305
  Calories from Fat 55
Total Fat . . . . 6.0 g
  Saturated Fat . . . . 2.3 g
  Trans Fat . . . . 0.0 g
Cholesterol . . . . 40 mg
Sodium . . . . 325 mg
Total Carbohydrate . . . 39 g
  Dietary Fiber . . . . 5 g
  Sugars . . . . 4 g
Protein . . . . 23 g

Tasty Baked Chicken

Serves 4   Serving size: 1/4 recipe

Nonstick cooking spray

1 lb boneless, skinless chicken breasts (trimmed of fat)

1/4 cup sugar-free apricot preserves

1/4 cup light Catalina salad dressing

Preheat oven to 350°F. Lightly spray a baking pan with nonstick cooking spray. Rinse the chicken and pat dry. Place chicken in pan. Combine preserves and salad dressing in a small bowl. Spoon over the chicken. Bake, uncovered, for 1 hour and 15 minutes or until chicken is tender and fully cooked.

Exchanges/Choices

1/2 Carbohydrate
3 Lean Meat

Basic Nutritional Values

Calories 165
  Calories from Fat 35
Total Fat . . . . 4.0 g
  Saturated Fat . . . . 0.9 g
  Trans Fat . . . . 0.0 g
Cholesterol . . . . 65 mg
Sodium . . . . 190 mg
Total Carbohydrate . . . 10 g
  Dietary Fiber . . . . 0 g
  Sugars . . . . 6 g
Protein . . . . 24 g

Summer Pasta Salad

Serves 4   Serving size: 1/4 recipe

1 **cup** pasta spirals (about 4 oz)

1 **cup** broccoli florets

1/2 **cup** sliced carrots

1 **cup** sliced yellow summer squash

3 **Tbsp** cider vinegar

1 **Tbsp** Smart Balance Omega oil

2 medium cloves garlic, minced

1/4 **tsp** pepper

3 **Tbsp** chopped basil leaves (or 1 tbsp dried)

2 **Tbsp** grated Parmesan cheese

Exchanges/Choices

1 1/2 Starch
1 Vegetable
1/2 Fat

Basic Nutritional Values

Calories 155
 Calories from Fat 35
Total Fat . . . . 4.0 g
 Saturated Fat . . . . 0.3 g
 Trans Fat . . . . 0.0 g
Cholesterol . . . . 0 mg
Sodium . . . . 20 mg
Total Carbohydrate . . . 25 g
 Dietary Fiber . . . . 2 g
 Sugars . . . . 3 g
Protein . . . . 5 g

In a stockpot or large saucepan, cook pasta using package directions. When pasta is nearly done (about 7 minutes), add broccoli and carrots; cook for 1 minute. Add squash; cook for 30 seconds. Immediately drain in a colander and run under cold water to cool; set aside. In a large bowl, whisk together all remaining ingredients. Stir cooled pasta mixture into dressing and gently toss. Refrigerate at least 15 minutes before serving.

Appendix One

Choose Your Foods: Exchange Lists for Diabetes

Healthy Eating Is the First Step in Taking Care of Your Diabetes

Carbohydrate, protein, and fat are found in the food you eat. They supply your body with energy, which is measured in calories. When you eat food, and especially carbohydrate, it is turned into glucose. Glucose is the energy source for the cells in your body. However, our body needs insulin to use this energy. Insulin is made in the pancreas. If you have diabetes, either your pancreas is no longer making insulin, it is not making enough insulin, or your body is resistant to insulin. In each case, insulin is not working properly, the glucose is not getting into the cells, and your blood glucose levels can get too high.

You can make a difference in your blood glucose control through your food choices. To keep your blood glucose levels near normal, you need to balance the food you eat (especially the carbohydrates), your physical activities, and the insulin your body makes or gets by injection. Blood glucose monitoring gives you information to help you with this balancing act. Near-normal blood glucose levels help you feel better and may reduce or prevent the complications of diabetes.

It is helpful for most people with diabetes to eat about the same amount of carbohydrate around the same time each day. However, if you take multiple daily injections of insulin to control your blood glucose levels, you have more freedom to choose your foods and mealtimes. Regardless of how you manage your diabetes, try to spread your meals throughout the day and do not skip meals. If you use insulin or some glucose-lowering medications, skipping meals may lead to low blood glucose levels and may make it harder to control your appetite. Snacks can also be an important part of many diabetes food plans. Your registered dietitian (RD) can help you decide the time and size of snacks that are right for you.

How This Works

There are three main groups of foods in this appendix. They are based on the three major nutrients: carbohydrates, protein (meat and meat substitutes), and fat. Each food list contains foods grouped together because they have similar nutrient content and serving sizes. Each serving of a food has about the same amount of carbohydrate, protein, fat, and calories as the other foods on the same list.

- Foods on the **Starch** list, **Fruits** list, **Milk** list, and **Sweets, Desserts, and Other Carbohydrates** list are similar because they contain 12 to 15 grams of carbohydrate per serving.
- Foods on the **Fat** list and **Meat and Meat Substitutes** list usually do not have carbohydrate (except for the plant-based meat substitutes such as beans and lentils).
- Foods on the **Starchy Vegetables** list (part of the **Starch** list and including foods such as potatoes, corn, and peas) contain 15 grams of carbohydrate per serving.
- Foods on the **Nonstarchy Vegetables** list (such as green beans, tomatoes, and carrots) contain 5 grams of carbohydrate per serving.
- Some foods have so little carbohydrate and calories that they are considered "free," if eaten in small amounts. You can find these foods on the **Free Foods** list.
- Foods that have different amounts of carbohydrates and calories are listed as **Combination Foods** (such as lasagna) or **Fast Foods**.

The Food Lists

The following chart shows the amount of nutrients in 1 serving from each list.

Food List	Carbohydrate (grams)	Protein (grams)	Fat (grams)	Calories
CARBOHYDRATES				
Starch: breads, cereals and grains; starchy vegetables; crackers, snacks; and beans, peas, and lentils	15	0–3	0–1	80
Fruits	15	—	—	60
Milk				
Fat-free, low-fat, 1%	12	8	0–3	100
Reduced-fat, 2%	12	8	5	120
Whole	12	8	8	160
Sweets, Desserts, and Other Carbohydrates	15	varies	varies	varies
Nonstarchy Vegetables	5	2	—	25
MEAT AND MEAT SUBSTITUTES				
Lean	—	7	0–3	45
Medium-fat	—	7	4–7	75
High-fat	—	7	8+	100
Plant-based proteins	varies	7	varies	varies
Fats	—	—	5	45
Alcohol (1 alcohol equivalent)	varies	—	—	100

Starch

Cereals, grains, pasta, breads, crackers, snacks, starchy vegetables, and cooked beans, peas, and lentils are starches. In general, 1 starch is:

- 1/2 cup of cooked cereal, grain, or starchy vegetable
- 1/3 cup of cooked rice or pasta
- 1 oz of a bread product, such as 1 slice of bread
- 3/4 oz to 1 oz of most snack foods (some snack foods may also have extra fat)

Nutrition Tips

- A choice on the Starch list has 15 grams of carbohydrate, 0–3 grams of protein, 0–1 gram of fat, and 80 calories.

Bread

Food	Serving Size
Bagel, large (about 4 oz)	1/4 (1 oz)
Biscuit, 2 1/2 inches across	1

Bread
  reduced-calorie
  white, whole-grain, pumpernickel, rye, unfrosted raisin
	
	2 slices (1 1/2 oz)
	1 slice (1 oz)

Chapatti, small, 6 inches across	1
Corn bread, 1 3/4-inch cube	1 (1 1/2 oz)
English muffin	1/2
Hot dog bun or hamburger bun	1/2 (1 oz)
Naan, 8 inches by 2 inches	1/4
Pancake, 4 inches across, 1/4 inch thick	1
Pita, 6 inches across	1/2
Roll, plain, small	1 (1 oz)
Stuffing, bread	1/3 cup
Taco shell, 5 inches across	2
Tortilla, corn, 6 inches across	1
Tortilla, flour, 6 inches across	1
Tortilla, flour, 10 inches across	1/3 tortilla
Waffle, 4-inch square or 4 inches across	1

Cereals and Grains

Food	Serving Size
Barley, cooked	1/3 cup

Bran, dry
  oat
  wheat
	
	1/4 cup
	1/2 cup

Bulgur (cooked)	1/2 cup

Cereals
  bran
  cooked (oats, oatmeal)
  puffed
  shredded wheat, plain
  sugar-coated
  unsweetened, ready-to-eat
	
	1/2 cup
	1/2 cup
	1 1/2 cups
	1/2 cup
	1/2 cup
	3/4 cup

Couscous	1/3 cup

Granola
  low-fat
  regular
	
	1/4 cup
	1/4 cup

(continued)

Cereals and Grains *(continued)*

Food	Serving Size
Grits, cooked	1/2 cup
Kasha	1/2 cup
Millet, cooked	1/3 cup
Muesli	1/4 cup
Pasta, cooked	1/3 cup
Polenta, cooked	1/3 cup
Quinoa, cooked	1/3 cup
Rice, white or brown, cooked	1/3 cup
Tabbouleh (tabouli), prepared	1/2 cup
Wheat germ, dry	3 Tbsp
Wild rice, cooked	1/2 cup

Starchy Vegetables

Food	Serving Size
Cassava	1/3 cup
Corn on cob, large	1/2 cup 1/2 cob (5 oz)
Hominy, canned	3/4 cup
Mixed vegetables with corn, peas, or pasta	1 cup
Parsnips	1/2 cup
Peas, green	1/2 cup
Plantain, ripe	1/3 cup

Potato
   baked with skin
   boiled, all kinds
   mashed, with milk and fat
   French fried (oven-baked)
	
	1/4 large (3 oz)
	1/2 cup or 1/2 medium (3 oz)
	1/2 cup
	1 cup (2 oz)

Pumpkin, canned, no sugar added	1 cup
Spaghetti/pasta sauce	1/2 cup
Squash, winter (acorn, butternut)	1 cup
Succotash	1/2 cup
Yam, sweet potato, plain	1/2 cup

Crackers and Snacks

Food	Serving Size
Animal crackers	8

Crackers
    round, butter-type
    saltine-type
    sandwich-style, cheese or peanut butter filling
    whole-wheat regular
    whole-wheat lower fat or crispbreads
	
	6
	6
	3
	2–5 (3/4 oz)
	2–5 (3/4 oz)

Graham cracker, 2 1/2 inch square	3
Matzoh	3/4 oz
Melba toast, about 2-inch by 4-inch piece	4 pieces
Oyster crackers	20

Popcorn
    with butter
    no fat added
    lower fat
	
	3 cups
	3 cups
	3 cups

Pretzels	3/4 oz
Rice cakes, 4 inches across	2

Snack chips
    fat-free or baked (tortilla, potato), baked pita chips
    regular (tortilla, potato)
	
	15–20 (3/4 oz)
	9–13 (3/4 oz)

Beans, Peas, and Lentils

The choices on this list count as 1 starch + 1 lean meat.

Food	Serving Size
Baked beans	1/3 cup
Beans, cooked (black, garbanzo, kidney, lima, navy, pinto, white)	1/2 cup
Lentils, cooked (brown, green, yellow)	1/2 cup
Peas, cooked (black-eyed, split)	1/2 cup
Refried beans, canned	1/2 cup

Fruits

Fresh, frozen, canned, and dried fruits and fruit juices are on this list. In general, 1 fruit choice is:

- 1/2 cup of canned or fresh fruit or unsweetened fruit juice
- 1 small fresh fruit (4 oz)
- 2 Tbsp of dried fruit

Nutrition Tips

■ A choice on the **Fruits** list has 15 grams of carbohydrate, 0 grams of protein, 0 grams of fat, and 60 calories.

■ Fresh, frozen, and dried fruits are good sources of fiber. Fruit juices contain very little fiber. Choose fruits instead of juices whenever possible.

■ Citrus fruits, berries, and melons are good sources of vitamin C.

Selection Tips

■ The weight listed includes skin, core, seeds, and rind.

■ Food labels for fruits may contain the words "no sugar added" or "unsweetened." This means that no table sugar (sucrose) has been added; it does not mean the food contains no sugar.

■ Fruit canned in "extra light syrup" has the same amount of carbohydrate per serving as canned fruit labeled "no sugar added" or "juice pack." All canned fruits on the **Fruits** list are based on one of these three types of pack. Avoid fruit canned in heavy syrup.

Fruit

Food	Serving Size
Apple, unpeeled, small	1 (4 oz)
Apples, dried	4 rings
Applesauce, unsweetened	1/2 cup
Apricots	
canned	1/2 cup
dried	8 halves
fresh	4 whole (5 1/2 oz)
Banana, medium	1 (4 oz)
Blackberries	3/4 cup
Blueberries	3/4 cup
Cantaloupe, small	1/3 melon or 1 cup cubed (11 oz)
Cherries	
sweet, canned	1/2 cup
sweet, fresh	12 (3 oz)
Dates	3
Dried fruits (blueberries, cherries, cranberries, mixed fruit, raisins)	2 Tbsp
Figs	
dried	1 1/2
fresh	1 1/2 large or 2 medium (3 1/2 oz)
Fruit cocktail	1/2 cup

(continued)

Fruit *(continued)*

Food	Serving Size

Grapefruit
    large
    sections, canned
	1/2 (11 oz)
	3/4 cup

Grapes, small	17 (3 oz)
Honeydew melon	1 slice or 1 cup cubed (10 oz)
Kiwi	1 (3 1/2 oz)
Mandarin oranges, canned	3/4 cup
Mango, small	1/2 fruit (5 1/2 oz) or 1/2 cup
Nectarine, small	1 (5 oz)
Orange, small	1 (6 1/2 oz)
Papaya	1/2 fruit or 1 cup cubed (8 oz)

Peaches
    canned
    fresh, medium
	1/2 cup
	1 (6 oz)

Pears
    canned
    fresh, large
	1/2 cup
	1/2 (4 oz)

Pineapple
    canned
    fresh
	1/2 cup
	3/4 cup

Plums
    canned
    dried (prunes)
    small
	1/2 cup
	3
	2 (5 oz)

Raspberries	1 cup
Strawberries	1 1/4 cup whole berries
Tangerines, small	2 (8 oz)
Watermelon	1 slice or 1 1/4 cup cubes (13 1/2 oz)

Fruit Juice

Food	Serving Size
Apple juice/cider	1/2 cup
Fruit juice blends, 100% juice	1/3 cup
Grape juice	1/3 cup
Grapefruit juice	1/2 cup
Orange juice	1/2 cup
Pineapple juice	1/2 cup
Prune juice	1/3 cup

Milk

Different types of milk and milk products are on this list. However, two types of milk products are found in other lists:

- Cheeses are on the **Meat and Meat Substitutes** list (because they are rich in protein).
- Cream and other dairy fats are on the **Fats** list.

Milks and yogurts are grouped in three categories based on the amount of fat they have: fat-free/(skim), low-fat (1%), reduced-fat (2%), or whole. The following chart shows you what 1 milk choice contains:

	Carbohydrate (grams)	Protein (grams)	Fat (grams)	Calories
Fat-free/nonfat (skim), low-fat (1%)	12	8	0–3	100
Reduced-fat (2%)	12	8	5	120
Whole	12	8	8	160

Nutrition Tips

- Milk and yogurt are good sources of calcium and protein.
- The higher the fat content of milk and yogurt, the more saturated fat and cholesterol it has.
- Children over the age of 2 and adults should choose lower-fat varieties, such as skim, 1%, or 2% milks or yogurts.

Selection Tips

- 1 cup equals 8 fluid oz or 1/2 pint.

Milk and Yogurts

Food	Serving Size	Count as
FAT-FREE/NONFAT (SKIM) OR LOW-FAT (1%)		
Milk, buttermilk, acidophilus milk, Lactaid	1 cup	1 fat-free milk
Evaporated milk	1/2 cup	1 fat-free milk
Yogurt, plain or flavored with an artificial sweetener	2/3 cup (6 oz)	1 fat-free milk
REDUCED-FAT (2%)		
Milk, acidophilus milk, kefir, Lactaid	1 cup	1 reduced-fat milk
Yogurt, plain	2/3 cup (6 oz)	1 reduced-fat milk

(continued)

Milk and Yogurts *(continued)*

Food	Serving Size	Count as
WHOLE		
Milk, buttermilk, goat's milk	1 cup	1 whole milk
Evaporated milk	1/2 cup	1 whole milk
Yogurt, plain	1 cup (8 oz)	1 whole milk

Dairy-Like Foods

Food	Serving Size	Count as
Chocolate milk fat-free	1 cup	1 fat-free milk + 1 carbohydrate
whole	1 cup	1 whole milk + 1 carbohydrate
Eggnog, whole milk	1/2 cup	1 carbohydrate + 2 fat
Rice drink flavored, low-fat	1 cup	2 carbohydrate
plain, fat-free	1 cup	1 carbohydrate
Smoothies, flavored, regular	10 oz	1 fat-free milk + 2 1/2 carbohydrate
Soy milk light	1 cup	1 carbohydrate + 1/2 fat
regular, plain	1 cup	1 carbohydrate + 1 fat
Yogurt and juice blends	1 cup	1 fat-free milk + 1 carbohydrate
low-carbohydrate (less than 6 grams carbohydrate per serving)	2/3 cup (6 oz)	1/2 fat-free milk
with fruit, low-fat	2/3 cup (6 oz)	1 fat-free milk + 1 carbohydrate

Sweets, Desserts, and Other Carbohydrates

Foods on this list have added sugars or fat. However, you can substitute food choices from this list for other carbohydrate-containing foods (such as those found on the **Starch**, **Fruit**, or **Milk** lists) in your meal plan.

Nutrition Tips

- A carbohydrate choice has 15 grams of carbohydrate and about 70 calories.

- The foods on this list do not have as many vitamins or minerals or as much fiber as the choices on the **Starch**, **Fruits**, and **Milk** lists. When choosing sweets, desserts, and other carbohydrate foods, you should also eat foods from other food lists to balance your meals.
- Many of these foods don't equal a single choice. Some will also count as one or more fat choices.
- If you are trying to lose weight, choose foods from this list less often.
- The serving sizes for these foods are small because of their fat content.

Beverages, Soda, and Energy/Sports Drinks

Food	Serving Size	Count as
Cranberry juice cocktail	1/2 cup	1 carbohydrate
Energy drink	1 can (8.3 oz)	2 carbohydrate
Fruit drink or lemonade	1 cup (8 oz)	2 carbohydrate
Hot chocolate regular	1 envelope added to 8 oz water	1 carbohydrate + 1 fat
sugar-free or light	1 envelope added to 8 oz water	1 carbohydrate
Soft drink (soda), regular	1 can (12 oz)	2 1/2 carbohydrate
Sports drink	1 cup (8 oz)	1 carbohydrate

Brownies, Cake, Cookies, Gelatin, Pie, and Pudding

Food	Serving Size	Count as
Brownie, small, unfrosted	1 1/4-inch square, 7/8-inch high (about 1 oz)	1 carbohydrate + 1 fat
Cake angel food, unfrosted	1/12 of cake (about 2 oz)	2 carbohydrate
frosted	2-inch square (about 2 oz)	2 carbohydrate + 1 fat
unfrosted	2-inch square (about 1 oz)	1 carbohydrate + 1 fat
Cookies chocolate chip	2 cookies (2 1/4 inches across)	1 carbohydrate + 2 fat
ginger snap	3 cookies	1 carbohydrate
sandwich, with crème filling	2 small (about 2/3 oz)	1 carbohydrate + 1 fat
sugar-free	3 small or 1 large (3/4–1 oz)	1 carbohydrate + 1–2 fat
vanilla wafer	5 cookies	1 carbohydrate + 1 fat

(continued)

Brownies, Cake, Cookies, Gelatin, Pie, and Pudding (continued)

Food	Serving Size	Count as
Cupcake, frosted	1 small (about 1 3/4 oz)	2 carbohydrate + 1–1 1/2 fat
Fruit cobbler	1/2 cup (3 1/2 oz)	3 carbohydrate + 1 fat
Gelatin, regular	1/2 cup	1 carbohydrate

Pie
   commercially prepared fruit, 2 crusts
   pumpkin or custard
	
	1/6 of 8-inch pie
	1/8 of 8-inch pie
		
		3 carbohydrate + 2 fat
		1 1/2 carbohydrate + 1 1/2 fat

Pudding
   regular (made with reduced-fat milk)
   sugar-free or sugar- and fat-free (made with nonfat milk)
	
	1/2 cup
	1/2 cup
		
		2 carbohydrate
		1 carbohydrate

Candy, Spreads, Sweets, Sweeteners, Syrups, and Toppings

Food	Serving Size	Count as
Candy bar, chocolate/peanut	2 "fun size" bars (1 oz)	1 1/2 carbohydrate + 1 1/2 fat
Candy, hard	3 pieces	1 carbohydrate
Chocolate "kisses"	5 pieces	1 carbohydrate + 1 fat

Coffee creamer
   dry, flavored
 	
   liquid, flavored
	
	4 tsp
	
	2 Tbsp
		
		1/2 carbohydrate + 1/2 fat
		
		1 carbohydrate

Fruit snacks, chewy (pureed fruit concentrate)	1 roll (3/4 oz)	1 carbohydrate
Fruit spreads, 100% fruit	1 1/2 Tbsp	1 carbohydrate
Honey	1 Tbsp	1 carbohydrate
Jam or jelly, regular	1 Tbsp	1 carbohydrate
Sugar	1 Tbsp	1 carbohydrate

Syrup
   chocolate
   light (pancake type)
   regular (pancake type)
	
	2 Tbsp
	2 Tbsp
	1 Tbsp
		
		2 carbohydrate
		1 carbohydrate
		1 carbohydrate

Condiments and Sauces

Food	Serving Size	Count as
Barbecue sauce	3 Tbsp	1 carbohydrate
Cranberry sauce, jellied	1/4 cup	1 1/2 carbohydrate
Gravy, canned or bottled	1/2 cup	1/2 carbohydrate + 1/2 fat
Salad dressing, fat-free, low-fat, cream-based	3 Tbsp	1 carbohydrate
Sweet and sour sauce	3 Tbsp	1 carbohydrate

Doughnuts, Muffins, Pastries, and Sweet Breads

Food	Serving Size	Count as
Banana nut bread	1-inch slice (2 oz)	2 carbohydrate + 1 fat
Doughnut cake, plain	1 medium (1 1/2 oz)	1 1/2 carbohydrate + 2 fat
yeast type, glazed	3 3/4 inches across (2 oz)	2 carbohydrate + 2 fat
Muffin (4 oz)	1/4 muffin (1 oz)	1 carbohydrate + 1/2 fat
Sweet roll or Danish	1 (2 1/2 oz)	2 1/2 carbohydrate + 2 fat

Frozen Bars, Frozen Desserts, Frozen Yogurt, and Ice Cream

Food	Serving Size	Count as
Frozen pops	1	1/2 carbohydrate
Fruit juice bars, frozen, 100% juice	1 bar (3 oz)	1 carbohydrate
Ice cream fat-free	1/2 cup	1 1/2 carbohydrate
light	1/2 cup	1 carbohydrate + 1 fat
no added sugar	1/2 cup	1 carbohydrate + 1 fat
regular	1/2 cup	1 carbohydrate + 2 fat
Sherbet, sorbet	1/2 cup	2 carbohydrate
Yogurt, frozen fat-free	1/3 cup	1 carbohydrate
regular	1/2 cup	1 carbohydrate + 0–1 fat

Granola Bars, Meal Replacement Bars/Shakes, and Trail Mix

Food	Serving Size	Count as
Granola or snack bar, regular or low-fat	1 bar (1 oz)	1 1/2 carbohydrate
Meal replacement bar	1 bar (1 1/3 oz)	1 1/2 carbohydrate + 0–1 fat
Meal replacement bar	1 bar (2 oz)	2 carbohydrate + 1 fat
Meal replacement shake, reduced calorie	1 can (10–11 oz)	1 1/2 carbohydrate + 0–1 fat
Trail mix candy/nut-based	1 oz	1 carbohydrate + 2 fat
dried fruit-based	1 oz	1 carbohydrate + 1 fat

Nonstarchy Vegetables

Vegetable choices include vegetables in this **Nonstarchy Vegetables** list and the **Starchy Vegetables** list found within the **Starch** list. Vegetables with small amounts of carbohydrate and calories are on the **Nonstarchy Vegetables** list. Vegetables contain important nutrients. Try to eat at least 2–3 nonstarchy vegetable choices each day (as well as choices from the **Starchy Vegetables** list). In general, 1 nonstarchy vegetable choice is:

- 1/2 cup of cooked vegetables or vegetable juice
- 1 cup of raw vegetables

Nutrition Tips

- A choice on this list (1/2 cup cooked or 1 cup raw) equals 5 grams of carbohydrate, 2 grams of protein, 0 grams of fat, and 25 calories.
- Fresh and frozen vegetables have less added salt than canned vegetables. Drain and rinse canned vegetables to remove some salt.
- Choose dark green and dark yellow vegetables each day. Spinach, broccoli, romaine, carrots, chilies, squash, and peppers are great choices.
- Brussels sprouts, broccoli, cauliflower, greens, peppers, spinach, and tomatoes are good sources of vitamin C.
- Eat vegetables from the cruciferous family several times each week. Cruciferous vegetables include bok choy, broccoli, Brussels sprouts, cabbage, cauliflower, collards, kale, kohlrabi, radishes, rutabaga, and turnips.

Nonstarchy Vegetables

- Amaranth or Chinese spinach
- Artichoke
- Artichoke hearts
- Asparagus
- Baby corn
- Bamboo shoots
- Bean sprouts
- Beans (green, wax, Italian)
- Beets
- Borscht
- Broccoli
- Brussels sprouts
- Cabbage (green, bok choy, Chinese)
- Carrots
- Cauliflower
- Celery
- Chayote
- Coleslaw, packaged, no dressing
- Cucumber
- Daikon
- Eggplant
- Gourds (bitter, bottle, luffa, bitter melon)
- Green onions or scallions
- Greens (collard, kale, mustard, turnip)
- Hearts of palm
- Jicama

- Kohlrabi
- Leeks
- Mixed vegetables (without corn, peas, or pasta)
- Mung bean sprouts
- Mushrooms, all kinds, fresh
- Okra
- Onions
- Pea pods
- Peppers (all varieties)
- Radishes
- Rutabaga
- Sauerkraut
- Soybean sprouts
- Spinach
- Squash (summer, crookneck, zucchini)
- Sugar snap peas
- Swiss chard
- Tomato
- Tomatoes, canned
- Tomato sauce
- Tomato/vegetable juice
- Turnips
- Water chestnuts
- Yard-long beans

Meat and Meat Substitutes

Meat and meat substitutes are rich in protein. Foods from this list are divided into four groups based on the amount of fat they contain. These groups are lean meat, medium-fat meat, high-fat meat, and plant-based proteins. The following chart shows you what one choice includes.

	Carbohydrate (grams)	Protein (grams)	Fat (grams)	Calories
Lean meat	—	7	0–3	45
Medium-fat meat	—	7	4–7	75
High-fat meat	—	7	8+	100
Plant-based protein	varies	7	varies	varies

Selection Tips

- Read labels to find foods low in fat and cholesterol. Try for 5 grams of fat or less per serving.
- Read labels to find "hidden" carbohydrate. For example, hot dogs actually contain a lot of carbohydrate. Most hot dogs are also high in fat, but are often sold in lower-fat versions.
- Whenever possible, choose lean meats.
  - Select grades of meat are the leanest.
  - Choice grades have a moderate amount of fat.
  - Prime cuts of meat have the highest amount of fat.
- Some types of fish, such as herring, mackerel, salmon, sardines, halibut, trout, and tuna, are rich in omega-3 fats, which may help reduce risk for heart disease.
- Bake, roast, broil, grill, poach, steam, or boil instead of frying.

- Trim off visible fat or skin.
- Roast, broil, or grill meat on a rack so the fat will drain off during cooking.

Lean Meats and Meat Substitutes

Serving sizes are based on cooked weight after bone and fat have been removed.

Food	Serving Size
Beef: Select or Choice grades trimmed of fat: ground round, roast (chuck, rib, rump), round, sirloin, steak (cubed, flank, porterhouse, T-bone), tenderloin	1 oz
Beef jerky	1/2 oz
Cheeses with 3 grams of fat or less per oz	1 oz
Cottage cheese	1/4 cup
Egg substitute, plain	1/4 cup
Egg whites	2
Fish, fresh or frozen, plain: catfish, cod, flounder, haddock, halibut, orange roughy, salmon, tilapia, trout, tuna	1 oz
Fish, smoked: herring or salmon (lox)	1 oz
Game: buffalo, ostrich, rabbit, venison	1 oz
Hot dog with 3 grams of fat or less per oz (8 dogs per 14-oz package) (Note: May be high in carbohydrate.)	1
Lamb: chop, leg, or roast	1 oz
Organ meats: heart, kidney, liver (Note: May be high in cholesterol.)	1 oz
Oysters, fresh or frozen	6 medium
Pork, lean Canadian bacon	1 oz
rib or loin chop/roast, ham, tenderloin	1 oz
Poultry, without skin: chicken, Cornish hen, domestic duck or goose (well drained of fat), turkey	1 oz
Processed sandwich meats with 3 grams of fat or less per oz: chipped beef, thin-sliced deli meats, turkey ham, turkey kielbasa, turkey pastrami	1 oz
Salmon, canned	1 oz
Sardines, canned	2 small
Sausage with 3 grams of fat or less per oz	1 oz
Shellfish: clams, crab, imitation shellfish, lobster, scallops, shrimp	1 oz
Tuna, canned in water or oil, drained	1 oz
Veal: loin chop, roast	1 oz

Medium-Fat Meat and Meat Substitutes

Serving sizes are based on cooked weight after bone and fat have been removed.

Food	Serving Size
Beef: corned beef, ground beef, meatloaf, Prime grades trimmed of fat (prime rib), short ribs, tongue	1 oz
Cheeses with 4–7 grams of fat per oz: feta, mozzarella, pasteurized processed cheese spread, reduced-fat cheeses, string	1 oz
Egg (Note: High in cholesterol, so limit to 3 per week.)	1
Fish, any fried type	1 oz
Lamb: ground, rib roast	1 oz
Pork: cutlet, shoulder roast	1 oz
Poultry: chicken with skin; dove, pheasant, wild duck, or goose; fried chicken; ground turkey	1 oz
Ricotta cheese	2 oz (1/4 cup)
Sausage with 4–7 grams of fat per oz	1 oz
Veal, cutlet (no breading)	1 oz

High-Fat Meat and Meat Substitutes

These foods are high in saturated fat, cholesterol, and calories and may raise blood cholesterol levels if eaten on a regular basis. Try to eat 3 or fewer servings from this group per week.

Food	Serving Size

Bacon
    pork
 	
    turkey
	2 slices (16 slices per lb or 1 oz each, before cooking)
	3 slices (1/2 oz each before cooking)

Cheese, regular: American, bleu, brie, cheddar, hard goat, Monterey jack, queso, and Swiss	1 oz
Hot dog: beef, pork, or combination (10 per 1 lb package)	1
Hot dog: turkey or chicken (10 per 1 lb package)	1
Pork: ground, sausage, spareribs	1 oz
Processed sandwich meats with 8 grams of fat or more per oz: bologna, hard salami, pastrami	1 oz
Sausage with 8 grams fat or more per oz: bratwurst, chorizo, Italian, knockwurst, Polish, smoked, summer	1 oz

Plant-Based Proteins

Because carbohydrate content varies among plant-based proteins, you should read the food label. A carbohydrate choice has 15 grams of carbohydrate and about 70 calories.

Food	Serving Size	Count as
"Bacon" strips, soy-based	3 strips	1 medium-fat meat
Baked beans	1/3 cup	1 starch + 1 lean meat
Beans, cooked: black, garbanzo, kidney, lima, navy, pinto, white	1/2 cup	1 starch + 1 lean meat
"Beef" or "sausage" crumbles, soy-based	2 oz	1/2 carbohydrate + 1 lean meat
"Chicken" nuggets, soy-based	2 nuggets (1 1/2 oz)	1/2 carbohydrate + 1 medium-fat meat
Edamame	1/2 cup	1/2 carbohydrate + 1 lean meat
Falafel (spiced chickpea and wheat patties)	3 patties (about 2 inches across)	1 carbohydrate + 1 high-fat meat
Hot dog, soy-based	1 (1 1/2 oz)	1/2 carbohydrate + 1 lean meat
Hummus	1/3 cup	1 carbohydrate + 1 high-fat meat
Lentils, brown, green, or yellow	1/2 cup	1 carbohydrate + 1 lean meat
Meatless burger, soy-based	3 oz	1/2 carbohydrate + 2 lean meat
Meatless burger, vegetable- and starch-based	1 patty (about 2 1/2 oz)	1 carbohydrate + 2 lean meat
Nut spreads: almond butter, cashew butter, peanut butter, soy nut butter	1 Tbsp	1 high-fat meat
Peas, cooked: black-eyed and split peas	1/2 cup	1 starch + 1 lean meat
Refried beans, canned	1/2 cup	1 starch + 1 lean meat
"Sausage" patties, soy-based	1 (1 1/2 oz)	1 medium-fat meat
Soy nuts, unsalted	3/4 oz	1/2 carbohydrate + 1 medium-fat meat
Tempeh	3/4 cup	1 medium-fat meat
Tofu	4 oz (1/2 cup)	1 medium-fat meat
Tofu, light	4 oz (1/2 cup)	1 lean meat

Fats

Fats are divided into three groups, based on the main type of fat they contain:

- **Unsaturated fats** (omega-3, monounsaturated, and polyunsaturated) are primarily vegetable and are liquid at room temperature. These fats have good health benefits.
    - Omega-3 fats are a type of polyunsaturated fat and can help lower triglyceride levels and the risk of heart disease.
    - Monounsaturated fats help lower total cholesterol levels and may help raise HDL (good) cholesterol levels.
    - Polyunsaturated fats can help lower cholesterol levels.
- **Saturated fats** have been linked with heart disease. They can raise LDL (bad) cholesterol levels and should be limited to small amounts. Saturated fats are solid at room temperature.
- *Trans* **fats** are made in a process that changes vegetable oils into semi-solid fats. These fats can raise blood cholesterol levels and should be limited to small amounts. Partially hydrogenated and hydrogenated fats are types of man-made *trans* fats and should be avoided. *Trans* fats are also found naturally occurring in some animal products, such as meat, cheese, butter, and dairy products.

Fats and oils have mixtures of unsaturated (polyunsaturated and monounsaturated) and saturated fats. Foods on the **Fats** list are grouped together based on the major type of fat they contain. In general, 1 fat choice equals:

- 1 tsp of regular margarine, vegetable oil, or butter
- 1 Tbsp of regular salad dressing

Nutrition Tips

- A choice on the **Fats** list contains 5 grams of fat and 45 calories.
- All fats are high in calories. Limit serving sizes for good nutrition and health.
- Limit the amount of fried foods you eat.
- Nuts and seeds are good sources of unsaturated fats if eaten in moderation. They have small amounts of fiber, protein, and magnesium.
- Good sources of omega-3 fatty acids include:
    - Fish, such as albacore tuna, halibut, herring, mackerel, salmon, sardines, and trout
    - Flaxseeds and English walnuts
    - Oils, such as canola, soybean, flaxseed, and walnut

Selection Tips

- When selecting regular margarine, choose a type that lists liquid vegetable oil as the first ingredient. Soft or tub margarines have less saturated fat than stick margarines and are a healthier choice. Look for *trans* fat–free soft margarines.
- When selecting reduced-fat or lower-fat margarines, look for types that have liquid vegetable oil (*trans* fat–free) as an ingredient. Water is usually the first ingredient.

Unsaturated/Monounsaturated Fats

Food	Serving Size
Avocado, medium	2 Tbsp (1 oz)
Nut butters (*trans* fat–free): almond butter, cashew butter, peanut butter (smooth or crunchy)	1 1/2 tsp
Nuts	
almonds	6 nuts
Brazil	2 nuts
cashews	6 nuts
filberts (hazelnuts)	5 nuts
macadamias	3 nuts
mixed (50% peanuts)	6 nuts
peanuts	10 nuts
pecans	4 halves
pistachios	16 nuts
Oil: canola, olive, peanut	1 tsp
Olives	
black (ripe)	8 large
green, stuffed	10 large

Unsaturated/Polyunsaturated Fats

Food	Serving Size
Margarine: lower-fat spread (30%–50% vegetable oil, *trans* fat–free)	1 Tbsp
Margarine: stick, tub (*trans* fat–free), or squeeze (*trans* fat–free)	1 tsp
Mayonnaise	
reduced-fat	1 Tbsp
regular	1 tsp
Mayonnaise-style salad dressing	
reduced-fat	1 Tbsp
regular	2 tsp
Nuts	
Pignolia (pine nuts)	1 Tbsp
walnuts, English	4 halves

(continued)

Unsaturated/Polyunsaturated Fats *(continued)*

Food	Serving Size
Oil: corn, cottonseed, flaxseed, grape seed, safflower, soybean, sunflower	1 tsp
Oil: made from soybean and canola oil—Enova	1 tsp
Plant stanol esters	
light	1 Tbsp
regular	2 tsp
Salad dressing reduced-fat (Note: May be high in carbohydrate.)	2 Tbsp
regular	1 Tbsp
Seeds	
flaxseed, whole	1 Tbsp
pumpkin, sunflower	1 Tbsp
sesame seeds	1 Tbsp
Tahini or sesame paste	2 tsp

Saturated Fats

Food	Serving Size
Bacon, cooked, regular, or turkey	1 slice
Butter	
reduced-fat	1 Tbsp
stick	1 tsp
whipped	2 tsp
Butter blends made with oil	
reduced-fat or light	1 Tbsp
regular	1 1/2 tsp
Chitterlings, boiled	2 Tbsp (1/2 oz)
Coconut, sweetened, shredded	2 Tbsp
Coconut milk	
light	1/3 cup
regular	1 1/2 Tbsp
Cream	
half and half	2 Tbsp
heavy	1 Tbsp
light	1 1/2 Tbsp
whipped	2 Tbsp
whipped, pressurized	1/4 cup
Cream cheese	
reduced-fat	1 1/2 Tbsp (3/4 oz)
regular	1 Tbsp (1/2 oz)

(continued)

Saturated Fats *(continued)*

Food	Serving Size
Lard	1 tsp
Oil: coconut, palm, palm kernel	1 tsp
Salt pork	1/4 oz
Shortening, solid	1 tsp
Sour cream reduced-fat or light regular	 3 Tbsp 2 Tbsp

Free Foods

A "free" food is any food or drink choice that has less than 20 calories and 5 grams or less of carbohydrate per serving.

Selection Tips

- Most foods on this list should be limited to 3 servings (as listed here) per day. Spread out the servings throughout the day. If you eat all 3 servings at once, it could raise your blood glucose level.
- Food and drink choices listed here without a serving size can be eaten whenever you like.

Low-Carbohydrate Foods

Food	Serving Size
Cabbage, raw	1/2 cup
Candy, hard (regular or sugar-free)	1 piece
Carrots, cauliflower, or green beans, cooked	1/4 cup
Cranberries, sweetened with sugar substitute	1/2 cup
Cucumber, sliced	1/2 cup
Gelatin dessert, sugar-free unflavored	
Gum	
Jam or jelly, light or no sugar added	2 tsp
Rhubarb, sweetened with sugar substitute	1/2 cup
Salad greens	
Sugar substitutes (artificial sweeteners)	
Syrup, sugar-free	2 Tbsp

Modified-Fat Foods with Carbohydrate

Food	Serving Size
Cream cheese, fat-free	1 Tbsp (1/2 oz)
Creamers 　nondairy, liquid 　nondairy, powdered	 1 Tbsp 2 tsp
Margarine spread 　fat-free 　reduced-fat	 1 Tbsp 1 tsp
Mayonnaise 　fat-free 　reduced-fat	 1 Tbsp 1 tsp
Mayonnaise-style salad dressing 　fat-free 　reduced-fat	 1 Tbsp 1 tsp
Salad dressing 　fat-free or low-fat 　fat-free, Italian	 1 Tbsp 2 Tbsp
Sour cream, fat-free or reduced-fat	1 Tbsp
Whipped topping 　light or fat-free 　regular	 2 Tbsp 1 Tbsp

Condiments

Food	Serving Size
Barbecue sauce	2 tsp
Catsup (ketchup)	1 Tbsp
Honey mustard	1 Tbsp
Horseradish	
Lemon juice	
Miso	1 1/2 tsp
Mustard	
Parmesan cheese, freshly grated	1 Tbsp
Pickle relish	1 Tbsp
Pickles 　dill 　sweet, bread and butter 　sweet, gherkin	 1 1/2 medium 2 slices 3/4 oz
Salsa	1/4 cup
Soy sauce, light or regular	1 Tbsp
Sweet and sour sauce	2 tsp

(continued)

Condiments *(continued)*

Food	Serving Size
Sweet chili sauce	2 tsp
Taco sauce	1 Tbsp
Vinegar	
Yogurt, any type	2 Tbsp

Drinks/Mixes

The foods on this list without a serving size provided can be consumed in any moderate amount.

- Bouillon, broth, consommé
- Bouillon or broth, low-sodium
- Carbonated or mineral water
- Club soda
- Cocoa powder, unsweetened (1 Tbsp)
- Coffee, unsweetened or with sugar substitute
- Diet soft drinks, sugar-free
- Drink mixes, sugar-free
- Tea, unsweetened or with sugar substitute
- Tonic water, diet
- Water
- Water, flavored, carbohydrate-free

Seasonings

Any food on this list can be consumed in any moderate amount.

- Flavoring extracts (for example, vanilla, almond, peppermint)
- Garlic
- Herbs, fresh or dried
- Hot pepper sauce
- Nonstick cooking spray
- Pimento
- Spices
- Wine, used in cooking
- Worcestershire sauce

Combination Foods

Many of the foods you eat are mixed together in various combinations, such as casseroles. These "combination" foods do not fit into any one choice list. This is a list of choices for some typical combination foods. A carbohydrate choice has 15 grams of carbohydrate and about 70 calories.

Entrees

Food	Serving Size	Count as
Casserole type (tuna noodle, lasagna, spaghetti with meatballs, chili with beans, macaroni and cheese)	1 cup (8 oz)	2 carbohydrate + 2 medium-fat meat
Stews (beef/other meats and vegetables)	1 cup (8 oz)	1 carbohydrate + 1 medium-fat meat + 0–3 fat
Tuna salad or chicken salad	1/2 cup (3 1/2 oz)	1/2 carbohydrate + 2 lean meat + 1 fat

Frozen Meals/Entrees

Food	Serving Size	Count as
Burrito (beef and bean)	1 (5 oz)	3 carbohydrate + 1 lean meat + 2 fat
Dinner-type meal	generally 14–17 oz	3 carbohydrate + 3 medium-fat meat + 3 fat
Entree or meal with less than 340 calories	about 8–11 oz	2–3 carbohydrate + 1–2 lean meat
Pizza cheese/vegetarian, thin crust meat topping, thin crust	1/4 of a 12-inch (4 1/2–5 oz) 1/4 of a 12-inch (5 oz)	2 carbohydrate + 2 medium-fat meat 2 carbohydrate + 2 medium-fat meat + 1 1/2 fat
Pocket sandwich	1 (4 1/2 oz)	3 carbohydrate + 1 lean meat + 1–2 fat
Pot pie	1 (7 oz)	2 1/2 carbohydrate + 1 medium-fat meat + 3 fat

Salads (Deli-Style)

Food	Serving Size	Count as
Coleslaw	1/2 cup	1 carbohydrate + 1 1/2 fat
Macaroni/pasta salad	1/2 cup	2 carbohdyrate + 3 fat
Potato salad	1/2 cup	1 1/2–2 carbohydrate + 1–2 fat

Soups

Food	Serving Size	Count as
Bean, lentil, or split pea	1 cup	1 carbohydrate + 1 lean meat
Chowder (made with milk)	1 cup (8 oz)	1 carbohydrate + 1 lean meat + 1 1/2 fat
Cream (made with water)	1 cup (8 oz)	1 carbohydrate + 1 fat
Instant with beans or lentils	6 oz prepared	1 carbohydrate
	8 oz prepared	2 1/2 carbohydrate + 1 lean meat
Miso soup	1 cup	1/2 carbohydrate + 1 fat
Ramen noodle	1 cup	2 carbohydrate + 2 fat
Rice (congee)	1 cup	1 carbohydrate
Tomato (made with water)	1 cup (8 oz)	1 carbohydrate
Vegetable beef, chicken noodle, or other broth-type	1 cup (8 oz)	1 carbohydrate

Fast Foods

The choices in the **Fast Foods** list are not specific fast food meals or items, but are estimates based on popular foods. You can get specific nutrition information for almost every fast food or restaurant chain. Ask the restaurant or check its website for nutrition information about your favorite fast foods. A carbohydrate choice has 15 grams of carbohydrate and about 70 calories.

Breakfast Sandwiches

Food	Serving Size	Count as
Egg, cheese, meat, English muffin	1 sandwich	2 carbohydrate + 2 medium-fat meat
Sausage biscuit sandwich	1 sandwich	2 carbohydrate + 2 high-fat meat + 3 1/2 fat

Main Dishes/Entrees

Food	Serving Size	Count as
Burrito (beef and beans)	1 (about 8 oz)	3 carbohydrate + 3 medium-fat meat + 3 fat
Chicken breast, breaded and fried	1 (about 5 oz)	1 carbohydrate + 4 medium-fat meat
Chicken drumstick, breaded and fried	1 (about 2 oz)	2 medium-fat meat

(continued)

Main Dishes/Entrees *(continued)*

Food	Serving Size	Count as
Chicken nuggets	6 (about 3 1/2 oz)	1 carbohydrate + 2 medium-fat meat + 1 fat
Chicken thigh, breaded and fried	1 (about 4 oz)	1/2 carbohydrate + 3 medium-fat meat + 1 1/2 fat
Chicken wings, hot	6 (5 oz)	5 medium-fat meat + 1 1/2 fat

Asian

Food	Serving Size	Count as
Beef/chicken/shrimp with vegetables in sauce	1 cup (about 5 oz)	1 carbohydrate + 1 lean meat + 1 fat
Egg roll, meat	1 (about 3 oz)	1 carbohydrate + 1 lean meat + 1 fat
Fried rice, meatless	1/2 cup	1 1/2 carbohydrate + 1 1/2 fat
Meat and sweet sauce (orange chicken)	1 cup	3 carbohydrate + 3 medium-fat meat + 2 fat
Noodles and vegetables in sauce (chow mein, lo mein)	1 cup	2 carbohydrate + 1 fat

Pizza

Food	Serving Size	Count as
Pizza cheese, pepperoni, regular crust	1/8 of a 14-inch (about 4 oz)	2 1/2 carbohydrate + 1 medium-fat meat + 1 1/2 fat
cheese/vegetarian, thin crust	1/4 of a 12-inch (about 6 oz)	2 1/2 carbohydrate + 2 medium-fat meat + 1 1/2 fat

Sandwiches

Food	Serving Size	Count as
Chicken sandwich, grilled	1	3 carbohydrate + 4 lean meat
Chicken sandwich, crispy	1	3 1/2 carbohydrate + 3 medium-fat meat + 1 fat
Fish sandwich with tartar sauce	1	2 1/2 carbohydrate + 2 medium-fat meat + 2 fat

(continued)

Sandwiches *(continued)*

Food	Serving Size	Count as
Hamburger large with cheese	1	2 1/2 carbohydrate + 4 medium-fat meat + 1 fat
regular	1	2 carbohydrate + 1 medium-fat meat + 1 fat
Hot dog with bun	1	1 carbohydrate + 1 high-fat meat + 1 fat
Submarine sandwich less than 6 grams fat	6-inch sub	3 carbohydrate + 2 lean meat
regular	6-inch sub	3 1/2 carbohydrate + 2 medium-fat meat + 1 fat
Taco, hard or soft shell (meat and cheese)	1 small	1 carbohydrate + 1 medium-fat meat + 1 1/2 fat

Salads

Food	Serving Size	Count as
Salad, main dish (grilled chicken type, no dressing or croutons)	Salad	1 carbohydrate + 4 lean meat
Salad, side (no dressing or cheese)	Small (about 5 oz)	1 vegetable

Sides/Appetizers

Food	Serving Size	Count as
French fries, restaurant style	small	3 carbohydrate + 3 fat
	medium	4 carbohydrate + 4 fat
	large	5 carbohydrate + 6 fat
Nachos with cheese	small (about 41/2 oz)	2 1/2 carbohydrate + 4 fat
Onion rings	1 serving (about 3 oz)	2 1/2 carbohydrate + 3 fat

Desserts

Food	Serving Size	Count as
Milkshake, any flavor	12 oz	6 carbohydrate + 2 fat
Soft-serve ice cream cone	1 small	2 1/2 carbohydrate + 1 fat

Alcohol

Nutrition Tips

▪ In general, 1 alcohol equivalent (1/2 oz absolute alcohol) has about 100 calories.

Selection Tips

▪ Women who choose to drink alcohol should limit themselves to 1 drink or less per day. The limit is 2 drinks or less per day for men.
▪ To reduce your risk of low blood glucose (hypoglycemia), especially if you take insulin or a diabetes pill that increases insulin, always drink alcohol with food.
▪ Although alcohol, by itself, does not directly affect blood glucose, be aware of the carbohydrate (for example, in mixed drinks, beer, and wine) that may raise your blood glucose.
▪ Check with your registered dietitian if you would like to fit alcohol into your meal plan.

Alcoholic Beverage	Serving Size	Count as
Beer light (4.2%)	12 fl oz	1 alcohol equivalent + 1/2 carbohydrate
regular (4.9%)	12 fl oz	1 alcohol equivalent + 1 carbohydrate
Distilled spirits: vodka, rum, gin, whiskey (80 or 86 proof)	1 1/2 fl oz	1 alcohol equivalent
Liqueur, coffee (53 proof)	1 fl oz	1/2 alcohol equivalent + 1 carbohydrate
Sake	1 fl oz	1/2 alcohol equivalent
Wine dessert (sherry)	3 1/2 fl oz	1 alcohol equivalent + 1 carbohydrate
dry, red or white (10%)	5 fl oz	1 alcohol equivalent

Appendix Two

Common Cooking Measurement Equivalents

These cooking measurement equivalents can make life easier when you're trying to figure out just how much of an ingredient you need. Remember that liquid or volume weights (such as fluid ounces) do not equal dry weights (such as ounces).

Common Abbreviations

c. (or C)	cup
fl. oz.	fluid ounce
g (or gm)	grams
gal	gallon
kg	kilogram
l	liter
lb	pound
ml (or mL)	milliliters
oz	ounce
pt	pint
qt	quart
Tbsp (or T)	tablespoon
tsp (or t)	teaspoon

Dry
Measurement Equivalents

3 tsp	1 Tbsp	1/2 oz
2 Tbsp	1/8 cup	1 oz
4 Tbsp	1/4 cup	2 oz
5 Tbsp + 1 tsp	1/3 cup	2.6 oz
8 Tbsp	1/2 cup	4 oz
12 Tbsp	3/4 cup	6 oz
16 Tbsp	1 cup	8 oz
32 Tbsp	2 cups	16 oz (or 1 lb)

Liquid (Volume)
Measurement Equivalents

2 Tbsp	1 fl. oz.
1/4 cup	2 fl. oz.
1/2 cup	4 fl. oz.
3/4 cup	6 fl. oz
1 cup	8 fl. oz.
1 pint (2 cups)	16 fl. oz.
1 quart (2 pints)	32 fl. oz.
1 gallon (4 quarts)	128 fl. oz.

Other Useful Equivalents

16 oz	1 lb
1 fl. oz.	29.57 milliliters
1 oz	28.35 grams
1 gram	.03 oz
14.2 grams	1/2 oz
28.3 grams	1 oz
1,000 grams	1 kilogram
1 kilogram	2.2 lbs
1,000 milliliters	1 liter
1 liter	1.06 quart
3.8 liters	1 gallon

Measurement Equivalents Chart

	teaspoon	tablespoon	fluid ounce	cup	pint	quart	gallon
teaspoon	—	1/3	1/6	—	—	—	—
tablespoon	3	—	1/2	1/16	—	—	—
ounce	6	2	—	1/8	1/16	—	—
cup	48	16	8	—	1/2	1/4	1/16
pint	96	32	16	2	—	1/2	1/8
quart	192	64	32	4	2	—	1/4
gallon	768	256	128	16	8	4	—

Index

Alphabetical List of Recipes

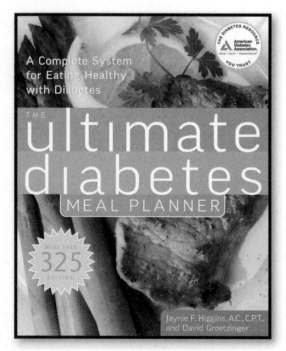

Other Titles from the American Diabetes Association

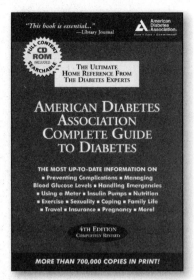

American Diabetes Association Complete Guide to Diabetes, 4th Edition
by American Diabetes Association

Have all the tips and information on diabetes that you need close at hand. The world's largest collection of diabetes self-care tips, techniques, and tricks for solving diabetes-related problems is back in its fourth edition, and it's bigger and better than ever before.
Order no. 4809-04; NEW LOW price $19.95

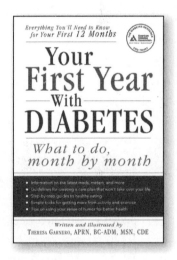

Your First Year with Diabetes
by Theresa Garnero, CDE, APRN, BC-ADM, MSN

Diabetes happens. It can happen to anyone—even you. If diabetes has left you feeling confused or angry, then it's time to turn to Theresa Garnero. Straightforward and easy to read, *Your First Year with Diabetes* will help you manage and deal with your diabetes—day to day, week to week, and month to month. You'll learn about medication, exercise, meal planning, and lifestyle and emotional issues at a pace that suits you.
Order no. 5024-01; Price $16.95

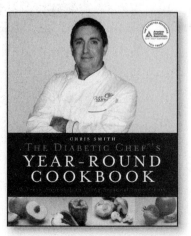

The Diabetic Chef's Year-Round Cookbook
by Chris Smith, The Diabetic Chef

Are you tired of uninspired, bland meals? Then you're ready for the creative dishes from The Diabetic Chef. Take advantage of seasonal foods available from month to month and enjoy a year of amazing, market-fresh meals. With *The Diabetic Chef's Year-Round Cookbook*, you'll enjoy perfect hors d'oeuvres to start off a dinner party and find the best entrees to delight your family on a weeknight.
Order no. 4667-01; Price $19.95

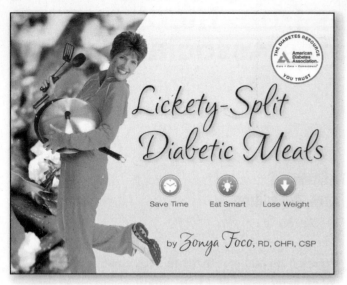

Lickety-Split Diabetic Meals
by Zonya Foco, RD, CHFI, CSP

Let Zonya Foco be your guide as you learn how to save time, eat smart, lose weight, and win the war against obesity, diabetes, and heart disease. You'll get over 175 recipes and meals that can be prepared in minutes. *Lickety-Split Diabetic Meals* is a one-of-a-kind resource for people with diabetes and can help you learn how to change the life you
have into the life you want.
Order no. 4669-01; Price $18.95

Diabetes & Heart Healthy Meals for Two
by the American Diabetes Association and the American Heart Association

If you or a loved one has diabetes, you need to eat heart-healthy meals. The simple, flavorful recipes were designed for those looking to improve or maintain their cardiovascular health. Each recipe is for two people, making this book perfect for adults without children in the house or for those who want to keep leftovers to a minimum. With over 170 recipes, there are countless options to keep your heart at its healthiest and your blood glucose under control.
Order no. 4673-01; Price $18.95

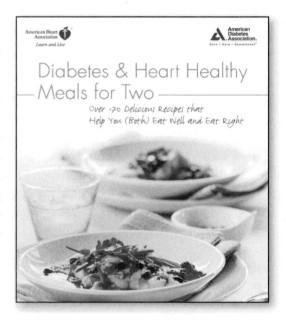

To order these and other great American Diabetes Association titles, call **1-800-232-6733** or visit *http://store.diabetes.org*. American Diabetes Association titles are also available in bookstores nationwide.